Series Editor

Prof. Dr. Michael J. Parnham
PLIVA
Research Institute
Prilaz baruna Filipovica 25
10000 Zagreb
Croatia

Published titles:
T Cells in Arthritis, P. Miossec, W. van den Berg, G. Firestein (Editors), 1998
Chemokines and Skin, E. Kownatzki, J. Norgauer (Editors), 1998
Medicinal Fatty Acids, J. Kremer (Editor), 1998
Inducible Enzymes in the Inflammatory Response, D.A. Willoughby, A. Tomlinson (Editors), 1999
Cytokines in Severe Sepsis and Septic Shock, H. Redl, G. Schlag (Editors), 1999
Fatty Acids and Inflammatory Skin Diseases, J.-M. Schröder (Editor), 1999
Immunomodulatory Agents from Plants, H. Wagner (Editor), 1999
Cytokines and Pain, L. Watkins, S. Maier (Editors), 1999
In Vivo *Models of Inflammation*, D. Morgan, L. Marshall (Editors), 1999
Pain and Neurogenic Inflammation, S.D. Brain, P. Moore (Editors), 1999
Anti-Inflammatory Drugs in Asthma, A.P. Sampson, M.K. Church (Editors), 1999
Apoptosis and Inflammation, J. D. Winkler (Editor), 1999
Novel Inhibitors of Leukotrienes, G. Folco, B. Samuelsson, R.C. Murphy (Editors), 1999

Forthcoming titles:
Metalloproteinases as Targets for Anti-Inflammatory Drugs, K.M.K. Bottomley, D. Bradshaw, J.S. Nixon (Editors), 1999
Free Radicals and Inflammation, P. Winyard, D. Blake, Ch. Evans (Editors), 1999
Gene Therapy in Inflammatory Diseases, Ch. Evans, P. Robbins (Editors), 1999

Vascular Adhesion Molecules and Inflammation

Jeremy D. Pearson

Editor

Springer Basel AG

Editor

Dr. Jeremy D. Pearson
Centre for Cardiovascular Biology and Medicine
School of Biomedical Sciences
King's College London
Guy's Campus
London SE1 9RT
UK

A CIP catalogue record for this book is available from the Library of Congress, Washington D.C., USA

Deutsche Bibliothek Cataloging-in-Publication Data
Vascular adhesion molecules and inflammation / ed. by Jeremy D.
Pearson. - Basel ; Boston ; Berlin : Birkhäuser, 1999
  (Progress in inflammation research)
    ISBN 978-3-0348-9753-2   ISBN 978-3-0348-8743-4 (eBook)
    DOI 10.1007/978-3-0348-8743-4

© 1999 Springer Basel AG
Originally published by Birkhäuser Verlag in 1999
Softcover reprint of the hardcover 1st edition 1999

Printed on acid-free paper produced from chlorine-free pulp. TCF ∞
Cover design: Markus Etterich, Basel
Cover illustration:

ISBN 978-3-0348-9753-2

9 8 7 6 5 4 3 2 1

Contents

List of contributors.   vii

Jeremy D. Pearson
How early studies of inflammation led to our current views on the roles
of vascular adhesion molecules.   1

Klaus Ley
Adhesion of leukocytes from flow: The selectins and their ligands.   11

C. Wayne Smith, Alan R. Burns and Scott I. Simon
Co-operative signaling between leukocytes and endothelium mediating
firm attachment.   39

Martha B. Furie
Production and presentation of chemokines by endothelial cells.   65

Diane E. Lorant, Thomas M. McIntyre, Stephen M. Prescott
and Guy A. Zimmerman
Platelet-activating factor: A signaling molecule for leukocyte adhesion.   81

James M. Staddon and Tetsuaki Hirase
Tight junctions and adherens junctions in endothelial cells:
structure and regulation 109

William A. Muller
The role of PECAM in leukocyte emigration. 125

Mark A. Jutila
Selective lymphocyte migration into secondary lymphoid organs and
inflamed tissues. 141

Xi-Lin Chen and Russell M. Medford
Oxidation-reduction sensitive regulation of vascular inflammatory
gene expression..161

Tanya Y. Huehns and Dorian O. Haskard
Quantification and imaging of vascular adhesion molecule expression
in inflammatory diseases *in vivo*.....................................179

Simon C. Robson and David Goodman
Leukocyte adhesion and activation in xenografts 197

Tak Yee Aw and D. Neil Granger
Control of leukocyte adhesion and activation in ischemia-reperfusion injury 221

Judith A. Berliner, Devendra K. Vora and Peggy T. Shih
Control of leukocyte adhesion and activation in atherogenesis 239

Index...257

List of contributors

Tak Yee Aw, Department of Molecular and Cellular Physiology, LSU Medical Center, PO Box 33932, 1501 Kings Highway, Shreveport, LA 71130-3932, USA

Judith A. Berliner, Departments of Medicine and Pathology, University of California, Los Angeles, CA 90095-1732, USA;
e-mail: jberline@pathology.medsch.ucla.edu

Alan R. Burns, Department of Medicine, Baylor College of Medicine, One Baylor Plaza, 512C, Houston, TX 77030, USA; e-mail: aburns@bmc.tmc.edu

Xi-Lin Chen, Division of Cardiology, Department of Medicine, Emory University School of Medicine, 1639 Pierce Drive, Atlanta, GA 30322, USA

Martha B. Furie, Department of Pathology, School of Medicine, State University of New York at Stony Brook, Stony Brook, NY 11794-8691, USA;
e-mail: mfurie@path.som.sunysb.edu

David Goodman, Department of Clinical Immunology & Nephrology, St Vincent's Hospital Melbourne, Fitzroy, Australia 3065; e-mail: goodman@svhm.org.au

D. Neil Granger, Department of Molecular and Cellular Physiology, LSU Medical Center, PO Box 33932, 1501 Kings Highway, Shreveport, LA 71130-3932, USA;
e-mail: dgrang@mail.sh.lsumc.edu

Dorian O. Haskard, BHF Cardiovascular Medicine Unit, National Heart and Lung Institute (Hammersmith Hospital), Imperial College School of Medicine, Du Cane Road, London W12 0NN, UK; e-mail: dhaskard@rpms.ac.uk

Tetusaki Hirase, 1st Department of Internal Medicine, School of Medicine, Kobe University, 7-5-2 Kusunoki-cho, Chuo-ku, Kobe-City 650, Japan;
e-mail: hirase@med.kobe-u.ac.jp

Tanya Y. Huehns, BHF Cardiovascular Medicine Unit, National Heart and Lung Institute (Hammersmith Hospital), Imperial College School of Medicine, Du Cane Road, London W12 0NN, UK

Mark A. Jutila, Veterinary Molecular Biology, Montana State University, Bozeman, MT 59717, USA; e-mail: uvsmj@montana.edu

Klaus Ley, University of Virginia School of Medicine, Department of Biomedical Engineering, Health Sciences Center, Box 377, Charlottesville, VA 22908, USA; e-mail: kfl3f@virginia.edu

Diane E. Lorant, University of Utah, CVRTI, 95 South 2000 East, Salt Lake City, UT 84112-5000, USA

Thomas M. McIntyre, University of Utah, CVRTI, 95 South 2000 East, Salt Lake City, UT 84112-5000, USA

Russell M. Medford, AtheroGenics, Inc., 8995 Westside Parkway, Alpharetta, GA 30004, USA; e-mail: rmedford@atherogenics.com

William A. Muller, Department of Pathology and the Center for Vascular Biology, Weill Medical College of Cornell University, 1300 York Avenue, New York, NY 10021, USA; e-mail: wamuller@mail.med.cornell.edu

Jeremy D. Pearson, Centre for Cardiovascular Biology and Medicine, School of Biomedical Sciences, King's College London, Guy's Campus, London SE1 9RT, UK; e-mail: jeremy.pearson@kcl.ac.uk

Stephen M. Prescott, University of Utah, CVRTI, 95 South 2000 East, Salt Lake City, UT 84112-5000, USA

Simon C. Robson, Department of Medicine, Beth Israel Deaconess Medical Center, Research North, Rm 370H, 99 Brookline Avenue, Boston, MA 02215, USA; e-mail: srobson@caregroup.harvard.edu

Peggy T. Shih, Departments of Medicine and Pathology, University of California, Los Angeles, CA 90095-1732, USA

Scott I. Simons, Children's Nutrition Research Center, 1100 Bates, Room 6014, Houston, TX 77030-2600, USA

C. Wayne Smith, Children's Nutrition Research Center, 1100 Bates, Room 6014, Houston, TX 77030-2600, USA; e-mail: cwsmith@bcm.tmc.edu

James M. Staddon, Eisai London Research Laboratories Ltd., Bernard Katz Building, University College London, Gower Street, London WC1E 6BT, UK; e-mail: James_Staddon@eisai.net

Devendra K. Vora, Departments of Medicine and Pathology, University of California, Los Angeles, CA 90095-1732, USA

Guy A. Zimmerman, University of Utah, CVRTI, 95 South 2000 East, Salt Lake City, UT 84112-5000, USA; e-mail: guy_zimmerman@gatormail.cvrti.utah.edu

How early studies of inflammation led to our current views on the roles of vascular adhesion molecules

Jeremy D. Pearson

Centre for Cardiovascular Biology and Medicine, School of Biomedical Sciences, King's College London, Guy's Campus, London SE1 9RT, UK

Dutrochet [1] is generally credited with the first observation, in 1824, that leukocytes could be seen to emigrate across the walls of small blood vessels, and the experimental induction of leukocyte diapedesis in response to tissue injury was first reported by Addison in 1843 [2]. The most elegant early experimental studies were carried out by Arnold in Heidelberg in the 1870s, examining leukocyte adhesion to, and demonstrating emigration between, endothelial cells in small blood vessels of the frog [3, 4]. He used silver staining to outline endothelial cell boundaries, and injection of cinnabar to detect sites of leakage. The resulting drawings (e.g. Fig. 1) accurately demonstrate the early stages of the acute inflammatory process in as much detail as many contemporary textbooks. He was also perspicacious enough to attribute emigration to a molecular process, writing:

> *"It is possible that chemical agents seep into interendothelial junctions and thereby attract pavemented leukocytes, but there is, as yet, no evidence for this concept".*

Arnold did not use the word "chemotaxis", probably only coined in the 1880s, and first unequivocally described for leukocytes, attracted into glass capillary tubes containing various chemicals placed in the cornea, by Leber in 1888 [5]. It was Metchnikoff in the 1890s who firmly established the importance of chemotaxis, together with phagocytosis, in leukocyte behaviour [6].

However, it is to Cohnheim [7] that we owe the first formulation of the importance of changes in the properties of the endothelium in initiating adhesion of leukocytes in the acute inflammatory process. In 1882 (published in translation in 1889) he stated:

> *"...we hold fast the conviction which was forced on us by our experiments and reflection that inflammation is the expression and consequence of a molecular alteration in the vessel walls. By it, adhesion between the vessel wall and the blood ... is increased."*

Vascular Adhesion Molecules and Inflammation, edited by J. D. Pearson
© 1999 Birkhäuser Verlag Basel/Switzerland

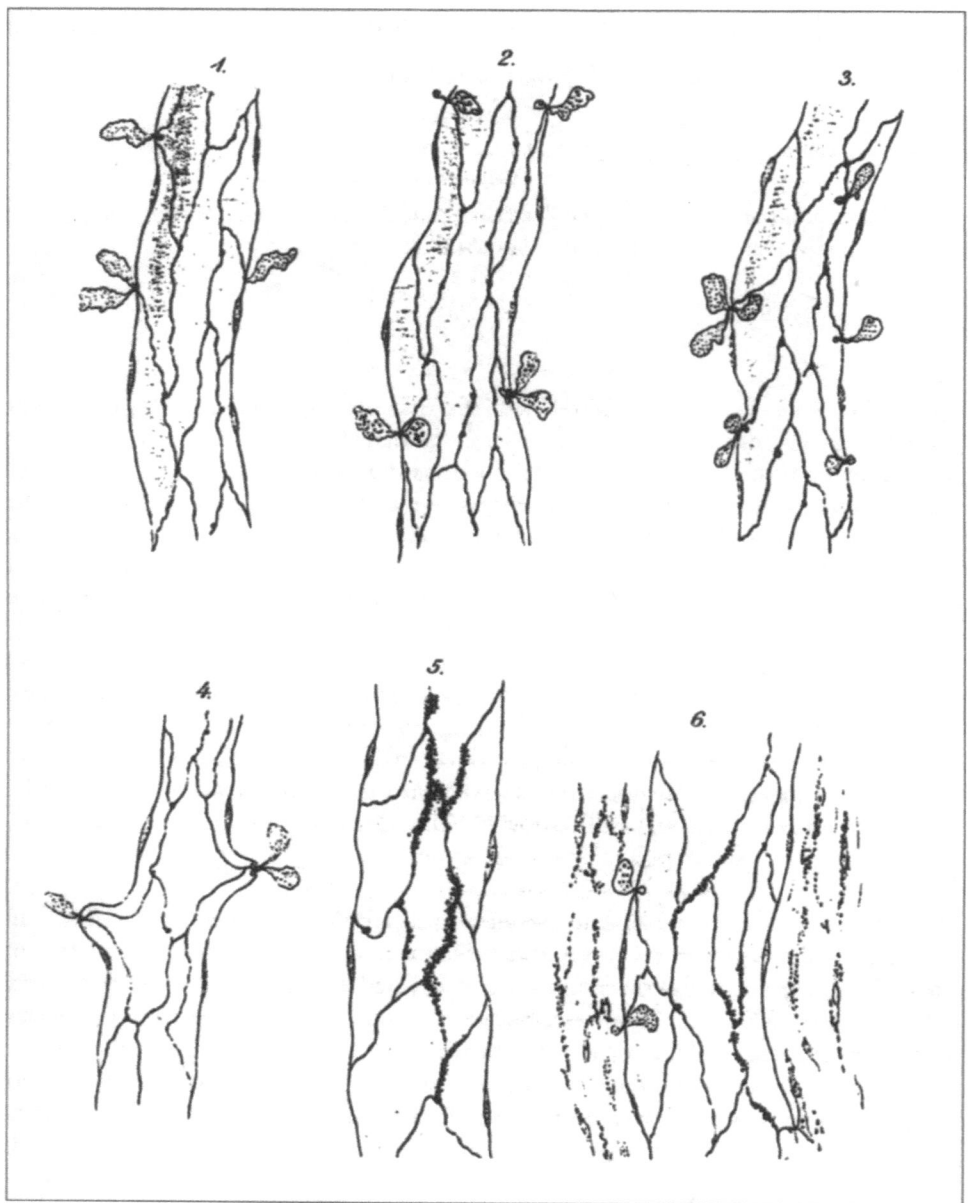

Figure 1
Drawings of leukocyte adhesion and emigration between endothelial cells of venules in frog blood vessels, in response to inflammatory stimuli. Endothelial cell junctions are silver stained, and leakage of injected particles (cinnabar) is depicted in panels 5–6. From [4].

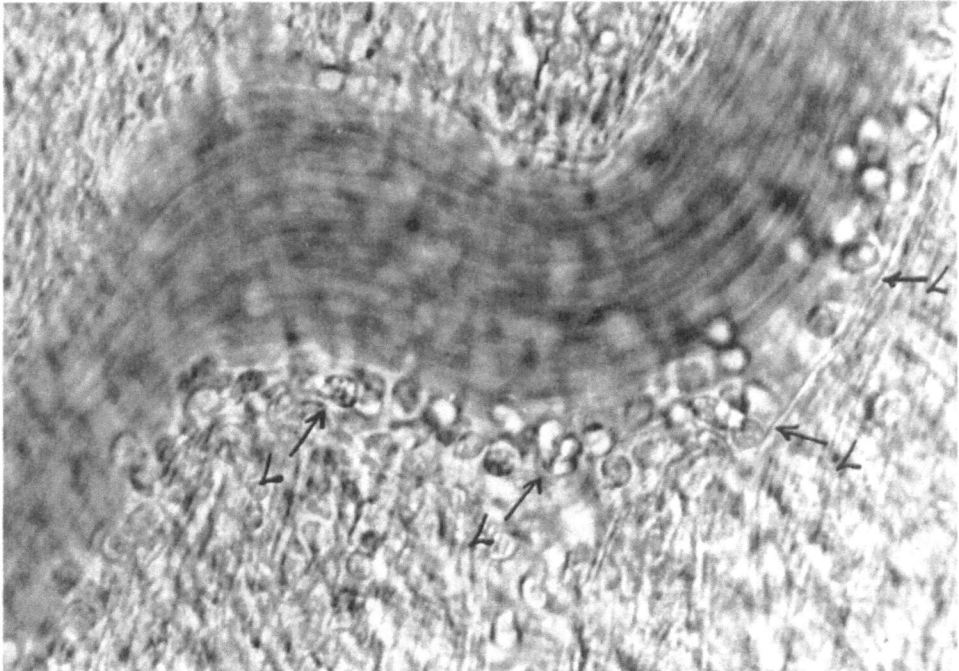

Figure 2
Light micrograph showing unilateral adhesion of leukocytes (L) to the side of a small vessel
nearest where thermal injury was applied 30 min previously. From [11] by copyright per-
mission of The Rockefeller University Press.

This conclusion was reinforced by the detailed studies of leukocyte adhesion and emigration in the rabbit ear chamber model used by Clark and Clark in the 1930s [8] and Zweifach in the 1940s (reviewed by Grant [9]). Zweifach additionally promoted the currently unfashionable idea that local activation of the coagulation process was an important component of the early inflammatory interactions between endothelial cells and leukocytes [10]; an idea that would bear re-examination *in vivo* with today's selective inhibitors. With the ear chamber, Allison et al. [11] first showed in 1955 that focal tissue injury led to initial leukocyte adhesion only on the side of the vessel nearest the injury (Fig. 2), providing further strong support for the primacy of changes in endothelial cell properties as a consequence of molecular signals from the injured tissue.

The nature of these changes remained obscure. Grant [9] summarised the state of knowledge in 1973 thus:

"Perhaps the most important single fact about white cell sticking is the unassailable one that when blood vascular endothelium is injured, it becomes 'sticky' [and loses] its 'non-wettable' character ... since 'sticky' and 'non-wettable' are literary, not scientific, terms they provide no insight into the mechanism of the phenomenon... One problem for the investigator, then, is to determine what factors are involved in alterations in the character of the endothelial cell. This is a rather difficult point to pin down, and the precise entry into this problem, at this time, is not obvious."

Experiments by Thompson et al. [12] as well as Atherton and Born [13], who first quantified leukocyte rolling and sticking in the cheek pouch and mesentery to show that chelation of Ca^{2+} abolished adhesion, led Ryan and Majno [14] in an influential review in 1977 to state that:

"Attempts have also been made to explain this stickiness by an invisible, molecular, change; it is possible that a local alteration of the cell membranes somehow permits calcium-bridging between the endothelium and the leukocyte..."

Attempts to understand how leukocyte adhesive behaviour could be modulated *in vitro* were first reported by Garvin in 1961 [15], using isolated cells and a glass bead column, and were extended and modified significantly by MacGregor in 1974 [16]. These kinds of study provided quantitative information about the effect of drugs on leukocyte adhesion to artificial surfaces, but could not necessarily shed light on whether similar effects would modulate leukocyte adhesion to endothelial cells. Routine culture of endothelial cells, achieved in the mid-1970s [17], opened up the possibility of doing such experiments.

Our group started to work on cultured endothelial cells at that time, initially concentrating on the control of platelet interactions with endothelium, and demonstrating that the newly discovered labile platelet-inhibitory prostaglandin, prostacyclin (PGI_2), was synthesised by endothelial cells [18]. Following the pioneering *in vitro* studies of neutrophil adhesion to fibroblasts by Armstrong and Lackie [19], and lymphocyte adhesion to endothelium by Lackie and De Bono [20], we set up quantitative studies of neutrophil adhesion to, and migration across, endothelial cell monolayers [21–23]. We noted that neutrophils adhered preferentially to endothelial cells rather than to other cell types or to artificial substrates in a highly shear-dependent manner. While this should have alerted us to the likelihood that specific adhesion molecules were involved – and, indeed, we had evidence from electron micrographs of very close cellular apposition and endothelial membrane organisation at sites of leukocyte adhesion (Fig. 3) – our view was influenced by the platelet studies and we concentrated, largely unsuccessfully, on seeking soluble endothelium-derived mediators that would modulate leukocyte adhesion. Similar findings were concurrently reported by two other groups [24, 25].

4

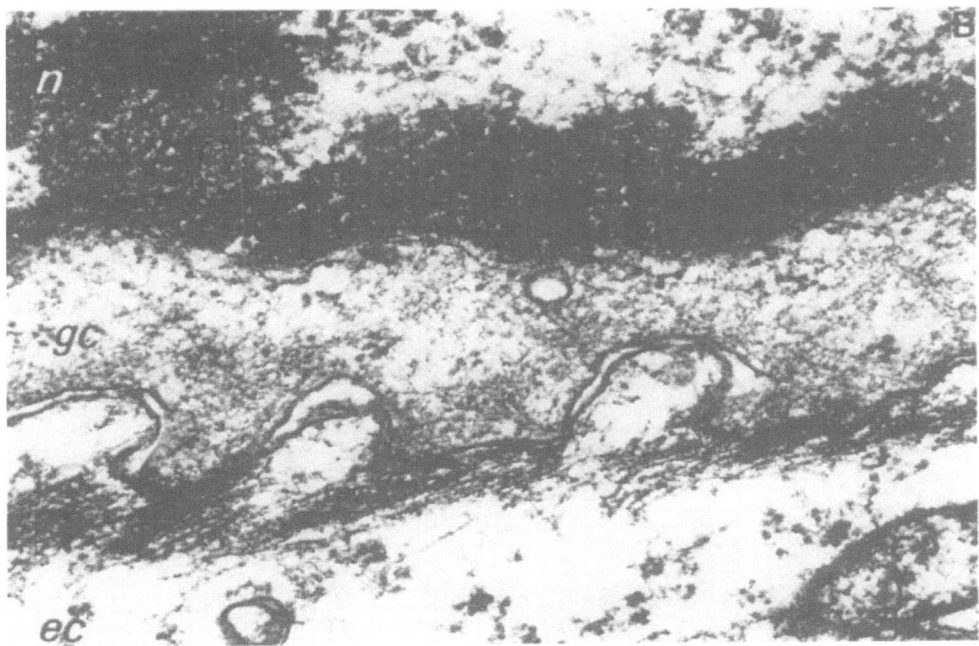

Figure 3
Electron micrograph showing selective microfilament organisation in the endothelial cell
cytoplasm beneath a tightly adherent neutrophil leukocyte. (n, granulocyte nucleus; gc, gran-
ulocyte cytoplasm; ec, endothelial cytoplasm). Final magnification $\cong \times$ 50,000. From [23]
with permission.

Classic work by Gowans' group in Oxford in the 1960s first demonstrated that the specialised "high" endothelial cells in lymph node venules were the site for the efficient adhesion and emigration required to enable lymphocytes to recirculate and encounter antigen [26, 27] (Fig. 4). The development in the 1970s of an adhesion assay using lymph node sections, by Stamper and Woodruff [28], showed that lymphocyte adhesion was highly selective to these endothelial cells, and Butcher et al. [29] then used a similar assay system to demonstrate that different lymphocyte subpopulations exhibited tissue-specific preferences in lymph node binding.

Thus by 1980 the concept that selective adhesion interactions were due to specific adhesion molecules expressed by leukocytes and/or endothelial cells was firmly established, but no such molecule had been identified, and nothing was known about the regulation of adhesion molecule expression or activity.

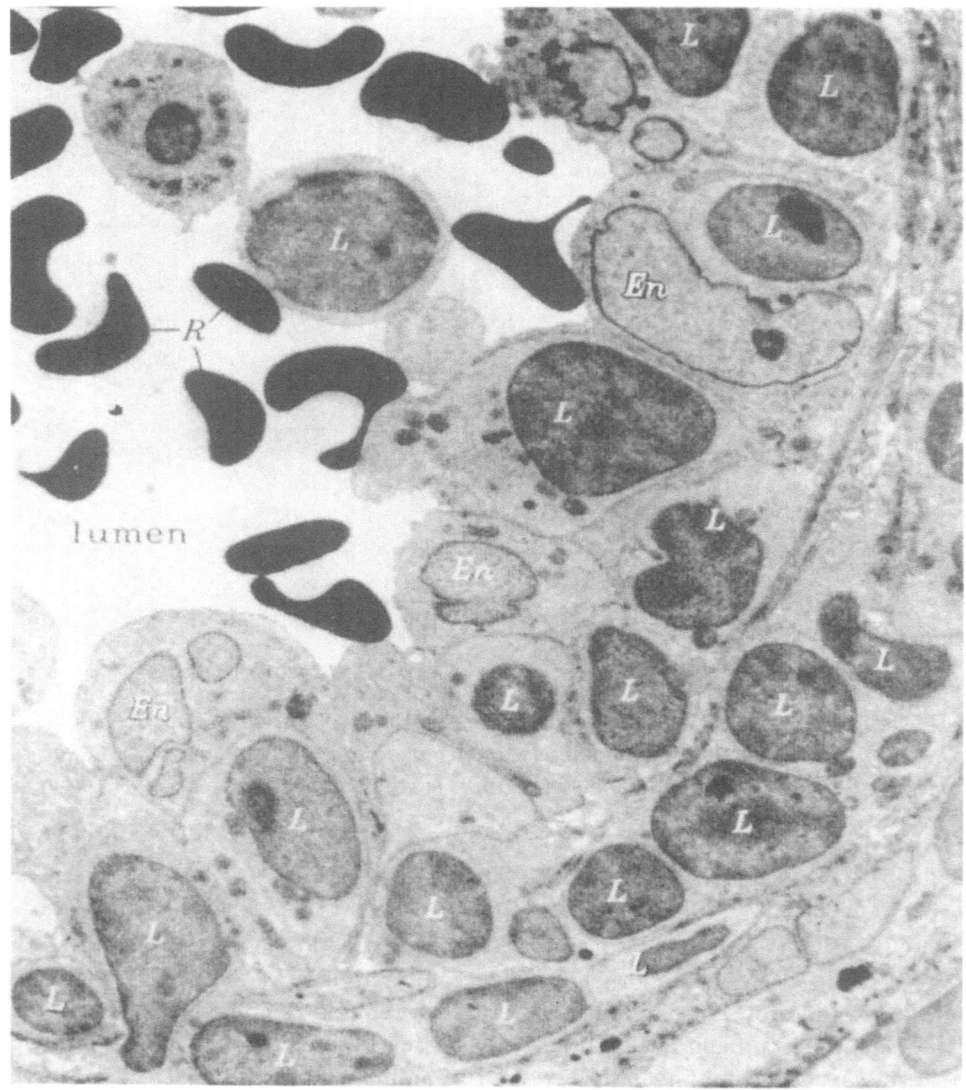

Figure 4
Electron micrograph showing emigrating lymphocytes in the post-capillary venule of a rat lymph node (L, lymphocyte; En, endothelial cell). From [27] with permission.

The first blocking antibody, Mel 14, that inhibited mouse lymphocyte adhesion to lymph nodes, was described by Gallatin et al. in 1983 [30]. In the early 1980s a series of leukocyte surface antigens was defined by monoclonal antibodies and in 1984 it was shown that one of these, LFA-1 (CD11a/CD18) was selectively missing from leukocytes in patients with the rare but debilitating Leukocyte Adhesion Deficiency disease [31]. The heterodimeric CD11/CD18 molecule proved to be an early member of the still expanding family of integrins, first implicated in the early 1980s in platelet adhesion and fibroblast-matrix adhesion [32]. The availability of CD11/CD18-deficient lymphocyte lines led to the discovery in 1986 by Rothlein et al. [33] of intercellular adhesion molecule-1 (ICAM-1), the ligand on these cells bound by CD11/CD18, and they also noted its presence on endothelium.

Simmons et al. [34] used the newly-developed technique of expression cloning to clone ICAM-1 and define it as a member of the immunoglobulin superfamily of adhesion molecules, subsequently joined by vascular cell adhesion molecule-1 (VCAM-1) [35]. A monoclonal antibody (H4/18), later found to recognise E-selectin, a member of the third group of vascular adhesion molecules, was first raised by Pober et al. [36], who then showed that H4/18 binding to endothelial cells increased in response to cytokines in parallel with increased leukocyte adhesion; they cloned E-selectin four years later [37]. At the same time the human homologue, LAM-1 (i.e. L-selectin), of the adhesion molecule recognised by Mel 14 was cloned [38] and several so-called addressins, responsible for tissue-selective lymphocyte homing, had been identified [39].

Thus, within a decade between 1980 and 1990, the burgeoning power of molecular biology had been used to identify many important vascular adhesion molecules. During the current decade their distinctive contributions to leukocyte pathophysiology have been explored in more depth. Counterligands and domain interactions have been better defined (in particular for the selectins, which recognise oligosaccharide rather than peptide domains of surface glycoproteins). The regulation of expression and activity of adhesion molecules by extracellular agonists such as cytokines, and the intracellular signalling pathways required, are being clarified. A multistep paradigm has been evolved [40] in which sequential molecular interactions have been assigned to: (i) the selectin-induced initial rolling and tethering of leukocytes to endothelium; (ii) the activation of leukocyte integrins by endothelium-bound chemokines or related molecules; (iii) firm adhesion and migration of leukocytes mediated by integrin-Ig superfamily interactions; and (iv) leukocyte emigration, in which another Ig superfamily member, platelet endothelial cell adhesion molecule-1 (PECAM-1), has been implicated (Fig. 5).

The following chapters in this book review our current knowledge of vascular adhesion molecules in each of these interactions, particularly highlighting their selective involvement in specific disease processes, and the potential use of reagents that detect or inhibit adhesion molecule expression to yield novel therapeutic possibilities in inflammatory diseases.

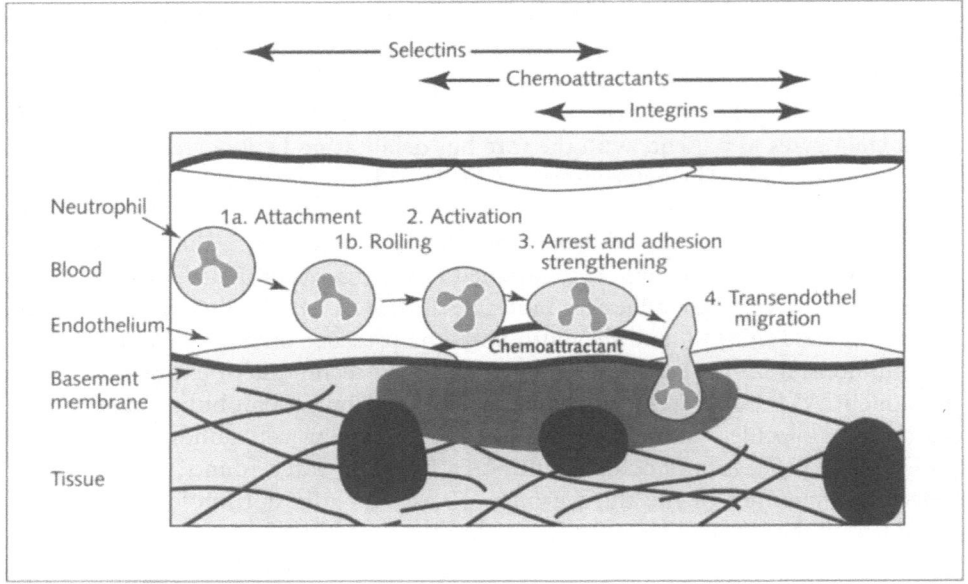

Figure 5
The multistep paradigm for neutrophil adhesion and emigration. From [40] with permission,
© *1995, by Annual Reviews.*

References

1   Dutrochet MH (1824) *Recherches anatomiques et physiologiques sur la structure intime des animaux et des végétaux, et sur leur motilité.* Baillière, Paris

2   Addison W (1843) Experimental and practical researches on the structure and function of blood corpuscles; on inflammation, and on the origin and nature of tubercles in the lungs. *Trans Provinc Med Surg Assoc* 11: 223–306

3   Arnold J (1873) Ueber Diapedesis, Eine experimentelle Studie. *Virchows Archiv* 58: 203–254

4   Arnold J (1875) Ueber das Verhalten der Wandungen der Blutgefässe bei der Emigration weisser Blutkörper. *Virchows Archiv* 62:487–503

5   Leber T (1888) Ueber die Entstehung der Entzündung und die Wirkung der entzündungserregenden Schädlichkeiten. *Fortschritte der Medizin* 4: 460

6   Metchnikoff E (1893) *Lectures on the comparative pathology of inflammation.* Kegan Paul, London

7   Cohnheim J (1889) *Lectures on general pathology,* vol 1. New Sydenham Society, London

8   Clark ER, Clark EL (1935) Observations on changes in blood vascular endothelium in the living animal. *Am J Anat* 57: 385–438

9   Grant L (1973) The sticking and emigration of white blood cells in inflammation. In: Zweifach BW, Grant L, McCluskey RT (eds): *The inflammatory process,* vol 2. Academic Press, London, 205–249

10 Chambers R, Zweifach BW (1947) Intercellular cement and capillary permeability. *Physiol Rev* 27: 436–463

11 Allison F, Smith MR, Wood WB (1955) Studies on the pathogenesis of acute inflammation I : The inflammatory reaction to thermal injury as observed in the rabbit ear chamber. *J Exp Med* 102: 655–668

12 Thompson PL, Papadimitriou JM, Walters MN-I (1967) Suppression of leukocyte sticking and emigration by chelation of calcium. *J Path Bact* 94: 389–396

13 Atherton A, Born GVR (1972) Quantitative investigations of the adhesiveness of circulating polymorphonuclear leukocytes to blood vessel walls. *J Physiol* 222: 447–474

14 Ryan GB, Majno G (1977) Acute inflammation. *Am J Pathol* 86: 185–276

15 Garvin JE (1961) Factors affecting the adhesiveness of human leukocytes and platelets *in vitro. J Exp Med* 114: 51–78

16 MacGregor RR, Spagnuolo PJ, Lentnek AL (1974) Inhibition of granulocyte adherence by ethanol, prednisolone and aspirin, measured with an assay system. *N Eng J Med* 291: 642–646

17 Jaffe EA, Nachman R, Becker C, Minick R (1973) Culture of human endothelial cells derived from umbilical vessels. Identification by morphologic and immunologic criteria. *J Clin Invest* 52: 2745–2756

18 MacIntyre DE, Pearson JD, Gordon JL (1978) Localisation and stimulation of prostacyclin production in vascular cells. *Nature* 271: 549–551

19 Armstrong PB, Lackie JM (1975) Studies on intercellular invasion in vitro using rabbit peritoneal neutrophil granulocytes. *J Cell Biol* 65: 439–462

20 Lackie JM, De Bono DP (1977) Interactions of neutrophil granulocytes and endothelium *in vitro. Microvasc Res* 13: 107–112

21 Beesley JE, Pearson JD, Carleton JS, Hutchings A, Gordon JL (1978) Interaction of leukocytes with vascular cells in culture. *J Cell Sci* 33: 85–101

22 Pearson JD, Carleton JS, Beesley JE, Hutchings A, Gordon JL (1979) Granulocyte adhesion to endothelium cells in culture. *J Cell Sci* 38: 225–235

23 Beesley JE, Pearson JD, Hutchings A, Carleton JS, Gordon JL (1979) Granulocyte migration though endothelial cells in culture. *J Cell Sci* 38: 237–248

24 Hoover RL, Briggs RT, Karnovsky MJ (1978) The adhesive interaction between polymorphonuclear leukocytes and endothelial cells *in vitro. Cell* 14: 423–428

25 MacGregor RR, Macarak EJ, Kefalides N (1978) Comparative adherence of granulocytes to endothelial monolayers and to nylon fibers. *J Clin Invest* 61: 697–702

26 Gowans JL, Knight EJ (1964) The route of re-circulation of lymphocytes in the rat. *Proc Roy Soc B* 159: 257–282

27 Marchesi VT, Gowans JL (1964) The migration of lymphocytes through the endotheli-

um of venules in lymph nodes : an electron microscope study. *Proc Roy Soc B* 159: 283–290

28 Stamper HB, Woodruff JJ (1976) Lymphocyte homing into lymph nodes: *in vitro* demonstration of the selective affinity of recirculating lymphocytes for high-endothelial venules. *J Exp Med* 144: 828–833

29 Butcher EC, Scollay RG, Weissman IL (1980) Organ specificity of lymphocyte migration: mediation by highly selective lymphocyte interaction with organ-specific determinants on high endothelial venules. *Eur J Immunol* 10: 556–561

30 Gallatin WM, Weissman IL, Butcher EL (1983) A cell surface molecule involved in organ-specific homing of lymphocytes. *Nature* 304: 30–34

31 Anderson DC, Springer TA (1987) Leukocyte adhesion deficiency: an inherited defect in the Mac-1, LFA-1 and p150, 95 glycoproteins. *Ann Rev Med* 38: 175–194

32 Hynes RO (1987) Integrins: a family of cell surface receptors. *Cell* 48: 549–554

33 Rothlein R, Dustin ML, Martin SD, Springer TA (1986) A human intercellular adhesion molecule (ICAM-1) distinct from LFA-1. *J Immunol* 137: 1270–1274

34 Simmons D, Makgoba MW, Seed B (1988) ICAM, an adhesion ligand of LFA-1, is homologous to the neural cell adhesion molecule NCAM. *Nature* 331: 624–627

35 Osborn L, Hession C, Tizard R, Vassallo C, Luhowskyj JS, Chi-Rosso G, Lobb R (1980) Direct cloning of vascular cell adhesion molecule 1 (VCAM-1), a cytokine-induced endothelial protein that binds to lymphocytes. *Cell* 59: 1203–1211

36 Pober JS, Bevilacqua MP, Mendrick DL, Lapierre LA, Fiers W, Gimbrone MA Jr (1986) Two distinct monokines, interleukin-1 and tumour necrosis factor, each independently induce biosynthesis and transient expression of the same antigen on the surface of cultured human vascular endothelial cells. *J Immunol* 136: 1680–1687

37 Bevilacqua MP, Stengelin S, Gimbrone MA Jr, Seed B (1989) Endothelial leukocyte adhesion molecule 1: an inducible receptor for neutrophils related to complement regulatory proteins and lectins. *Science* 243: 1160–1165

38 Tedder TF, Issacs CM, Ernst TJ, Demetri GD, Adler DA, Disteche CM (1989) Isolation and chromosomal localization of cDNAs encoding a novel human lymphocyte cell surface molecule, LAM-1. *J Exp Med* 170: 123–133

39 Berg EL, Goldstein LA, Jutila MA, Nakache M, Picker LJ, Streeter PR, Wu NW, Zhou D, Butcher EC (1989) Homing receptors and vascular addressins: cell adhesion molecules that direct lymphocyte traffic. *Immunol Rev* 108: 5–18

40 Springer TA (1995) Traffic signals on endothelium for lymphocyte recirculation and leukocyte emigration. *Ann Rev Physiol* 57: 857–87

Adhesion of leukocytes from flow:
The selectins and their ligands

Klaus Ley

University of Virginia School of Medicine, Department of Biomedical Engineering, Health Sciences Center, Box 377, Charlottesville, VA 22908, USA

The multistep process of leukocyte adhesion in inflammation

Leukocyte adhesion is a hallmark of the inflammatory process. Their recruitment to a site of inflammation encompasses a remarkable sequence of events necessary to efficiently and specifically arrest leukocytes on the vascular endothelium and direct their transmigration [1–6]. In most inflammatory settings, leukocyte recruitment is restricted to postcapillary venules with diameters between 10 and 300 μm. Typical blood flow velocities in such vessels range from 1 to 10 mm/s, allowing for blood transit times on the order of 0.1 to 0.01 s for a 100 μm segment of venule. This time interval is too short to ensure activation and attachment of leukocytes suspended in the flowing blood.

Early work on leukocyte recruitment focused on the role of margination, defined as a process by which the leukocyte is brought into close proximity with the endothelium [7]. As long as the leukocyte is not in physical contact with the endothelium, margination depends entirely on rheological forces exerted on the leukocyte. In small venules (diameter ~ 10 μm), red blood cells can travel slightly faster than white blood cells because of their larger deformability and consequently smaller hydrodynamic cross section. Therefore, red blood cells tend to overtake white blood cells in small postcapillary venules [8], thereby pushing the leukocyte closer to the vessel wall. Additional rheological margination mechanisms exist [9, 10], which depend on the tendency of red blood cells to reversibly aggregate with each other, especially under inflammatory conditions. However, even a maximally marginated leukocyte (diameter, 7 μm) that almost touches the vessel wall travels at a velocity ranging between 14% and 51% of the blood flow velocity in vessels with diameters of 100 μm and 20 μm, respectively. This velocity has been termed critical velocity [11] or hydrodynamic velocity [12] and is an accurate criterion for distinguishing rolling from freely flowing leukocytes in microvessels *in vivo* [13] and in flow chambers *in vitro* [12].

Leukocyte rolling is initiated by a distinguishing event called tethering [14] or capture [15]. Capture is defined as the formation of the first molecular bond

Vascular Adhesion Molecules and Inflammation, edited by J. D. Pearson
© 1999 Birkhäuser Verlag Basel/Switzerland

between the flowing leukocyte and the vascular endothelium. This step obviously requires very rapid bond formation and exceptional bond strength for an initial period until more bonds are formed. Capture is distinguishable from stable leukocyte rolling and is mediated by an overlapping but distinct set of adhesion molecules. In model experiments using parallel-plate flow chambers, the capture event is often initiated by an interaction between flowing and already adherent leukocytes [16], a phenomenon called secondary tethering or capture as opposed to primary capture between the leukocyte and the substrate proper. Attachment through secondary capture appears to be favored by the geometry of parallel-plate flow chambers, absence of red blood cells, and the gravitational force causing sedimentation of flowing leukocytes prior to attachment. In inflamed venules *in vivo*, only a small percentage of leukocyte attachment appears to involve secondary capture [17].

If leukocyte capture is followed by the formation of new molecular bonds before the initial molecular bonds dissociate, a stable rolling movement ensues [18, 19]. Rolling is defined as a flow-driven downstream movement of a cell traveling below the critical velocity and being in continuous contact with the vessel wall. Rolling does not require metabolic energy, because it can proceed in the presence of inhibitors of metabolism [20] and even when the leukocytes are fixed [21]. Even beads coated with appropriate adhesion molecules can roll on immobilized adhesion molecules [22] or on activated endothelial cells [23] *in vitro*. However, the velocity of leukocyte rolling is modulated by proteolytic shedding of at least one of the adhesion molecules involved, L-selectin. Blocking L-selectin shedding reduces the velocity of rolling leukocytes *in vitro* [23a] and *in vivo* [23b]. Rolling has at least two distinct consequences for the cell, (i) rolling may facilitate stable leukocyte arrest (firm adhesion), and (ii) rolling drastically reduces the leukocyte velocity (to between 1 and 100 µm/s) and hence increases the leukocyte transit time during which the leukocyte is exposed to chemoattractants presented on the endothelial surface.

After a rolling leukocyte encounters an appropriate activating signal, usually in the form of a chemoattractant or chemokine molecule binding to a heptahelical transmembrane receptor on the leukocyte surface, leukocyte activation ensues which is necessary for firm adhesion [3, 5, 24]. In flow chamber systems, this process can be exceptionally rapid [24a,b], but neutrophil activation during rolling *in vivo* may require as much as ~ 80 s and ~ 300 µm of rolling distance [83]. Firm adhesion is thought to require binding between integrin receptors in their active conformation and their endothelial ligands. The details of this process are described in the chapter by Smith et al. in this volume.

The selectins

The selectins are a family of mammalian lectins expressed on the surface of leukocytes, endothelial cells, and platelets [25–27]. The three selectins share about 50%

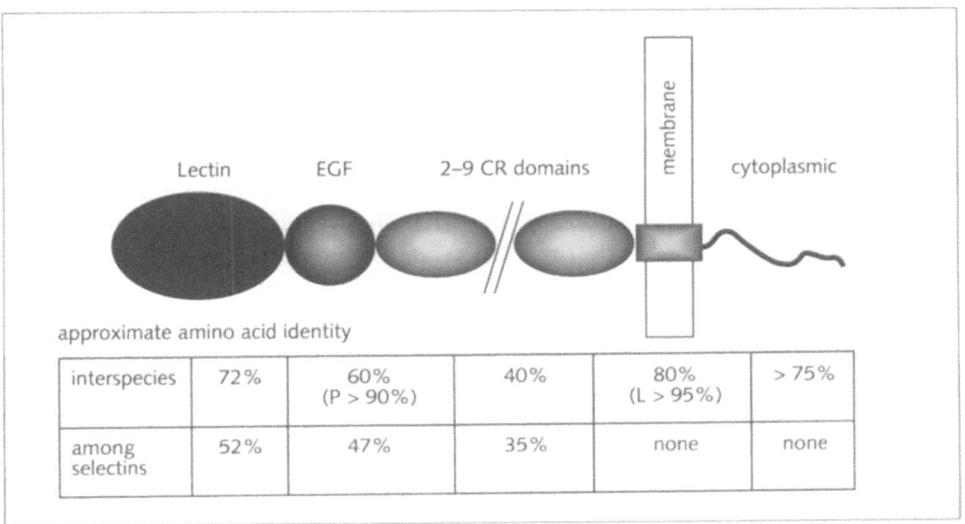

Lectin   EGF   2–9 CR domains   membrane   cytoplasmic

approximate amino acid identity

	Lectin	EGF	2–9 CR domains	membrane	cytoplasmic
interspecies	72%	60% (P > 90%)	40%	80% (L > 95%)	> 75%
among selectins	52%	47%	35%	none	none

Figure 1
Schematic representation of the modular structure of the selectins. Lectin, C-type lectin domain; EGF, domain with homology to epidermal growth factor; CR, consensus repeats with homology to complement regulatory proteins (only 2 are shown, but more may be present, indicated by slashes); transmembrane domain shown inserted in cell membrane. Approximate amino acid identities for the same selectin among species (top) and among the different selectins within one species (bottom) indicated. P, P-selectin; L, L-selectin. Modified from [27].

sequence homology among the extracellular portions of the molecule, but not in the transmembrane and cytoplasmic domains [27, 28]. Figure 1 shows a schematic representation of the modular structure of the selectins. The N-terminal lectin domain is followed by a domain with homology to epidermal growth factor (EGF) and two (L-selectin), six (E-selectin) or nine (P-selectin) domains with sequence homology to complement regulatory proteins. These domains are also called short consensus repeats (CR). The domain boundaries coincide with exon boundaries in the selectin genes, which are all located on chromosome 1 and have evolved by gene duplication [28]. Although the primary structure of each of the selectins encodes for a single membrane-spanning domain and does not predict oligomerization, it is not clear whether the selectins exert their physiological function as monomers. The structure of the selectins is highly conserved among species, but the number of CR domains can vary slightly.

L-selectin is expressed on most peripheral blood leukocytes where its expression is developmentally regulated. Whereas all mature neutrophils, eosinophils, and monocytes express L-selectin, lymphocytes appear to express L-selectin preferentially in the naïve state. L-selectin is expressed on some, but not all memory T and B cells and a subset of natural killer cells [27]. L-selectin is expressed by many immature hematopoietic cells in the bone marrow. On neutrophils, the level of L-selectin expression correlates negatively with the age of the individual cell, suggesting that neutrophils may lose L-selectin as they mature in the bone marrow [29] and age in the circulation [30]. Although most lymphocytes in the cortex of secondary lymphoid organs express L-selectin, the activated cells in the germinal centers do not [27]. This corresponds to reduced or absent L-selectin expression in activated lymphocytes. L-selectin disappears from the cell surface through the action of an unidentified metalloproteinase which catalyzes the cleavage of L-selectin at an extracellular site between K283 and S284 of the mature protein, close to the membrane [31–33]. Proteolytic cleavage leads to shedding of L-selectin into the suspending fluid. The shedding metalloproteinase [34] is activated after chemoattractant or other activation of the leukocytes [35–37]. For neutrophils, activating agents that induce shedding include chemokines such as interleukin-8 (IL-8), complement factors like C5a, bacterial peptides such as formyl-methionyl-leucyl-phenylalanine (fMLP), and lipid mediators like platelet activating factor (PAF) or leukotriene B_4 (LTB_4) [38]. Lymphocytes in culture shed L-selectin when they are stimulated with phorbol esters, or by cross-linking of CD3 [39]. *In vivo*, shed L-selectin is present in the plasma at high concentrations [40] and may further increase under inflammatory conditions [41], but clear correlations remain to be established. The level of L-selectin in the plasma correlates with a negative outcome in acute myeloid leukemia [41a]. On leukocytes, L-selectin is preferentially expressed on the tips of microprocesses [42], and this location has been shown to be critical for cell capture under flow conditions, but no longer necessary once rolling is established [43]. The mechanism of L-selectin localization to microprocesses is not understood. L-selectin binds to cytoskeletal α-actinin via its cytoplasmic tail [44]. L-selectin lacking most of its cytoplasmic tail fails to bind α-actinin [44] and fails to support leukocyte adhesion under flow [45], but is still sorted to microprocesses in lymphoid cells [44].

P-selectin is constitutively synthesized by megakaryocytes and endothelial cells, but not expressed on the surface of resting platelets or endothelial cells. Rather, P-selectin is stored in secretory vesicles called Weibel-Palade bodies in endothelial cells and α-granules in platelets through the regulated secretion pathway [46, 47]. P-selectin is expressed on the cell surface after these granules fuse with the plasma membrane, which is promoted by activators like histamine, thrombin, complement C5a, calcium ionophores, and adenosine diphosphate (ADP) [46–49]. Maximal expression of P-selectin at the cell surface is detected within a few minutes, after which expression is reduced by rapid internalization and degradation [46]. Some P-selectin is also shed from the cell surface and can be measured as soluble protein in the blood plasma [50]. In the mouse, cytokine activation of endothelial cells induces a more prolonged surface expression of P-selectin through transcriptional regulation

[51–53]. In humans, P-selectin expression is not induced by cytokine stimulation, which may be based on structural differences in the promoter region [53a,b].

E-selectin is expressed by endothelial cells activated by interleukin-1 (IL-1) or tumor necrosis factor α (TNFα) [54, 55], but is not expressed by platelets. Its expression is under the control of nuclear factor κB (NFκB), which is dissociated from its cytoplasmic inhibitor, IκB, via the proteasome pathway [56]. E-selectin expression on cultured endothelial cells is transient with a maximum between 2 and 6 hours. E-selectin is re-internalized and also shed from the endothelial surface [57]. E-selectin expression *in vivo* appears to be more prolonged at least in some organs [58]. Soluble E-selectin in blood plasma is a useful marker for the activity of some inflammatory diseases [59].

Selectin function: Adhesion under flow

All three selectins are involved in trafficking of granulocytes and lymphocytes to sites of inflammation and immune activity. Selectins specialize in cell capture from flow, which requires the rapid formation of the first molecular bond to initiate capture, eventually followed by stable rolling (Fig. 2). The selectins bind to their ligands with moderate affinities, exhibiting equilibrium dissociation constants in the nanomolar range [60]. Importantly, the selectins appear to be endowed with exceptionally rapid forward reaction rates (on-rates) [61], although direct measurements have not been reported so far. Since the equilibrium binding dissociation constant is

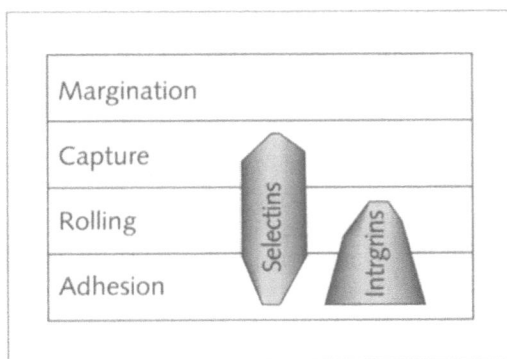

Figure 2
Role of selectins and integrins in leukocyte adhesion under flow. The selectins initiate capture (L,P), mediate rolling (P,E) and support the transition to firm adhesion (E). Some integrins (α₄) support rolling or reduce rolling velocity (β₂), and are responsible for firm adhesion.

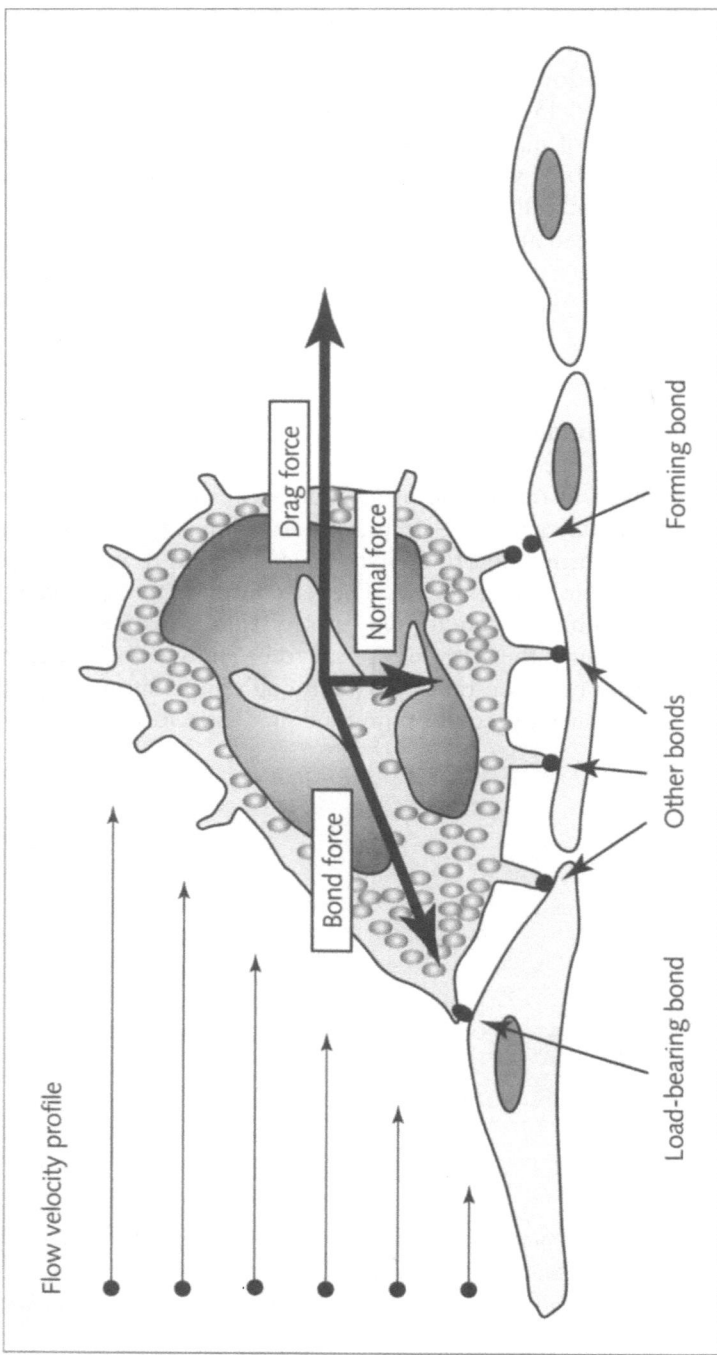

Figure 3

Forces acting on a rolling leukocyte. The flowing blood exerts a drag force (arrow) in the direction parallel to the flow, which is roughly equal to three times the exposed surface area times the wall shear stress [177]. This force is partially balanced by the bond force (arrow) exerted by selectin bonds at the trailing end of the leukocyte [18]. The resulting normal force (vertical arrow) pushes the leukocyte toward the underlying substrate and is balanced by a reaction force of equal size and opposite direction (not shown). New bonds form at the leading edge where the leukocyte first makes contact with the substrate. Shape of rolling leukocyte based on in vivo measurements [18,178]. Bonds outside the trailing edge are thought to not bear load, but this has not been measured directly.

the ratio of the off-and on-rates, on-rates can indirectly be estimated by measuring off-rates as observed for individual bonds under flow. This idea was pioneered by Kaplanski and Bongrand [62] for E-selectin and later applied to P-selectin [63] and L-selectin [64]. These experiments suggest that E-selectin has a slightly slower off-rate than P-selectin, and L-selectin may have the highest off-rate ([63, 64] and M.B. Lawrence, unpublished observations). In addition to the selectin dissociation rate under no-load conditions [64a], the bond response to mechanical load is very important, because the selectin bonds bear essentially all of the drag force exerted on the rolling leukocyte by the flowing blood (Fig. 3). Modeling studies have predicted that the off-rate of selectins would increase with mechanical load [18]. This property was recently confirmed experimentally for P-selectin [63] and L-selectin [64].

Although the selectins all serve functions in leukocyte recruitment under flow, each selectin plays a distinctive role in the physiological sequence of events, and the importance of each selectin varies among models of inflammation. Importantly, L-selectin serves a mandatory role in lymphocyte homing to peripheral lymph nodes [65] and an accessory role in lymphocyte homing to Peyer's patches, a component of the gut-associated lymphatic tissue [65], as described in the chapter by Jutila, this volume. High endothelial venules (HEV) in these tissues constitutively express functional ligands for L-selectin on their surface. The important role of L-selectin in lymphocyte homing is emphasized by the absence of normal-sized lymph nodes in L-selectin knockout mice [65] and a delay in lymphocyte homing to Peyer's patches [65]. Here, L-selectin appears to synergize with β_7 integrins, because absence of both L-selectin and β_7 integrins completely abrogates lymphocyte homing to Peyer's patches [66, 66a].

L-selectin also plays an important role in recruiting neutrophils and other cells to sites of inflammation [67, 68]. This is most clearly illustrated by the substantial inflammatory defects seen in L-selectin deficient mice [65, 69]. Although several reports have shown that neutrophils and monocytes can bind to activated endothelial cells through L-selectin [70–72], the molecular nature of L-selectin ligand(s) on endothelial cells has remained elusive. L-selectin ligand directly mediates leukocyte rolling on inflamed endothelium [74, 76, 77] *in vivo*. L-selectin-mediated leukocyte binding appears to peak at ~8 h of TNFα treatment [73], well past the peak of expression of E-selectin. After prolonged stimulation with TNFα, L-selectin can also support neutrophil rolling in venules of E-selectin and P-selectin double mutant mice [74]. Recently, a posttranslational modification recognized by an antibody to the cutaneous lymphocyte antigen has been shown to be important for L-selectin ligand activity on inflamed endothelial cells [77a]. L-selectin is also involved in mediating leukocyte-leukocyte interactions [16, 75]. Although leukocyte-leukocyte interactions appear to be of little significance for neutrophil accumulation under at least some inflammatory conditions *in vivo* [17], they may facilitate recruitment of L-selectin-bearing monocytes and lymphocytes to sites of inflammation.

Rolling mediated by L-selectin occurs at much higher velocities (typically ~ 100 µm/s) than rolling through P- or E-selectin [76, 78]. Under conditions of mild stimulation *in vivo*, smooth rolling is not observed at physiological wall shear rates when E- and P-selectins are not present or not functional [78]. Rather, L-selectin mediated rolling appears to be a succession of capture and detachment events, resulting in intermittent rolling, or "skipping". When the velocity is averaged over a fixed distance or time period, the velocities of these skipping cells are determined to be smaller than the critical velocity, confirming the presence of intermittent adhesive interactions. These findings support the concept that L-selectin is particularly apt at mediating capture events. However, after long-term stimulation with TNFα, L-selectin can also mediate much slower rolling (~ 20 µm/s), suggesting that more or different L-selectin ligands can be induced on inflamed endothelium [74]. Although L-selectin is necessary for this rolling after prolonged TNFα treatment, other integrin-dependent adhesion mechanisms may also help to slow down rolling leukocytes under these conditions since TNFα activated endothelium expresses various chemoattractants that may activate rolling leukocytes to engage integrin-mediated adhesion. In support of this concept, gene-targeted mice lacking the receptor for a major endogenous chemoattractant, IL-8, show elevated leukocyte rolling velocities [79]. Similarly, blocking the CD18 subunit of β_2 integrins [80, 81] or eliminating CD18 by gene targeting [82] results in elevated rolling velocities on inflamed endothelium *in vivo* [83]. The interplay between selectins and integrin-mediated adhesion in leukocyte rolling and adhesion is an emerging theme and requires further studies to fully understand the implications of this interaction.

During inflammation, endogenous inflammatory mediators including histamine and thrombin promote fusion of the Weibel-Palade bodies with the plasma membrane [46, 47], leading to rapid and robust surface expression of P-selectin [53]. Intravital microscopic experiments in many laboratories have shown that P-selectin is responsible for "spontaneous" leukocyte rolling [77, 84–87]. Rolling is not truly spontaneous, because P-selectin expression is induced by the minimal trauma associated with careful preparation for intravital microscopy [53, 77, 85, 88–90], and this induction is at least partially dependent on mast cell degranulation [89, 91, 92]. Under these conditions, expression of P-selectin is limited to venules [53], which coincides with the site of leukocyte rolling [13, 90]. After cytokine stimulation with TNFα, some leukocyte rolling and concomitant P-selectin expression are also seen on the endothelial lining of arterioles, which is completely absent in P-selectin deficient mice [93]. In P-selectin deficient mice, leukocyte rolling is initially also absent in venules of all tissues studied [77, 84], but leukocyte rolling is induced to various degrees at later time points [77] after treatment with inflammatory cytokines such as TNFα [77, 94, 95], or in the dorsal skin fold chamber [96]. In addition, endothelial P-selectin apparently binds to an unidentified ligand on platelets to mediate platelet rolling in inflamed venules *in vivo* [97]. Activated platelets can bind to monocytes and other leukocytes through P-selectin [98, 99] and may be able to direct lymphocytes to high endothelial venules independent of L-selectin [100].

Although the defect of leukocyte rolling in P-selectin deficient mice is very impressive, neutrophil recruitment to sites of inflammation is only delayed by about 2 h, but not abolished [84, 94, 101, 102]. This finding prompted investigations into the potential overlapping nature of selectin function. Leukocyte recruitment to mouse peritonitis was blocked when both P- and L-selectin [103] or both P- and E-selectin [102, 104–106] were blocked by monoclonal antibodies or gene targeting. Mice lacking both P- and E-selectins do not only lack efficient neutrophil recruitment to sites of inflammation, but also show more than ten-fold elevated circulating neutrophil counts, spontaneous dermatitis, and other inflammation-related pathologies [104, 105]. It will be important to determine whether the large numbers of circulating neutrophils, high levels of chemokines, and elevated immunoglobulin concentrations are secondary to these inflammatory pathologies [104] or primary disturbances of the hematopoietic system [105]. Recently, mice lacking E- and P-selectin have been found to have a homing defect of hematopoietic stem cells to bone marrow [105a]. Interestingly, IL-8 receptor knockout mice, which also have high circulating leukocyte counts [107], revert to normal counts when kept under strictly germ-free conditions [108]. It is not clear whether eliminating or blocking all three selectins would have additional effects beyond those seen in P- and E-selectin double mutant mice. Recent data suggest that residual L-selectin dependent rolling occurs in mice lacking both P- and E-selectin after prolonged (6–8 h) cytokine treatment, and accounts for significant neutrophil accumulation [74]. Although mice lacking all three selectins show even less leukocyte rolling [108a], they have lower circulating leukocyte counts than mice lacking only E- and P-selectin, and do not show spontaneous disease [108b].

Although P- and E-selectin have overlapping functions in mediating rolling, distinctive properties can be identified for each molecule. As suggested by *in vitro* experiments [12, 21], P-selectin mediated rolling occurs at about five times higher velocities than E-selectin mediated rolling in venules *in vivo* [95]. It is not clear whether this can be attributed to a slower dissociation rate of E-selectin because the number of selectin molecules per unit surface area may not be equivalent for P- and E-selectin in venules. The slow rolling velocity of leukocytes rolling on E-selectin facilitates the induction of firm leukocyte adhesion in response to local chemoattractant [109]. However, it appears that E-selectin is not required for leukocyte recruitment in at least some models of inflammation because E-selectin deficient mice recruit normal or supra-normal numbers of neutrophils into peritonitis models [104, 106]. Interestingly, E-selectin deficient mice succumb to systemic infection with *Streptococcus pneumoniae* [110], suggesting that efficient elimination of some organisms may require E-selectin.

Although many *in vitro* studies have shown that ligation of L-selectin [111–115] or selectin ligands [116–118] can activate leukocytes, there is no direct evidence that such signaling contributes to leukocyte activation relevant to leukocyte recruitment. Importantly, neutrophils rolling over a substrate containing both P-selectin and intercellular adhesion molecule-1 (ICAM-1), a ligand for β_2 integrins, do not show signs of activation and do not adhere firmly, whereas introduction of a soluble chemoattractant into the system rapidly leads to firm adhesion [12]. Similarly, lymphocytes roll over a surface coated with a mixture of partially purified L-selectin ligand and ICAM-1 without becoming activated, unless a chemoattractant is also presented [119]. *In vivo*, rolling can be maintained for hours without leading to significant leukocyte attachment or transmigration [13, 90]. Taken together, these data suggest that engaging selectins during physiological rolling may be insufficient to trigger activating signals. However, selectin-mediated activation may augment chemokine-induced activation and may be important in other settings including antigen presentation in secondary lymphoid organs.

Selectin ligands

After sialylated and fucosylated oligosaccharides such as sialyl-Lewis^x were shown to possess binding activity for all three selectins [120–122], a search for high-affinity ligands revealed that specific glycoproteins with appropriate post-translational modifications are necessary for high-affinity binding of selectins [123–125]. To date, the best-characterized selectin ligand is P-selectin glycoprotein ligand-1 (PSGL-1) [124, 126] (Fig. 4). PSGL-1 is a type 1 surface glycoprotein which is expressed on microprocesses of essentially all leukocytes [127]. PSGL-1 requires post-translational modifications to function as a P-selectin ligand. Critical modifications include tyrosine sulfation [128, 129], sialylation [130], decoration with core 2 oligosaccarides [131] and, perhaps most importantly, fucosylation [126]. Although PSGL-1 appears to be tyrosine-sulfated and sialylated on most or all leukocytes, fucosylation is regulated by specific, inducible fucosyl transferases (FT). Fucosyl transferase VII (FTVII) plays a key role in producing functional PSGL-1 [131–134] and other functional selectin ligands [134–136]. Mice lacking FTVII show severe restrictions of neutrophil trafficking [137], although they do not develop spontaneous disease as do mice lacking both E- and P-selectins [104, 105]. The expression of FTVII in lymphocytes appears to be regulated, enabling effector T cells to express functional P- and E-selectin ligands [135, 138, 139]. FTVII is constitutively expressed in neutrophils, monocytes and eosinophils [132, 133]. Another fucosyl transferase, FTIV, is also expressed in leukocytes, although at lower levels of activity [140]. PSGL-1 can also bind L-selectin [141, 142] and appears to be responsible for a portion, although not all [16, 143], of the interaction between flowing and already adherent leukocytes. Biochemical data have suggested that PSGL-1 can serve as a ligand for E-selectin [23, 144], but functional data using transfected cell lines and various mutants [27, 134] suggest that PSGL-1 is not relevant for mediating E-selectin

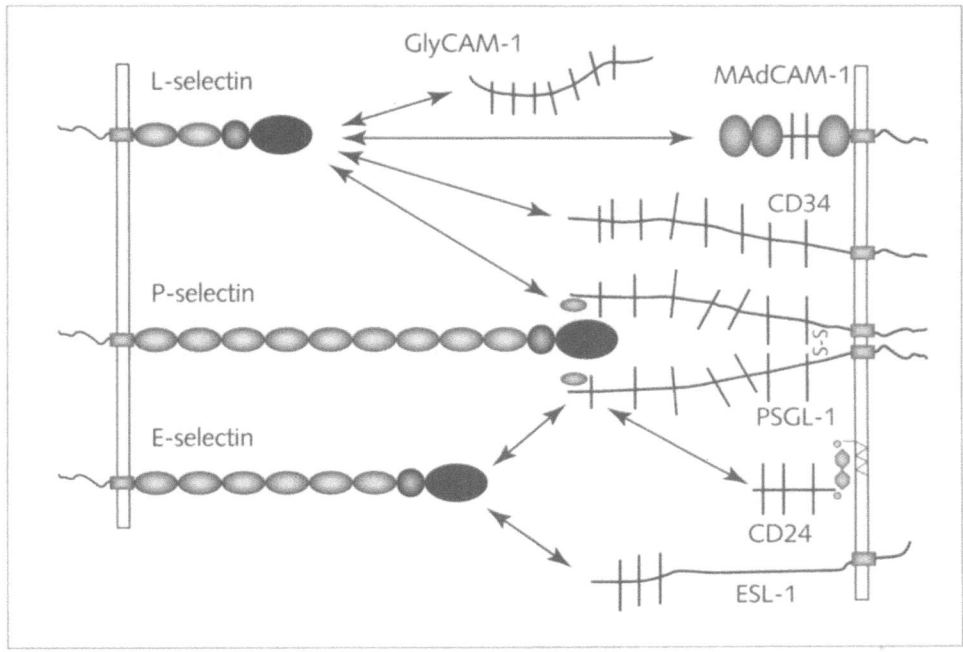

Figure 4

Selectins (left) and their ligands (right). The domains of the selectins are represented as in Figure 1. All selectin ligands possess oligosaccharide side chains (vertical lines). GlyCAM-1, glycosylation-dependent cell adhesion molecule-1 (secreted); MAdCAM-1, mucosal addressin adhesion molecule-1; immunoglobulin domains shown as filled circles; PSGL-1, P-selectin glycoprotein ligand-1, shown as dimer (S-S); tyrosine sulfate shown as small ovals; ESL-1, E-selectin ligand-1. Double headed arrows indicate interactions, not all of which may be relevant to leukocyte adhesion under flow.

dependent rolling under physiological conditions. *In vivo*, the role for PSGL-1 in binding to P-selectin has been directly demonstrated [145, 146], but potential roles of PSGL-1 in binding to L- and E-selectin await investigation. A second ligand for P-selectin is the glycosyl-phosphatidyl-inositol (GPI)-linked mucin CD24, which is expressed on most blood cells and many other cells. Again, P-selectin binding function appears to be regulated by post-translational modifications because CD24 from some, but not all, cells supports P-selectin-dependent binding [147, 148]. In myeloid cells which also express PSGL-1, CD24 appears to play a very minor, if any, role in P-selectin binding [149]. However, under near-physiological flow conditions, CD24 appears to account for most P-selectin binding in tumor cells which are negative for PSGL-1 [148, 149].

Several glycoproteins have been proposed to serve as ligands for L-selectin. Glycosylation-dependent cell adhesion molecule-1 (GlyCAM-1) was initially identified as sgp50 by immunopurification from sulfate-labeled mouse lymph nodes [125] and was subsequently cloned and sequenced ([150]; see also the chapter by Jutila, this volume). Since GlyCAM-1 does not possess a transmembrane domain and is secreted into plasma [151] and milk [152], it probably does not serve as an adhesion molecule under physiological conditions. Recent experiments have suggested that GlyCAM-1 binding to L-selectin may specifically activate naïve lymphocytes and promote their adhesion and transmigration in lymph node microvessels [153, 154]. A second L-selectin binding molecule identified in the same manner is CD34 [155], a transmembrane mucin expressed broadly on endothelium and hematopoietic cells [156]. CD34 is contained in a mixture of glycoproteins called peripheral node addressin (PNAd) that can be purified from lymph nodes or tonsils using the carbohydrate-binding monoclonal antibody MECA-79 [157, 158]. CD34 appears to account for about one half of the L-selectin binding activity of PNAd [159]. It is unlikely that CD34 plays a major role in L-selectin mediated lymphocyte homing to peripheral lymph nodes since gene-targeted mice lacking CD34 have no defect in lymphocyte homing [160, 161], which is in contrast to L-selectin deficient mice [65]. Very discrete inflammatory defects are seen in CD34 deficient mice [160, 161], whereas substantial deficiencies are observed in L-selectin deficient mice [65, 69, 77]. Mice lacking GlyCAM-1 or both GlyCAM-1 and CD34 do not show obvious defects in lymphocyte homing or inflammation (L.A. Lasky, unpublished data). A third putative L-selectin ligand, sgp200, also isolated from lymph node tissue [158], awaits sequencing and further characterization. Recently, a podocalysin-like sialomucin present in high endothelial venules has been shown to support lymphocyte rolling in a flow chamber assay [161a]. Several studies have shown that sulfatides [111, 162] and heparan sulfate proteoglycans [163, 164] can bind to L-selectin, but a physiological role of these potential L-selectin ligands has yet to be demonstrated. As mentioned above, PSGL-1 [141, 142] and other mucin-like molecules expressed on neutrophils and hematopoietic cells [16, 143] can bind to L-selectin and may serve to initiate leukocyte rolling by nucleating capture events [16]. The physiological role of selectin-dependent interactions among neutrophils [16, 75, 165], monocytes [16] and lymphocytes [16, 166] remains to be explored. Interestingly, L-selectin ligands on inflamed endothelium have repeatedly been characterized functionally both *in vitro* [70, 72] and *in vivo* [76, 85], but no candidate molecules have been identified which could serve as endothelial L-selectin ligands in inflammation. A recent report [16] suggested that secondary capture may be responsible for the apparent role of L-selectin in binding to endothelium, but such L-selectin dependent binding also occurs in conditions where few [74, 76] or no [77] adherent leukocytes are present, indicating that primary capture and rolling on endothelium through L-selectin occurs *in vivo*. L-selectin ligand(s) on inflamed human endothelium appear to require a carbohydrate epitope recognized by an antibody to cutaneous lymphocyte antigen [77a]. A further ligand for L-selectin is mucosal addressin adhesion molecule-1 (MAdCAM-1), an adhesion molecule expressed on the surface of high endothelial venules of Peyer's patches and mucosal lymph nodes [167, 168]. MAd-CAM-1 immunopurified from mesenteric lymph nodes of young mice supports L-selectin dependent lymphocyte rolling in a flow chamber assay [169]. Intravital microscopic evidence shows a role for L-selectin in lymphocyte rolling in Peyer's patch high endothelial venules, but it is not clear whether all L-selectin ligand activity in this system is attributable to MAdCAM-1 [66, 66a, 170].

E-selectin was initially reported to bind to sialyl Lewis[x] and related oligosaccharides [120, 121], but high-affinity binding of E-selectin may also require specific glycoproteins. Candidate molecules include a 250 kDa molecule precipitated from bovine γδ T lymphocytes [171] and E-selectin Ligand-1 (ESL-1), a molecule with homology to fibroblast growth factor receptors [172]. Although an ESL-1-IgG construct has been shown to support adhesion of E-selectin transfectants [172], neither ESL-1 nor the 250 kDa molecule have been shown to serve as functional E-selectin ligands under truly physiological conditions [144]. Interestingly, ESL-1 is expressed at high copy number in the Golgi [172] and at lower concentrations on the cell surface with a propensity for distribution to cellular processes [173]. A third candidate ligand for E-selectin is L-selectin isolated from human neutrophils [42, 174]. Since neutrophils constitutively express sialyl-transferases and fucosyl-transferase VII (FTVII), many of their surface glycoproteins including L-selectin are decorated with sialyl Lewis[x] oligosaccharides. L-selectin from human, but not from mouse neutrophils can bind to E-selectin in biochemical assays [174]. Again, it is not clear whether this interaction is of physiological significance. Cells expressing E- and/or P-selectin ligands do not require L-selectin for binding in flow assays *in vitro* [76, 175] or in venules *in vivo* [76, 85]. Conversely, L-selectin transfectants lacking the ability to bind E- or P-selectin can attach to activated endothelial cells *in vitro* independently of P- or E-selectin, and can roll in venules *in vivo*, although less efficiently than neutrophils [76, 85, 176]. Taken together, these data suggest that the true E-selectin ligands may not have been identified so far, and further research is needed to clarify this issue.

Summary

The selectins are firmly established as the main adhesion receptors mediating leukocyte capture and rolling *in vitro* and *in vivo*. Binding to selectins requires sialylated, fucosylated glycoproteins on the surface of the partner cell, which are fucosylated mainly by FTVII on leukocytes. Other post-translational modifications may be required for selectin binding, as demonstrated by the tyrosine sulfation requirement for PSGL-1 binding to P-selectin. Although several candidate selectin ligands have been described, PSGL-1 is the only selectin ligand for which physiological significance has been firmly established. Selectins achieve capture and rolling by rapidly binding to their ligands. The selectin-mediated interactions are transient, caused by their inherently high dissociation rate which is further increased by mechanical load. The selectin binding kinetics decrease in a sequence from L-selectin (fastest) to P-selectin (intermediate) to E-selectin (slowest). In mouse models of inflammation, absence of both E- and P-selectin causes the most severe inflammatory defects, followed by absence of FTVII (severe), L-selectin alone (intermediate), P-selectin alone (moderate), or E-selectin alone (slight). Organ- and disease-specific variations in the importance of individual selectins are beginning to be explored and offer a rich field for further investigation.

References

1   Arfors K-E, Lundberg C, Lindbom L, Lundberg K, Beatty PG, Harlan JM (1987) A monoclonal antibody to the membrane glycoprotein complex CD18 inhibits polymorphonuclear leukocyte accumulation and plasma leakage *in vivo*. *Blood* 69: 338–340

2   Ley K, Lundgren E, Berger EM, Arfors K-E (1989) Shear-dependent inhibition of granulocyte adhesion to cultured endothelium by dextran sulfate. *Blood* 73: 1324–1330

3   Ley K (1989) Granulocyte adhesion to microvascular and cultured endothelium. *Studia Biophys* 134: 179–184

4   von Andrian UH, Chambers JD, McEvoy LM, Bargatze RF, Arfors K-E, Butcher EC (1991) Two step model of leukocyte-endothelial cell interaction in inflammation: Distinct roles for LECAM-1 and the leukocyte β_2 integrins *in vivo*. *Proc Natl Acad Sci USA* 88: 7538–7542

5   Butcher EC (1991) Leukocyte-endothelial cell recognition – Three (or more) steps to specificity and diversity. *Cell* 67: 1033–1036

6   Springer TA (1995) Traffic signals on endothelium for lymphocyte recirculation and leukocyte emigration. *Annu Rev Physiol* 57: 827–872

7   Vejlens G (1938) The distribution of leukocytes in the vascular system. *Acta Pathol Microbiol Scand* (Suppl) 33: 1–239

8   Schmid-Schönbein GW, Usami S, Skalak R, Chien S (1980) The interaction of leukocytes and erythrocytes in capillary and postcapillary vessels. *Microvasc Res* 19: 45–70

9   Nobis U, Pries AR, Cokelet GR, Gaehtgens P (1985) Radial distribution of white cells during blood flow in small tubes. *Microvasc Res* 29: 295–304

10 Goldsmith HL, Spain S (1984) Margination of leukocytes in blood flow through small tubes. *Microvasc Res* 27: 204–222

11 Ley K, Cerrito M, Arfors K-E (1991) Sulfated polysaccharides inhibit leukocyte rolling in rabbit mesentery venules. *Am J Physiol* 260: H1667–H1673

12 Lawrence MB, Springer TA (1991) Leukocytes roll on a selectin at physiologic flow rates: Distinction from and prerequisite for adhesion through integrins. *Cell* 65: 859–873

13   Ley K, Gaehtgens P (1991) Endothelial, not hemodynamic differences are responsible for preferential leukocyte rolling in venules. *Circ Res* 69: 1034–1041

14   Zimmerman GA, Prescott SM, McIntyre TM (1992) Endothelial cell interactions with granulocytes -tethering and signaling molecules. *Immunol Today* 13: 93–100

15   Ley K, Tedder TF (1995) Leukocyte interactions with vascular endothelium: New insights into selectin-mediated attachment and rolling. *J Immunol* 155: 525–528

16   Alon R, Fuhlbrigge RC, Finger EB, Springer TA (1996) Interactions through L-selectin between leukocytes and adherent leukocytes nucleate rolling adhesions on selectins and VCAM-1 in shear flow. *J Cell Biol* 135: 849–865

17   Kunkel EJ, Chomas JE, Ley K (1998) Role of primary and secondary capture for leuko-cyte accumulation *in vivo*. *Circ Res* 82: 30–38

18   Tözeren A, Ley K (1992) How do selectins mediate leukocyte rolling in venules? *Bio-phys J* 63: 700–709

19   Hammer DA, Apte SM (1992) Simulation of cell rolling and adhesion on surfaces in shear flow: general results and analysis of selectin-mediated neutrophil adhesion. *Bio-phys J* 63: 35–57

20   Lalor PF, Clements JM, Pigott R, Humphries MJ, Spragg JH, Nash GB (1997) Associ-ation between receptor density, cellular activation, and transformation of adhesive behavior of flowing lymphocytes binding to VCAM-1. *Eur J Immunol* 27: 1422–1426

21   Lawrence MB, Springer TA (1993) Neutrophils roll on E-selectin. *J Immunol* 151: 6338–6346

22   Brunk DK, Hammer DA (1997) Quantifying rolling adhesion with a cell-free assay – E-selectin and its carbohydrate ligands. *Biophys J* 72: 2820–2833

23   Goetz DJ, Greif DM, Ding H, Camphausen RT, Howes S, Comess KM, Snapp KR, Kansas GS, Luscinskas FW (1997) Isolated P-Selectin Glycoprotein Ligand-1 mediates dynamic adhesion to P- and E-selectin. *J Cell Biol* 137: 509–519

23a Walcheck B, Kahn J, Fisher JM, Wang BB, Fisk RS, Payan DG, Feehan C, Betageri R, Darlak K, Spatola AF et al (1996) Neutrophil rolling altered by inhibition of L-selectin shedding *in vitro*. *Nature* 380: 720–723

23b Hafezi-Moghadam A, Ley K (1999) Relevance of L-selectin shedding for leukocyte rolling *in vivo*. *J Exp Med* 189: 939–948

24   Lorant DE, Patel KD, McIntyre TM, McEver RP, Prescott SM, Zimmerman GA (1991) Coexpression of GMP-140 and PAF by endothelium stimulated by histamine or throm-bin: A juxtacrine system for adhesion and activation of neutrophils. *J Cell Biol* 115: 223–224

24a Rainger GE, Fisher AC, Nash GB (1997) Endothelial-borne platelet-activating factor and interleukin-8 rapidly immobilize rolling neutrophils. *Am J Physiol – Heart Circul Physiol* 41: H114–H122

24b Campbell JJ, Hedrick J, Zlotnik A, Siani MA, Thompson DA, Butcher EC (1998) Chemokines and the arrest of lymphocytes rolling under flow conditions. *Science* 279: 381–384

25   Bevilacqua MP, Butcher EC, Furie B, Furie BC, Gallatin WM, Gimbrone MA Jr, Har-

lan JM, Kishimoto TK, Lasky LA, McEver RP et al (1991) Selectins – a family of adhesion receptors. *Cell* 67: 233

26 Vestweber D (ed) (1997) *The selectins.* Harwood Academic Publishers, Amsterdam

27 Kansas GS (1996) Selectins and their ligands: current concepts and controversies. *Blood* 88: 3259–3287

28 Bevilacqua MP, Nelson RM (1993) Selectins. *J Clin Invest* 91: 379–387

29 Van Eeden S, Miyagashima R, Haley L, Hogg JC (1995) L-selectin expression increases on peripheral blood polymorphonuclear leukocytes during active marrow release. *Am J Respir Crit Care Med* 151: 500–507

30 Vaneeden SF, Bicknell S, Walker BAM, Hogg JC (1997) Polymorphonuclear leukocytes' L-selectin expression decreases as they age in circulation. *Am J Physiol – Heart Circul Physiol* 41: H 401–H 408

31 Kahn J, Ingraham RH, Shirley F, Migaki GI, Kishimoto TK (1994) Membrane proximal cleavage of L-selectin: Identification of the cleavage site and a 6-kD transmembrane peptide fragment of L-selectin. *J Cell Biol* 125: 461–470

32 Chen A, Engel P, Tedder TF (1995) Structural requirements regulate endoproteolytic release of the L-selectin (CD62L) adhesion receptor from the cell surface of leukocytes. *J Exp Med* 182: 519–530

33 Migaki GI, Kahn J, Kishimoto TK (1995) Mutational analysis of the membrane-proximal cleavage site of L-selectin: relaxed sequence specificity surrounding the cleavage site. *J Exp Med* 182: 549–557

34 Feehan C, Darlak K, Kahn J, Walcheck B, Spatola AF, Kishimoto TK (1996) Shedding of the lymphocyte L-selectin adhesion molecule is inhibited by a hydroxamic acid-based protease inhibitor – Identification with an L-selectin-alkaline phosphatase reporter. *J Biol Chem* 271: 7019–7024

35 Jutila MA, Rott L, Berg EL, Butcher EC (1989) Function and regulation of the neutrophil MEL-14 antigen *in vivo*: Comparison with LFA-1 and Mac-1. *J Immunol* 143: 3318–3324

36 Kishimoto TK, Jutila MA, Berg EL, Butcher EC (1989) Neutrophil Mac-1 and MEL-14 adhesion proteins inversely regulated by chemotactic factors. *Science* 245: 1238–1241

37 Walzog B, Seifert R, Zakrzewicz A, Gaehtgens P, Ley K (1994) Cross-linking of CD18 in human neutrophils induces an increase of intracellular free Ca^{2+}, exocytosis of azurophilic granules, quantitative up-regulation of CD18, shedding of L-selectin, and actin polymerization. *J Leukocyte Biol* 56: 625–635

38 Jutila KL, Kishimoto TK, Butcher EC (1990) Regulation and lectin activity of the human neutrophil peripheral lymph node homing receptor. *Blood* 76: 178–183

39 Bührer C, Berlin C, Thiele H-G, Hamann A (1990) Lymphocyte activation and expression of the human leukocyte-endothelial cell adhesion molecule 1 (Leu8/TQ1 antigen). *Immunology* 71: 442–448

40 Schleiffenbaum B, Spertini O, Tedder TF (1992) Soluble L-selectin is present in human plasma at high levels and retains functional activity. *J Cell Biol* 119: 229–238

41   Suguri T, Kikuta A, Iwagaki H, Yoshino T, Tanaka N, Orita K (1996) Increased plasma GlyCAM-1, a mouse L-selectin ligand, in response to an inflammatory stimulus. *J Leukocyte Biol* 60: 593–597

41a   Extermann M, Bacchi M, Monai N, Fopp M, Fey M, Tichelli A, Schapira M, Spertini O (1998) Relationship between cleaved L-selectin levels and the outcome of acute myeloid leukemia. *Blood* 92: 3115–3122

42   Picker LJ, Warnock RA, Burns AR, Doerschuk CM, Berg EL, Butcher EC (1991) The neutrophil selectin LECAM-1 presents carbohydrate ligands to the vascular selectins ELAM-1 and GMP-140. *Cell* 66: 921–933

43   von Andrian UH, Hasslen SR, Nelson RD, Erlandsen SL, Butcher EC (1995) A central role for microvillous receptor presentation in leukocyte adhesion under flow. *Cell* 82: 989–999

44   Pavalko FM, Walker DM, Graham L, Goheen M, Doerschuk CM, Kansas GS (1995) The cytoplasmic domain of L-selectin interacts with cytoskeletal proteins via α-actinin: Receptor positioning in microvilli does not require interaction with α-actinin. *J Cell Biol* 129: 1155–1164

45   Kansas GS, Ley K, Munro JM, Tedder TF (1993) Regulation of leukocyte rolling and adhesion to endothelium by the cytoplasmic domain of L-selectin. *J Exp Med* 177: 833–838

46   McEver RP, Beckstead JH, Moore KL, Marshall-Carlson L, Bainton DF (1989) GMP 140, a platelet alpha-granule membrane protein, is also synthesized by vascular endothelial cells and is localized in Weibel-Palade bodies. *J Clin Invest* 84: 92–99

47   Berman CL, Yeo EL, Wencel-Drake JD, Furie BC, Ginsberg MH, Furie B (1986) A platelet alpha granule membrane protein that is associated with the plasma membrane after activation. Characterization and subcellular localization of platelet activation-dependent granule-external membrane protein. *J Clin Invest* 78: 130–137

48   Geng JG, Bevilacqua MP, Moore KL, McIntyre TM, Prescott SM, Kim JM, Bliss GA, Zimmerman GA, McEver RP (1990) Rapid neutrophil adhesion to activated endothelium mediated by GMP-140. *Nature* 343: 757–760

49   Foreman KE, Vaporciyan AA, Bonish BK, Jones ML, Johnson KJ, Glovsky MM, Eddy SM, Ward PA (1994) C5a-induced expression of P-selectin in endothelial cells. *J Clin Invest* 94: 1147–1155

50   Wong CS, Gamble JR, Skinner MP, Lucas CM, Berndt MC, Vadas MA (1991) Adhesion protein GMP140 inhibits superoxide anion release by human neutrophils. *Proc Natl Acad Sci USA* 88: 2397–2401

51   Sanders WE, Wilson RW, Ballantyne CM, Beaudet AL (1992) Molecular cloning and analysis of *in vivo* expression of murine P-selectin. *Blood* 80: 795–800

52   Gotsch U, Jäger U, Dominis M, Vestweber D (1994) Expression of P-selectin on endothelial cells is upregulated by LPS and TNF-α *in vivo. Cell Adh Commun* 2: 7–14

53   Jung U, Ley K (1997) Regulation of E-selectin, P-selectin and ICAM-1 expression in mouse cremaster muscle vasculature. *Microcirculation* 4: 311–319

53a   Pan JL, Xia LJ, Yao LB, McEver RP (1998) Comparison of promoters for the murine and human P-selectin genes suggests species-specific and conserved mechanisms for transcriptional regulation in endothelial cells. *J Biol Chem* 273: 10058–10067

53b Pan JL, Xia LJ, Yao LB, McEver RP (1998) Tumor necrosis factor-alpha- or lipopolysaccharide-induced expression of the murine P-selectin gene in endothelial cells involves novel kappa-B sites and a variant activating transcription factor cAMP response element. *J Biol Chem* 273: 10068–10077

54 Bevilacqua MP, Pober JS, Mendrick DL, Cotran RS, Gimbrone MA Jr (1987) Identification of an inducible endothelial-leukocyte adhesion molecule. *Proc Natl Acad Sci USA* 84: 9238–9242

55 Bevilacqua MP, Stengelin S, Gimbrone MA Jr, Seed B (1989) Endothelial leukocyte adhesion molecule-1: An inducible receptor for neutrophils related to complement regulatory proteins and lectins. *Science* 243: 1160–1165

56 Read MA, Neish AS, Luscinskas FW, Palombella VJ, Maniatis T, Collins T (1995) The proteasome pathway is required for cytokine-induced endothelial-leukocyte adhesion molecule expression. *Immunity* 2: 493–506

57 Subramaniam M, Koedam JA, Wagner DD (1993) Divergent fates of P- and E-selectins after their expression on the plasma membrane. *Mol Biol Cell* 4: 791–801

58 Henseleit U, Steinbrink K, Goebeler M, Roth J, Vestweber D, Sorg C, Sunderkotter C (1996) E-selectin expression in experimental models of inflammation in mice. *J Pathol* 180: 317–325

59 Gearing AJ, Newman W (1993) Circulating adhesion molecules in disease. *Immunol Today* 14: 506–512

60 Ushiyama S, Laue TM, Moore KL, Erickson HP, McEver RP (1993) Structural and functional characterization of monomeric soluble P-selectin and comparison with membrane P-selectin. *J Biol Chem* 268: 15229–15237

61 Moore KL, Varki A, McEver RP (1991) GMP-140 binds to a glycoprotein receptor on human neutrophils: Evidence for a lectin-like interaction. *J Cell Biol* 112: 491–499

62 Kaplanski G, Farnarier C, Tissot O, Pierres A, Benoliel A-M, Alessi M-C, Kaplanski S, Bongrand P (1993) Granulocyte-endothelium initial adhesion. Analysis of transient binding events mediated by E-selectin in a laminar shear flow. *Biophys J* 64: 1922–1933

63 Alon R, Hammer DA, Springer TA (1995) Lifetime of the P-selectin-carbohydrate bond and its response to tensile force in hydrodynamic flow. *Nature* 374: 539–542

64 Alon R, Chen SQ, Puri KD, Finger EB, Springer TA (1997) The kinetics of L-selectin tethers and the mechanics of selectin-mediated rolling. *J Cell Biol* 138: 1169–1180

64a Mehta P, Cummings RD, McEver RP (1998) Affinity and kinetic analysis of P-selectin binding to P-selectin glycoprotein ligand-1. *J Biol Chem* 273: 32506–32513

65 Arbones ML, Ord DC, Ley K, Ratech H, Maynard-Curry C, Otten G, Capon DJ, Tedder TF (1994) Lymphocyte homing and leukocyte rolling and migration are impaired in L-selectin-deficient mice. *Immunity* 1: 247–260

66 Wagner N, Löhler J, Kunkel EJ, Ley K, Leung E, Krissansen G, Rajewsky K, Müller W (1996) Critical role for β_7 integrins in formation of the gut-associated lymphoid tissue. *Nature* 382: 366–370

66a   Kunkel EJ, Ramos CL, Steeber DA, Muller W, Wagner N, Tedder TF, Ley K (1998) The roles of L-selectin, β_7 integrins and P-selectin in leukocyte rolling and adhesion in high endothelial venules of Peyers patches. *J Immunol* 161: 2449–2456

67   Lewinsohn DM, Bargatze RF, Butcher EC (1987) Leukocyte-endothelial cell recognition: Evidence of a common molecular mechanism shared by neutrophils, lymphocytes, and other leukocytes. *J Immunol* 138: 4313–4321

68   Watson SR, Fennie C, Lasky LA (1991) Neutrophil influx into an inflammatory site inhibited by soluble homing receptor-IgG chimaera. *Nature* 349: 164–167

69   Tedder TF, Steeber DA, Pizcueta P (1995) L-selectin deficient mice have impaired leukocyte recruitment into inflammatory sites. *J Exp Med* 181: 2259–2264

70   Spertini O, Luscinskas FW, Kansas GS, Munro JM, Griffin JD, Gimbrone MA Jr, Tedder TF (1991) Leukocyte adhesion molecule-1 (LAM-1) interacts with an inducible endothelial cell ligand to support leukocyte adhesion. *J Immunol* 147: 2565–2573

71   Spertini O, Luscinskas FW, Gimbrone MA Jr, Tedder TF (1992) Monocyte attachment to activated human vascular endothelium *in vitro* is mediated by Leukocyte Adhesion Molecule-1 (L-selectin) under nonstatic conditions. *J Exp Med* 175: 1789–1792

72   Brady HR, Spertini O, Jimenez W, Brenner BM, Marsden PA, Tedder TF (1992) Neutrophils, monocytes, and lymphocytes bind to cytokine-activated kidney glomerular endothelial cells through L-selectin (LAM-1) *in vitro*. *J Immunol* 149: 2437–2444

73   Zakrzewicz A, Grafe M, Terbeek D, Bongrazio M, Auch-Schwelk W, Walzog B, Graf K, Fleck E, Ley K, Gaehtgens P (1997) L-selectin-dependent leukocyte adhesion to microvascular but not to macrovascular endothelial cells of the human coronary system. *Blood* 89: 3228–3235

74   Jung U, Ramos CL, Bullard DC, Ley K (1998) Gene-targeted mice reveal the importance of L-selectin-dependent rolling for neutrophil adhesion. *Am J Physiol* 274: H1785– H1791

75   Bargatze RF, Kurk S, Butcher EC, Jutila MA (1994) Neutrophils roll on adherent neutrophils bound to cytokine-induced endothelial cells via L-selectin on the rolling cells. *J Exp Med* 180: 1785–1792

76   Ley K, Tedder TF, Kansas GS (1993) L-selectin can mediate leukocyte rolling in untreated mesenteric venules *in vivo* independent of E- or P-selectin. *Blood* 82: 1632–1638

77   Ley K, Bullard DC, Arbones ML, Bosse R, Vestweber D, Tedder TF, Beaudet AL (1995) Sequential contribution of L- and P-selectin to leukocyte rolling *in vivo*. *J Exp Med* 181: 669–675

77a   Tu L, Delahunty MD, Ding H, Luscinskas FW, Tedder TF (1999) The cutaneous lymphocyte antigen is an essential component of the L-selectin ligand induced on human vascular endothelial cells. *J Exp Med* 189: 241–252

78   Jung U, Bullard DC, Tedder TF, Ley K (1996) Velocity difference between L-selectin and P-selectin dependent neutrophil rolling in venules of the mouse cremaster muscle *in vivo*. *Am J Physiol* 271: H2740–H2747

79   Morgan SJ, Moore MW, Cacalano G, Ley K (1997) Reduced leukocyte adhesion

response and absence of slow leukocyte rolling in interleukin-8 (IL-8) receptor deficient mice. *Microvasc Res* 54: 188–191

80   Perry MA, Granger DN (1991) Role of CD11/CD18 in shear rate-dependent leukocyte-endothelial cell interactions in cat mesenteric venules. *J Clin Invest* 87: 1798–1804

81   Gaboury JP, Kubes P (1994) Reductions in physiologic shear rates lead to CD11/CD18-dependent, selectin-independent leukocyte rolling *in vivo*. *Blood* 83: 345–350

82   Scharffetter-Kochanek K, Lu H, Norman KE, van Nood N, Munoz F, Grabbe S, McArthur M, Lorenzo I, Kaplan S, Ley K et al (1998) Spontaneous skin ulceration and defective T cell function in CD18 null mice. *J Exp Med* 188: 119–131

83   Jung U, Norman KE, Ramos CL, Scharffetter-Kochanek K, Beaudet AL, Ley K (1998) Transit time of leukocytes rolling through venules controls cytokine-induced inflammatory cell recruitment *in vivo*. *J Clin Invest* 102: 1526–1533

84   Mayadas TN, Johnson RC, Rayburn H, Hynes RO, Wagner DD (1993) Leukocyte rolling and extravasation are severely compromised in P selectin-deficient mice. *Cell* 74: 541–554

85   Ley K, Zakrzewicz A, Hanski C, Stoolman LM, Kansas GS (1995) Sialylated O-glycans and L-selectin sequentially mediate myeloid cell rolling *in vivo*. *Blood* 85: 3727–3735

86   Nolte D, Schmid P, Jäger U, Botzlar A, Roesken F, Hecht R, Uhl E, Messmer K, Vestweber D (1994) Leukocyte rolling in venules of striated muscle and skin is mediated by P-selectin, not by L-selectin. *Am J Physiol* 267: H1637–H1642

87   Dore M, Korthuis RJ, Granger DN, Entman ML, Smith CW (1993) P-selectin mediates spontaneous leukocyte rolling *in vivo*. *Blood* 82: 1308–1316

88   Fiebig E, Ley K, Arfors K-E (1991) Rapid leukocyte accumulation by "spontaneous" rolling and adhesion in the exteriorized rabbit mesentery. *Int J Microcirc: Clin Exp* 10: 127–144

89   Ley K (1994) Histamine can induce leukocyte rolling in rat mesenteric venules. *Am J Physiol* 267: H1017–H1023

90   Atherton A, Born GVR (1972) Quantitative investigations of the adhesiveness of circulating polymorphonuclear leukocytes to blood vessels. *J Physiol* (London) 222: 447–474

91   Kubes P, Kanwar S (1994) Histamine induces leukocyte rolling in post-capillary venules: A P-selectin mediated event. *J Immunol* 152: 3570–3577

92   Kubes P, Kanwar S, Niu X-F, Gaboury JP (1993) Nitric oxide synthesis inhibition induces leukocyte adhesion via superoxide and mast cells. *FASEB J* 7: 1293–1299

93   Kunkel EJ, Jung U, Ley K (1997) TNF-α induces selectin-dependent leukocyte rolling in mouse cremaster muscle arterioles. *Am J Physiol* 272: H1391–H1400

94   Johnson RC, Mayadas TN, Frenette PS, Mebius RE, Subramaniam M, Lacasce A, Hynes RO, Wagner DD (1995) Blood cell dynamics in P-selectin deficient mice. *Blood* 86: 1106–1114

95   Kunkel EJ, Ley K (1996) Distinct phenotype of E-selectin deficient mice: E-selectin is required for slow leukocyte rolling *in vivo*. *Circ Res* 79: 1196–1204

96   Yamada S, Mayadas TN, Yuan F, Wagner DD, Hynes RO, Melder RJ, Jain RK (1995)

Rolling in P-selectin deficient mice is reduced but not eliminated in the dorsal skin. *Blood* 86: 3487–3492

97   Frenette PS, Johnson RC, Hynes MR, Wagner DD (1995) Platelets roll on stimulated endothelium *in vivo*: an interaction mediated by endothelial P-selectin. *Proc Natl Acad Sci USA* 92: 7450–7454

98   Larsen E, Palabrica T, Sajer S, Gilbert GE, Wagner DD, Furie BC (1990) PADGEM-dependent adhesion of platelets to monocytes and neutrophils is mediated by a lineage-specific carbohydrate, LNF III (CD15). *Cell* 63: 467–474

99   Buttrum SM, Hatton R, Nash GB (1993) Selectin-mediated rolling of neutrophils on immoblized platelets. *Blood* 82: 1165–1174

100   Diacovo TG, Puri KD, Warnock RA, Springer TA, von Andrian UH (1996) Platelet-mediated lymphocyte delivery to high endothelial venules. *Science* 273: 252–255

101   Subramaniam M, Saffaripour S, Watson SR, Mayadas TN, Hynes RO, Wagner DD (1995) Reduced recruitment of inflammatory cells in a contact hypersensitivity response in P-selectin deficient mice. *J Exp Med* 181: 2277–2282

102   Staite ND, Justen JM, Sly LM, Beaudet AL, Bullard DC (1996) Inhibition of delayed-type contact hypersensitivity in mice deficient in both E-selectin and P-selectin. *Blood* 88: 2973–2979

103   Bosse R, Vestweber D (1994) Only simultaneous blocking of the L- and P-selectin completely inhibits neutrophil migration into mouse peritoneum. *Eur J Immunol* 24: 3019–3024

104   Bullard DC, Kunkel EJ, Kubo H, Hicks MJ, Lorenzo I, Doyle NA, Doerschuk CM, Ley K, Beaudet AL (1996) Infectious susceptibility and severe deficiency of leukocyte rolling and recruitment in E-selectin and P-selectin double mutant mice. *J Exp Med* 183: 2329–2336

105   Frenette PS, Mayadas TN, Rayburn H, Hynes RO, Wagner DD (1996) Susceptibility to infection and altered hematopoiesis in mice deficient in both P- and E-selectins. *Cell* 84: 563–574

105a Frenette PS, Subbarao S, Mazo IB, von Andrian UH, Wagner DD (1998) Endothelial selectins and vascular cell adhesion molecule-1 promote hematopoietic progenitor homing to bone marrow. *Proc Natl Acad Sci USA* 95: 14423–14428

106   Labow MA, Norton CR, Rumberger JM, Lombard-Gillooly KM, Shuster DJ, Hubbard J, Bertko R, Knaack PA, Terry RW, Harbison ML et al (1994) Characterization of E-selectin-deficient mice: demonstration of overlapping function of the endothelial selectins. *Immunity* 1: 709–720

107   Cacalano G, Lee J, Kikly K, Ryan AM, Pitts-Meek S, Hultgren B, Wood WI, Moore MW (1994) Neutrophil and B cell expansion in mice that lack the murine IL-8 receptor homolog. *Science* 265: 682–684

108   Shuster DE, Kehrli ME Jr, Ackermann MR (1995) Neutrophilia in mice that lack the murine IL-8 receptor homolog. *Science* 269: 1590–1591

108a Jung U, Ley K (1999) Mice lacking two or all three selectins demonstrate overlapping and distinct functions of each selectin. *J Immunol* 162: 6755–6762

108b Collins RG, Jung U, Bullard DC et al (1999) Viable phenotype but impaired leukocyte rolling and peritoneal emigration in triple selectin (E, L and P) null mice. *Keystone Symposia* C4: 39 (Abstract)

109 Ley K, Allietta M, Bullard DC, Morgan SJ (1998) The importance of E-selectin for firm leukocyte adhesion *in vivo*. *Circ Res* 83: 287–294

110 Munoz FM, Hawkins EP, Bullard DC, Beaudet AL, Kaplan SL (1997) Host defense against infection with s. pneumoniae is impaired in E-, P- and E-/P-selectin deficient mice. *J Clin Invest* 100: 2099–2106

111 Laudanna C, Constantin G, Baron P, Scardini E, Scarlato G, Cabrini G, Dechecchi C, Rossi F, Cassatella MA, Berton G (1994) Sulfatides trigger increase of cytosolic free calcium and enhanced expression of tumor necrosis factor α and interleukin-8 messenger RNA in human neutrophils – evidence for a role of L-selectin as a signaling molecule. *J Biol Chem* 269: 4021–4026

112 Waddell TK, Fialkow L, Chan CK, Kishimoto TK, Downey GP (1994) Potentiation of the oxidative burst of human neutrophils. A signaling role for L-selectin. *J Biol Chem* 269: 18485–18491

113 Crockett-Torabi E, Sulenbarger B, Smith CW, Fantone JC (1995) Activation of human neutrophils through L-selectin and Mac-1 molecules. *J Immunol* 154: 2291–2302

114 Brenner B, Gulbins E, Schlottmann K, Koppenhoefer U, Busch GL, Walzog B, Steinhausen M, Coggeshall KM, Linderkamp O, Lang F (1996) L-selectin activates the Ras pathway via the tyrosine kinase p56lck. *Proc Nat Acad Sci USA* 93: 15376–15381

115 Steeber DA, Engel P, Miller AS, Sheetz MP, Tedder TF (1997) Ligation of L-selectin through conserved regions within the lectin domain activates signal transduction pathways and integrin function in human, mouse, and rat leukocytes. *J Immunol* 159: 952–963

116 Cooper D, Butcher CM, Berndt MC, Vadas MA (1994) P-selectin interacts with a β_2-integrin to enhance phagocytosis. *J Immunol* 153: 3199–3209

117 Hidari KIPJ, Weyrich AS, Zimmerman GA, McEver RP (1997) Engagement of P-Selectin Glycoprotein Ligand-1 enhances tyrosine phosphorylation and activates mitogen-activated protein kinases in human neutrophils. *J Biol Chem* 272: 28750–28756

118 Elstad MR, La Pine TR, Cowley FS, McEver RP, McIntyre TM, Prescott SM, Zimmerman GA (1995) P-selectin regulates platelet-activating factor synthesis and phagocytosis by monocytes. *J Immunol* 155: 2109–2122

119 Campbell JJ, Hedrick J, Zlotnik A, Siani MA, Thompson DA, Butcher EC (1998) Chemokines and the arrest of lymphocytes rolling under flow conditions. *Science* 279: 381–384

120 Phillips ML, Nudelman ED, Gaeta FCA, Perez M, Singhal AK, Hakomori S, Paulson JC (1990) ELAM-1 mediates cell adhesion by recognition of a carbohydrate ligand, sialyl-Le^x. *Science* 250: 1130–1132

121 Walz G, Aruffo A, Kolanus W, Bevilacqua MP, Seed B (1990) Recognition by ELAM-1 of the sialyl-Le^x determinant on myeloid and tumor cells. *Science* 250: 1132–1135

122 Foxall C, Watson SR, Dowbenko D, Fennie C, Lasky LA, Kiso M, Hasegawa A, Asa

D, Brandley BK (1992) The three members of the selectin receptor family recognize a common carbohydrate epitope, the sialyl Lewis^x oligosaccharide. *J Cell Biol* 117: 895–902

123 Zhou Q, Moore KL, Smith DF, Varki A, McEver RP, Cummings RD (1991) The selectin GMP-140 binds to sialylated, fucosylated lactosaminoglycans on both myeloid and nonmyeloid cells. *J Cell Biol* 115: 557–564

124 Moore KL, Stults NL, Diaz S, Smith DF, Cummings RD, Varki A, McEver RP (1992) Identification of a specific glycoprotein ligand for P-selectin (CD62) on myeloid cells. *J Cell Biol* 118: 445–456

125 Imai Y, Singer MS, Fennie C, Lasky LA, Rosen SD (1991) Identification of a carbohydrate-based endothelial ligand for a lymphocyte homing receptor. *J Cell Biol* 113: 1213–1221

126 Sako D, Chang X-J, Barone KM, Vachino G, White HM, Shaw G, Veldman GM, Bean KM, Ahern TJ, Furie B et al (1993) Expression cloning of a functional glycoprotein ligand for P-selectin. *Cell* 75: 1179–1186

127 Moore KL, Patel KD, Breuhl RE, Fugang L, Johnson DA, Lichenstein HS, Cummings RD, Bainton DF, McEver RP (1995) P-selectin glycoprotein ligand-1 mediates rolling of human neutrophils on P-selectin. *J Cell Biol* 128: 661–671

128 Pouyani T, Seed B (1995) PSGL-1 recognition of P-selectin is controlled by a tyrosine sulfation consensus at the PSGL-1 amino terminus. *Cell* 83: 333–343

129 Sako D, Comess KM, Barone KM, Camphausen RT, Cumming DA, Shaw GD (1995) A sulfated peptide segment at the amino terminus of PSGL-1 is critical for P-selectin binding. *Cell* 83: 323–331

130 Norgard KE, Moore KL, Diaz S, Stults NL, Ushiyama S, McEver RP, Cummings RD, Varki A (1993) Characterization of a specific ligand for P-selectin on myeloid cells. A minor glycoprotein with sialylated O-linked oligosaccharides. *J Biol Chem* 268: 12764–12774

131 Li F, Wilkins PP, Crawley S, Weinstein J, Cummings RD, McEver RP (1996) Post-translational modifications of recombinant P-selectin glycoprotein ligand-1 required for binding to P- and E-selectin. *J Biol Chem* 271: 3255–3264

132 Sasaki K, Kurata K, Funayama K, Nagata M, Watanabe E, Ohta S, Hanai N, Nishi T (1994) Expression cloning of a novel alpha 1,3-fucosyltransferase that is involved in biosynthesis of the sialyl Lewis^x carbohydrate determinants in leukocytes. *J Biol Chem* 269: 14730–14737

133 Natsuka S, Gersten KM, Zenita K, Kannagi R, Lowe JB (1994) Molecular cloning of a cDNA encoding a novel human leukocyte alpha-1,3-fucosyltransferase capable of synthesizing the sialyl Lewis x determinant. *J Biol Chem* 269: 20806:

134 Snapp KR, Wagers AJ, Craig R, Stoolman LM, Kansas GS (1997) P-selectin glycoprotein ligand-1 (PSGL-1) is essential for adhesion to P-selectin but not E-selectin in stably transfected hematopoietic cell lines. *Blood* 89: 896–901

135 Knibbs RN, Craig RA, Natsuka S, Chang A, Cameron M, Lowe JB, Stoolman LM

(1996) The fucosyltransferase FucT-VII regulates E-selectin ligand synthesis in human T cells. *J Cell Biol* 133: 911–920

136 Smith PL, Gersten KM, Petryniak B, Kelly RJ, Rogers C, Natsuka Y, Alford JA, III, Scheidegger EP, Natsuka S, Lowe JB (1996) Expression of the α(1,3)fucosyltransferase Fuc-TVII in lymphoid aggregate high endothelial venules correlates with expression of L-selectin ligands. *J Biol Chem* 271: 8250–8259

137 Maly P, Thall AD, Petryniak B, Rogers CE, Smith PL, Marks RM, Kelly RJ, Gersten KM, Cheng G, Saunders TL et al (1996) The α(1,3)fucosyltransferase Fuc-TVII controls leukocyte trafficking through an essential role in L-, E-, and P-selectin ligand biosynthesis. *Cell* 86: 643–653

138 Wagers AJ, Lowe JB, Kansas GS (1996) An important role for the alpha-1,3 fucosyltransferase, FucT-VII, in leukocyte adhesion to E-selectin. *Blood* 88: 2125–2132

139 Austrup F, Vestweber D, Borges E, Lohning M, Brauer R, Herz U, Renz H, Hallmann R, Scheffold A, Radbruch A et al (1997) P- and E-selectin mediate recruitment of T-helper-1 but not T-helper-2 cells into inflamed tissues. *Nature* 385: 81–83

140 Goelz SE, Hession C, Goff D, Griffiths B, Tizard R, Newman B, Chi-Rosso G, Lobb RR (1990) ELFT: A gene that directs the expression of an ELAM-1 ligand. *Cell* 63: 1349–1356

141 Spertini O, Cordey AS, Monai N, Giuffre L, Schapira M (1996) P-Selectin Glycoprotein Ligand 1 is a ligand for L-selectin on neutrophils, monocytes, and CD34⁺ hematopoietic progenitor cells. *J Cell Biol* 135: 523–531

142 Walcheck B, Moore KL, McEver RP, Kishimoto TK (1996) Neutrophil-neutrophil interactions under hydrodynamic shear stress involve L-selectin and PSGL-1 – A mechanism that amplifies initial leukocyte accumulation on P-selectin *in vitro*. *J Clin Invest* 98: 1081–1087

143 Ramos CL, Smith MJ, Snapp KR, Kansas GS, Stickney GW, Ley K, Lawrence MB (1998) Functional characterization of L-selectin ligands on human neutrophils and leukemia cell lines: Evidence for mucin-like ligand activity distinct from P-selectin Glycoprotein Ligand-1. *Blood* 91: 1067–1075

144 Jones WM, Watts GM, Robinson MK, Vestweber D, Jutila MA (1997) Comparison of E-selectin-binding glycoprotein ligands on human lymphocytes, neutrophils, and bovine gamma-delta T cells. *J Immunol* 159: 3574–3583

145 Norman KE, Moore KL, McEver RP, Ley K (1995) Leukocyte rolling *in vivo* is mediated by P-Selectin Glycoprotein Ligand-1. *Blood* 86: 4417–4421

146 Borges E, Eytner R, Moll T, Steegmaier M, Campbell MA, Ley K, Mossmann H, Vestweber D (1997) The P-selectin glycoprotein ligand-1 is important for recruitment of neutrophils into inflamed mouse peritoneum. *Blood* 90: 1934–1942

147 Aigner S, Ruppert M, Hubbe M, Sammar M, Sthoeger Z, Butcher EC, Vestweber D, Altevogt P (1995) Heat stable antigen (mouse CD24) supports myeloid cell binding to endothelial and platelet P-selectin. *Int Immunol* 7: 1557–1565

148 Aigner S, Sthoeger ZM, Fogel M, Weber E, Zarn J, Ruppert M, Zeller Y, Vestweber D,

Stahel R, Sammar M et al (1997) CD24, a mucin-type glycoprotein, is a ligand for P-selectin on human tumor cells. *Blood* 89: 3385–3395

149 Aigner S, Ramos CL, Hafezi-Moghadam A, Lawrence MB, Altevogt P, Ley K (1998) CD24 mediates rolling of breast carcinoma cells on P-selectin. *FASEB J* 12: 1241–1251

150 Lasky LA, Singer MS, Dowbenko D, Imai Y, Henzel WJ, Grimley C, Fennie C, Gillett N, Watson SR, Rosen SD (1992) An endothelial ligand for L-selectin is a novel mucin-like molecule. *Cell* 69: 927–938

151 Brustein M, Kraal G, Mebius RE, Watson SR (1992) Identification of a soluble form of a ligand for the lymphocyte homing receptor. *J Exp Med* 176: 1415–1419

152 Dowbenko D, Kikuta A, Fennie C, Gillett N, Lasky LA (1993) Glycosylation-dependent cell adhesion molecule 1 (GlyCAM 1) mucin is expressed by lactating mammary gland epithelial cells and is present in milk. *J Clin Invest* 92: 952–960

153 Hwang ST, Singer MS, Giblin PA, Yednock TA, Bacon KB, Simon SI, Rosen SD (1996) Glycam-1, a physiologic ligand for L-selectin, activates β_2 integrins on naive peripheral lymphocytes. *J Exp Med* 184: 1343–1348

154 Giblin PA, Hwang ST, Katsumoto TR, Rosen SD (1997) Ligation of L-selectin on T lymphocytes activates β_1 integrins and promotes adhesion to fibronectin. *J Immunol* 159: 3498–3507

155 Baumhueter S, Singer MS, Henzel W, Hemmerich S, Renz M, Rosen SD, Lasky LA (1993) Binding of L-selectin to the vascular sialomucin CD34. *Science* 262: 436–438

156 Simmons DL, Satterthwaite AB, Tenen DG, Seed B (1992) Molecular cloning of a cDNA encoding CD34, a sialomucin of human hematopoietic stem cells. *J Immunol* 148: 267–271

157 Streeter PR, Rouse BTN, Butcher EC (1988) Immunohistologic and functional characterization of a vascular addressin involved in lymphocyte homing into peripheral lymph nodes. *J Cell Biol* 107: 1853–1862

158 Hemmerich S, Butcher EC, Rosen SD (1994) Sulfation-dependent recognition of high endothelial venules (HEV)-ligands by L-selectin and MECA 79, an adhesion-blocking monoclonal antibody. *J Exp Med* 180: 2219–2226

159 Puri KD, Finger EB, Gaudernack G, Springer TA (1995) Sialomucin CD34 is the major L-selectin ligand in human tonsil high endothelial venules. *J Cell Biol* 131: 261–270

160 Suzuki A, Andrew DP, Gonzalo J-A, Fukumoto M, Spellberg J, Hashiyama M, Suda T, Takimoto H, Gerwin N, Webb J et al (1996) CD34 deficient mice have reduced eosinophil accumulation after allergen exposure and reveal a novel crossreactive 90 kD protein. *Blood* 87: 3550–3562

161 Cheng J, Baumhueter S, Cacalano G, Carver-Moore K, Thibodeaux H, Thomas R, Broxmeyer HE, Cooper S, Hague N, Moore M et al (1996) Hematopoietic defects in mice lacking the sialomucin CD34. *Blood* 87: 479–490

161a Sassetti C, Tangemann K, Singer MS, Kershaw DB, Rosen SD (1998) Identification of podocalyxin-like protein as a high endothelial venule ligand for L-selectin – parallels to CD34. *J Exp Med* 187: 1965–1975

162 Alon R, Feizi T, Yuen C-T, Fuhlbrigge RC, Springer TA (1995) Glycolipid ligands for

selectins support leukocyte tethering and rolling under physiologic flow conditions. *J Immunol* 154: 5356–5366

163 Norgard-Sumnicht KE, Varki NM, Varki A (1993) Calcium-dependent heparin-like ligands for L-selectin in nonlymphoid endothelial cells. *Science* 261: 480–483

164 Nelson RM, Cecconi O, Roberts WG, Aruffo A, Linhardt RJ, Bevilacqua MP (1993) Heparin oligosaccharides bind L- and P-selectin and inhibit acute inflammation. *Blood* 82: 3253–3258

165 Simon SI, Chambers JD, Butcher EC, Sklar LA (1992) Neutrophil aggregation is β_2-integrin- and L-selectin-dependent in blood and isolated cells. *J Immunol* 149: 2765–2771

166 Snapp KR, Ding H, Atkins K, Warnke R, Luscinskas FW, Kansas GS (1998) A novel P-Selectin Glycoprotein Ligand-1 monoclonal antibody recognizes an epitope within the tyrosine sulfate motif of human PSGL-1 and blocks recognition of both P- and L-selectin. *Blood* 91: 154–164

167 Berlin C, Berg EL, Briskin MJ, Andrew DP, Kilshaw PJ, Holzmann B, Weissman IL, Hamann A, Butcher EC (1993) $\alpha_4\beta_7$ integrin mediates lymphocyte binding to the mucosal vascular addressin MAdCAM-1. *Cell* 74: 185–195

168 Briskin MJ, McEvoy LM, Butcher EC (1993) MAdCAM-1 has homology to immunoglobulin and mucin-like adhesion receptors and to IgA1. *Nature* 363: 461–464

169 Berg EL, McEvoy LM, Berlin C, Bargatze RF, Butcher EC (1993) L-selectin-mediated lymphocyte rolling on MAdCAM-1. *Nature* 366: 695–698

170 Bargatze RF, Jutila MA, Butcher EC (1995) Distinct roles of L-selectin and integrins $\alpha_4\beta_7$ and LFA-1 in lymphocyte homing to Peyer's patch-HEV in situ: the multistep model confirmed and refined. *Immunity* 3: 99–108

171 Walcheck B, Watts G, Jutila MA (1993) Bovine gamma/δ T cells bind E-selectin via a novel glycoprotein receptor: First characterization of a lymphocyte/E-selectin interaction in an animal model. *J Exp Med* 178: 853–863

172 Steegmaier M, Levinovitz A, Isenmann S, Borges E, Lenter M, Kocher HP, Kleuser B, Vestweber D (1995) The E-selectin-ligand ESL-1 is a variant of a receptor for fibroblast growth factor. *Nature* 373: 615–620

173 Steegmaier M, Borges E, Berger J, Schwarz H, Vestweber D (1997) The E-selectin-ligand ESL-1 is located in the Golgi as well as on microvilli on the cell surface. *J Cell Sci* 110: 687–694

174 Zöllner O, Lenter MC, Blanks JE, Borges E, Steegmaier M, Zerwes HG, Vestweber D (1997) L-selectin from human, but not from mouse neutrophils binds directly to E-selectin. *J Cell Biol* 136: 707–716

175 Wagers AJ, Stoolman LM, Kannagi R, Craig R, Kansas GS (1997) Expression of leukocyte fucosyltransferases regulates binding to E-selectin: relationship to previously implicated carbohydrate epitopes. *J Immunol* 159: 1917–1929

176 von Andrian UH, Chambers JD, Berg EL, Michie SA, Brown DA, Karolak D, Ramezani L, Berger EM, Arfors K-E, Butcher EC (1993) L-selectin mediates neutrophil rolling in

inflamed venules through sialyl Lewis^x-dependent and -independent recognition pathways. *Blood* 82: 182–191

177 Brooks SB, Tözeren A (1996) Flow past an array of cells that are adherent to the bottom plate of a flow channel. *J Computers and Fluids* 25: 741–757

178 Damiano ER, Westheider J, Tözeren A, Ley K (1996) Variation in the velocity, deformation, and adhesion energy density of leukocytes rolling within venules. *Circ Res* 79: 1122–1130

Co-operative signaling between leukocytes and endothelium mediating firm attachment

C. Wayne Smith[1,2], Alan R. Burns[1,3] and Scott I. Simon[1]

[1]Section of Leukocyte Biology, Department of Pediatrics, [2]Department of Microbiology and Immunology, [3]Section of Cardiovascular Sciences, Department of Medicine, Baylor College of Medicine, Houston, TX 77030-2600, USA

This chapter focuses on the interactions of leukocytes and endothelial cells that are necessary for adhesion sufficiently stable to withstand the shear forces of flowing blood. Some aspects of the interplay between shear rates and the functions of specific adhesion molecules will be discussed, as will possible signaling steps in the cascade of events leading to stable adhesion (though signaling pathways will not be discussed). In addition, simple observations of cell interactions will be presented to emphasize the potential influence of surface topography on the sequence of events that control firm adhesion and its localization.

Introduction: Background to the concepts of leukocyte/endothelial adhesion

Early descriptions document dynamic interactions between leukocytes and endothelial cells at inflammatory sites in numerous species and tissues [1]. Observations in rabbit ear chambers [2] have revealed leukocytes rolling along endothelial cells at rates much lower than the velocity of flowing erythrocytes. Atherton and Born [3] were the first to systematically quantify this rolling phenomenon, and they reported that, "...the rolling granulocyte count is itself the most sensitive criterion of vascular inflammation." Using direct microscopic examination of venules in the hamster cheek pouch, they found that superfusion of vessels with phlogistic agents not only increased leukocyte rolling, but stimulated firm adhesion of leukocytes to the endothelium and migration through the vessel wall into the surrounding tissue. They stated [4] that chemotactic agents, "...change the walls of the venules in some way so that they become selectively adhesive to circulating granulocytes which happen to touch them." Marchesi and Florey [5] performed the first systematic electron microscopic evaluations of leukocyte transendothelial migration and concluded that granulocytes emigrate through endothelial intercellular junctions.

The first insight into the specific adhesion molecules needed for leukocyte localization at inflammatory sites came from studies of a child with marked susceptibility to bacterial infection [6]. This syndrome, now known as leukocyte adhesion deficiency I (LAD I), is characterized by almost complete absence of neutrophil emigration at sites of infection, and life-threating bacterial infections beginning shortly after birth. LAD I is caused by mutations in the gene for CD18 (the β_2 subunit) that lead to exceedingly low or absent expression of the β_2 integrins. Two members of the β_2 integrin family, CD11a/CD18 (LFA-1) and CD11b/CDl8 (Mac-l), are critically important to the process of transendothelial migration [7] and interact with intercellular adhesion molecule-I (ICAM-1, CD54) on the surface of endothelial cells [7–9]. Monoclonal antibodies that block the function of CD18 or ICAM-1 in animal models of inflammation result in marked reductions in leukocyte emigration at inflamed sites [10].

Lawrence et al. [11, 12] developed an *in vitro* model of leukocyte-endothelial interactions under conditions of flow at shear rates similar to those in post-capillary venules, and were the first to show that isolated neutrophils would roll, adhere and transmigrate through IL-1 stimulated endothelial monolayers. Since this stimulation was known to induce surface expression of ICAM-1 [8], these investigators examined the contributions of the CD18/ICAM-1 adhesion pathway, and found that neutrophils from patients with LAD I formed rolling adhesions on endothelial cells, but failed to adhere firmly or transmigrate. Monoclonal antibodies that blocked the functions of ICAM-1 and CD18 induced the same behavior in normal neutrophils indicating that the rolling phenomenon was supported by a different set of adhesion molecules. This experimental model was used to show that L-selectin (CD62L) [13, 14] supports primary rolling adhesion to endothelial cells under flow conditions, that E-selectin (CD62E) [15] expressed on cytokine-stimulated endothelial cells supports rolling adhesion of neutrophils [16], and that P-selectin (CD62P) [17], when mobilized by histamine-stimulation of endothelial cells, supports rolling of neutrophils under flow [18]. The background to these observations and associated experimental work relating to these findings have been reviewed in detail (see chapter by Ley, this volume, and [19, 20]).

Numerous studies using blocking monoclonal antibodies in animal models of inflammation (reviewed in [10]) and mice with targeted deletions of specific adhesion molecules [21] have confirmed the initial observations made *in vitro*, that selectins are necessary for neutrophil localization because they serve as a primary capture mechanism under conditions of flow, and the CD18/ICAM-1 adhesion pathway, though unable to function at the shear rates of blood flowing in venules, will arrest rolling leukocytes and support adherence-dependent leukocyte locomotion necessary for leukocyte migration.

The transition from rolling to firm adhesion can be stimulated by chemotactic factors *in vitro*. Kishimoto et al. [22] demonstrated that chemotactic stimulation results in rapid shedding of L-selectin coincident with increases in the surface level of CD11b/CD18 integrin. In addition, avidity changes can be seen in CD11b/CD18 within 10 s after stimulation [23], and shedding of L-selectin is almost complete within 4–5 min [13]. Such stimulation appears to be the result of chemotactic agents synthesized by endothelial cells and presented on the luminal surface of the endothelium [24, 25]. IL-8 and platelet activating factor (PAF) apparently play such roles *in vitro* [26, 27]. In this model, both timing and location of leukocyte stimulation are critical. Neutrophils exposed to chemotactic factors prior to contacting activated endothelium have markedly reduced ability to initiate primary adhesion under conditions of flow [13, 28], though they show CD18 integrin-dependent adhesion. Under conditions of flow at venular shear rates, CD18-integrin-dependent adhesion is ineffective in mediating cell capture without selectin-dependent adhesion [13].

Intravital microscopy in the mesenteric or cremasteric vascular beds has revealed that leukocytes typically adhere to the endothelium in the post capillary venules, where shear rates have been estimated to be from less than 100 s^{-1} up to 1000 s^{-1}, depending on the blood flow and vessel diameter. Key factors that influence leukocyte adhesion include drag forces that drive the cell motion, and the frequency and duration of collisions between cells and the vessel wall [29].

Neutrophil adhesion to neutrophils – hydrodynamics and specific adhesion molecules

Neutrophils will adhere to each other when stimulated with soluble chemotactic factors such as complement component C5a. This process has been used as a model of neutrophil adhesion *in vitro*, and it reflects a potentially pathogenic process, a mechanism for additional leukocyte recruitment at sites of inflammation. Leukocyte aggregates have been observed in the blood and microvessels following complement activation (e.g. hemodialysis, systemic lupus erythematosus, and myocardial infarction) [30–34]. Leukocyte-platelet aggregates have been observed *in vivo* following systemic inflammatory activation induced by cigarette smoke, a process linked to the induction of oxidized phospholipids that stimulate cells through one of the chemotactic receptors (the PAF receptor) [35], and during coronary ischemic episodes [36]. Neutrophil-neutrophil adhesion may also provide an additional recruitment mechanism in the multistep adhesion cascade at sites of inflammation. Neutrophils rolling on a substrate in a parallel plate flow chamber *in vitro* can serve as sites for homotypic adhesion, marginating leukocytes at shear rates typical of venular blood flow [37–40]. Recent evidence shows this process proceeds as a sequence of events involving several classes of adhesion molecules.

The concept of a multistep cascade of molecular recognition, cell activation, and transition to firm adhesion that characterizes leukocyte adhesion under shear stress to endothelium in systemic venules also applies to neutrophil adhesion to neutrophils [41]. The primary mechanism of capture is mediated by a selectin on one cell binding to sialylated and fucosylated ligands on another [40]. Many of the same stimuli (e.g. PAF and IL-8) activate high avidity integrin binding and enable firm adhesion in both homotypic and heterotypic (i.e. to endothelium) adhesion [42, 43].

Early studies on neutrophil aggregation were conducted in a platelet aggregometer where leukocyte suspensions were mixed with a magnetic stir bar. Aggregation was shown to correlate with an increase in light transmittance through the turbid cell suspension [30–33]. These studies provided poor sensitivity and often required non-physiological stimulus conditions. Also, shear fields in these mixing conditions are too complex to allow precise calculations of shear rate. Recently, rotational viscometry has been used to apply precise and uniform shear rates to cell suspensions, and intercellular adhesion has been detected by flow cytometry. This technique affords a marked increase in sensitivity for resolving the size distribution of aggregates. The kinetics of aggregate formation can be mathematically modeled based on a theory that describes the interaction of spherical particles mixed in a linear shear field [44]. These approaches have enabled analysis of aggregation and disaggregation in terms of fluid shear rate (G) and shear stress (viscosity × G), and the kinetics of adhesion receptor activation and binding. In this experimental setting, three phases of adhesion can be defined [45, 46]. The first is detected within seconds of the addition of an agonist (e.g. a chemotactic factor such as formyl peptide). Adhesion peaks within 30 seconds under optimum conditions, and the rate and extent of adhesion is a function of the shear rate[46,47]. The efficiency of this adhesion is remarkably high. At optimum shear rates of 400–800 s^{-1}, a peak efficiency of 40% (4 out of 10 collisions resulting in aggregation) occurs over the first phase of aggregation. At higher (3000 s^{-1}) or lower (100 s^{-1}) shear rates, the efficiency is significantly reduced.

The second phase of homotypic adhesion is a steady state plateau observed over a period of 1–2 min in which aggregates remain stable to much higher shear rates (e.g. 3000 s^{-1}) than those that allow an optimum level of adhesion (400 s^{-1}). The third phase is characterized by a rapid transition to disaggregation, and its rate is directly proportional to the magnitude of the shear stress applied [47]. The mechanism of detachment appears to involve both active cell shape change associated with cell locomotion and a decrease in adhesion. The cells adopt a bipolar shape by the 2 min time point [47, 48], and this is accompanied by a three-fold reduction in the area of cell-cell contact and a concomitant increase in the tensile stress [49]. Following these changes, the strength of intercellular adhesion is exceeded by the hydrodynamic forces. The consistency with which the three phases occur is a remarkable aspect of neutrophil function.

Leukocytes from patients deficient in CD18-integrin (LAD I) [10] fail to adhere to each other, and blocking monoclonal antibodies demonstrate a requirement for CD11b/CD18 (Mac-1, complement receptor type 3) [50, 51]. Simon et al. [52] found that antibodies to L-selectin were as effective as those against CD18 in blocking aggregation. It appears that L-selectin is essential for transient adhesion, while CD18-integrin serves to stabilize adhesive interactions and enable aggregation [46, 52]. Experimental results support the concept of a multistep process in which L-selectin is essential for the initial step in the formation of neutrophil aggregates.

Additional studies indicate that P-selectin glycoprotein ligand-1 (PSGL-1) serves as a single counter-structure for L-selectin [38, 53]. Activated CD18-integrins then stabilize the otherwise transient cell contacts, a process that is complete within 30 seconds.

The events just described (see Fig. 1) occur at shear rates where homotypic adhesion is most efficient (i.e. between 400 and 800 s^{-1}). The contribution of L-selectin to neutrophil-neutrophil adhesion or in neutrophil capture to a substrate [54] is closely linked to the level of shear thereby revealing an intriguing feature of this molecule. L-selectin adhesion exhibits a shear threshold [54–56]. Adhesion at low shear rates (e.g. 100 s^{-1}) is independent of L-selectin since the tethering function of this molecule is only demonstrable at shear rates > 200 s^{-1}. Adhesion at low shear rates requires expression and activation of the CD18-integrins. The role of Mac-1, LFA-1 and ICAM-3 in supporting neutrophil homotypic adhesion have been studied using blocking MAbs [57]. ICAM-3 is expressed on neutrophils and has been shown to be a ligand for LFA-1 on resting and activated T cells [58]. When neutrophils are preincubated with either anti-LFA-1 or anti-Mac-1 the efficiency of aggregation is inhibited by 40%. Preincubation with a combination of MAbs to both LFA-1 and Mac-1 decreases adhesion efficiency to zero. Preincubation of neutrophils with anti-ICAM-3 also inhibits aggregation by 30%. In a series of blocking studies, the paradigm that has emerged is that homotypic aggregation at low shear is supported by LFA-1 interacting with ICAM-3, and by Mac-1, but the ligands recognized by Mac-1 remain to be discovered.

At shear rates optimal for homotypic adhesion (400 s^{-1}), the estimated duration of cell contact in the absence of firm adhesion is 6 msec. This interval is insufficient for adhesion mediated through binding of Mac-1 and LFA-1 alone to ligands on opposing neutrophils. However, given sufficient bonding time (e.g. at a shear rate of 100 s^{-1} corresponding to an encounter duration of ~ 25 msec) CD18-integrin-dependent adhesion can withstand high tensile stress (> 10 dynes/cm^2). At shear rates greater than 400 s-1 the encounter duration should still be well within the molecular association rate reported for selectins (~ 10^7 s^{-1}). Therefore, a critical function of the L-selectin bond, which has been reported to have a lifetime of 150 msec [37], is to enable sufficient Mac-1 and LFA-1 bonds to form stable adhesion. Considering leukocyte recruitment to a vessel wall [29] at a venular shear rate of 100 s^{-1}, the encounter duration in the absence of adhesion is approximately 1 ms, much shorter than the estimate for integrin-dependent adhesion.

A second potentially important mechanism supporting adhesion is through ligation of L-selectin, a process that triggers rapid activation of CD18-integrins and neutrophil adhesion [57, 59, 60]. There is evidence that this signaling pathway acts synergistically with that of chemotactic stimulation [59, 60].

These studies indicate that contact duration limits neutrophil adhesion efficiency at shear rates above 400 s^{-1} in sheared cell suspensions. The implications for neutrophil recruitment *in vivo* are that hydrodynamics and collisional geometries influ-

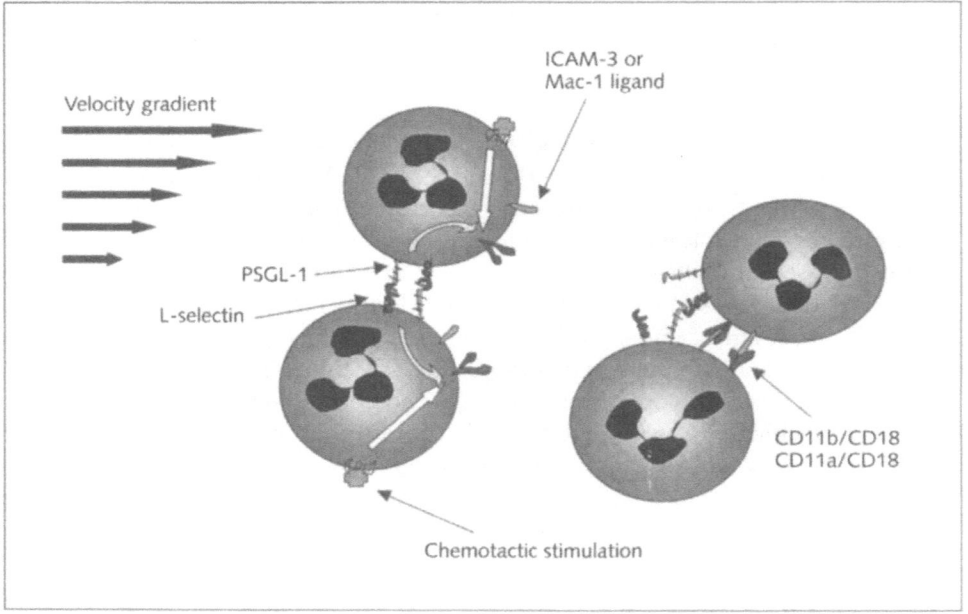

Figure 1

Homotypic neutrophil adhesion. Upon chemotactic stimulation with agents such as C5a, IL-8 or f-Met-Leu-Phe, neutrophils will adhere to each other under conditions of flow at shear rates between 100 s^{-1} and 3000 s^{-1}. At optimum shear rates between 400 and 800 s^{-1}, a sequence of adhesive interactions is required. The initial step is illustrated by the two neutrophils at the left, where chemotactic stimulation is occurring and L-selectin and PSGL-1 are interacting, a lectin based adhesion with a very rapid on rate. Both chemotactic stimulation and cross-linking of L-selectin synergistically signal a change in the avidity of CD18 (β_2) integrins. Mac-1 (CD11b/CD18) binds to an as yet unknown ligand on the opposing cell, and LFA-1 (CD11a/CD18) binds to ICAM-3. The avidity change allows the second step in the adhesion cascade, firm adhesion between the neutrophils as illustrated by the two neutrophils on the right.

ence targeting of cells to sites of inflammation. In this regard, the duration of a cell collision occurring parallel to the endothelium in flowing blood is much too short for integrin-dependent tethering. This concept has been corroborated by observations *in vivo* under very low flow conditions in which a shift towards integrin-dependent adhesion is observed [61, 62]. The binding kinetics and function of integrins and selectins are thus optimized to mediate adhesion within discrete ranges of shear rates and stress.

Factors contributing to firm adhesion of neutrophils rolling on endothelial monolayers

The following experiments address mechanisms that lead to stable adhesion of neutrophils under conditions of flow. We have approached this question using an experimental model *in vitro*. Human umbilical vein endothelial cell (HUVEC) monolayers have been used by a number of investigators as a model endothelial surface, and have revealed many of the mechanisms important to the functions of post-capillary venular endothelial cells *in vivo*. HUVEC monolayers grown to confluence and placed in a parallel plate flow chamber were stimulated with IL-1β for 4 h. These cells were then exposed to isolated neutrophils at shear rates comparable to those found *in vivo*. The analysis of adhesion is illustrated in Figure 2, showing that individual neutrophils were followed from the time they tethered on the endothelial monolayer until they stopped rolling or rolled beyond the field of view. This allowed the following data to be collected from videotaped phase contrast images – the number of cells accumulating in the field of view and their behavior (rolling, firm adhesion, velocity and distance of rolling, and the rate and extent of transendothelial migration). The last parameter is measurable since transmigrating neutrophils become phase dark after passing beneath the monolayer. Typical results in this model when flow rates are adjusted to produce a wall shear stress of 2 dynes/cm^2 are the linear accumulation of neutrophils on the monolayer over the first ten minutes of observation, with a high percentage of tethered cells firmly adhering before migrating beneath the monolayer (Fig. 3). While it has been well known that tethering in this model is dependent on L-selectin and E-selectin, and firm adhesion requires CD18 integrins, the relative contributions of Mac-1 (CD11b/CD18) and LFA-1 (CD11a/CD18) have not been defined. As shown in Figure 3, monoclonal antibodies to either of these integrins fails to block firm adhesion, and they fail to increase significantly the rolling distance before neutrophils arrest. In addition, they fail to reduce the number of adherent cells that undergo transendothelial migration. Only when both Mac-1 and LFA-1 are inhibited by monoclonal antibodies is firm adhesion reduced to the extent produced by anti-CD18. This combination of antibodies also leads to a marked increase in the distance neutrophils roll before stopping, and though not shown on the figure, the number of rolling cells is concomitantly increased. Inhibiting ICAM-1 caused a small but significant reduction in ability of neutrophils to arrest under flow. Others have observed that while Mac-1 can recognize ICAM-1, it also recognizes other ligands on the endothelial cell surface [63]. Thus, it appears that either LFA-1 or Mac-1 is sufficient to stop rolling cells, and while ICAM-1 plays a role, other ligands on the endothelial cells are of potential importance. In addition, the contributions of these adhesion molecules to the number of transmigrated neutrophils may be at the level of promoting firm adhesion, since an equally high percentage of neutrophils that stop under each experimental condition are able to transmigrate (Fig. 3).

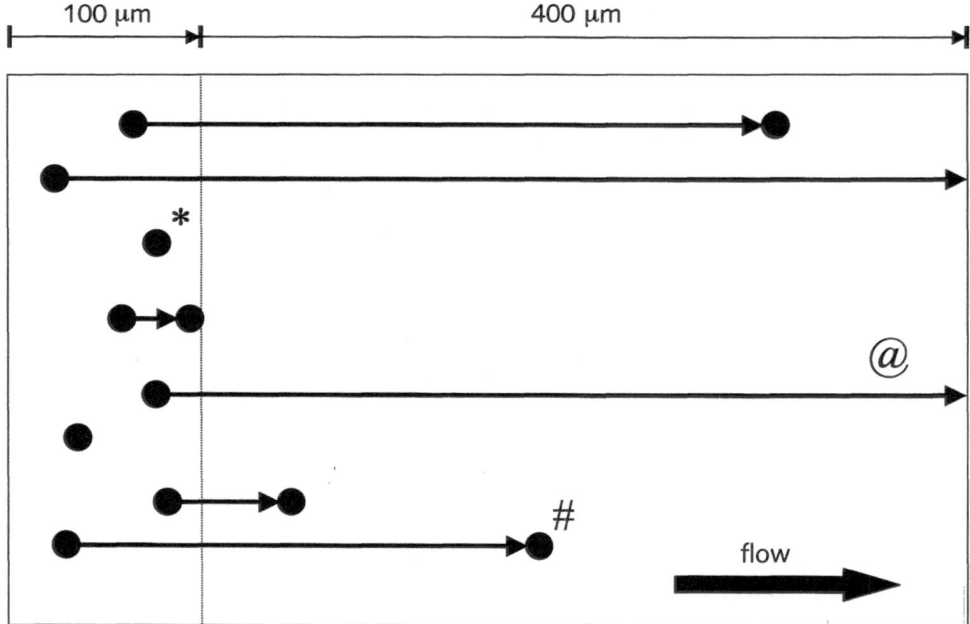

Figure 2
Assessment of leukocyte rolling and firm adhesion under conditions of flow. Under phase contrast videomicroscopy, individual leukocytes tethering to the HUVEC monolayer within the first 100 µm of the observation field are followed. Leukocytes may abruptly arrest from the flow stream (*), tether and roll through the length of the observation field (@), or roll for a time before coming to firm arrest (#). The rolling velocity can be calculated from these observations.

These observations are not entirely consistent with results of neutrophil adhesion to endothelial cells under static conditions. In this setting, there seems to be a necessary cooperative role of LFA-1 and Mac-1 for optimum adhesion [7]. Additionally, LFA-1 and ICAM-1 play distinctly dominant roles in transendothelial migration in the static setting [64] as shown in Figure 4. Note that neutrophils from patients with complete CD18 deficiency ("Severe LAD") [65] on this figure exhibit a marked inability to transmigrate, while cells from patients with a partial deficiency ("Mod. LAD") exhibit only partial reduction.

Which model (static or flow) reveals the relative physiological role of LFA-1 and Mac-1 in the processes of leukocyte emigration? The answer is still unclear, but there are a number of interesting published results that add insight. Issukutz et al. [66], Rutter et al. [67], and Graf et al. [68] in rat and rabbit models of inflamma-

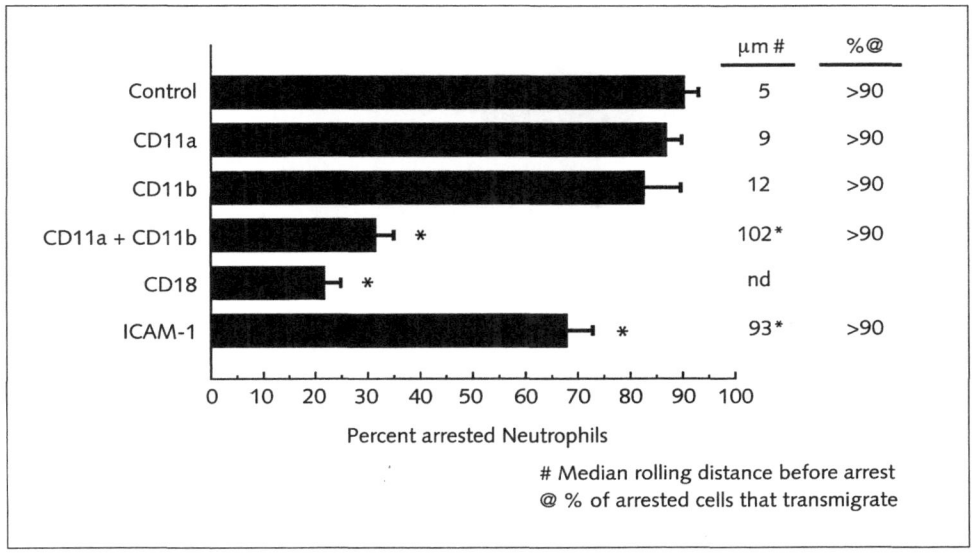

Figure 3
The percentage of neutrophils arresting on IL-1-stimulated endothelial monolayers. HUVEC monolayers were stimulated for 4 h with IL-1, placed in a parallel plate flow chamber and exposed to a wall shear stress of 2 dynes/cm². Isolated human neutrophils entered the flow stream and contacted the monolayers for a period of 9.5 min. At the end of this time the percentage of neutrophils on the monolayer that were firmly attached to the apical surface of the monolayer or transmigrated beneath the monolayer was determined by counting cells in several randomly selected fields. Neutrophils were incubated with or without concentrations of blocking monoclonal antibodies [7,13] to either CD11a, CD11b, both CD11a and CD11b or CD18 before passing through the flow chamber. The antibodies were retained with the leukocytes throughout the flow period. The endothelial cells were incubated either with or without a concentration of blocking monoclonal antibody to ICAM-1 [8] before passing a suspension of isolated neutrophils through the chamber. The anti-ICAM-1 concentration was maintained throughout the flow period. Two additional parameters were assessed: The median leukocyte rolling distance (μm) before firm adhesion was determined for 30 leukocytes in three experiments, and the mean percentage (%) of firmly adherent neutrophils that transmigrated during the observation period was also determined.
*p < 0.01 compared to control values.

tion have provided evidence that LFA-1 plays a dominant role in neutrophil emigration. Tang et al. [69], in a mouse model of peritoneal inflammation, found that neutrophil inhibitory factor (NIF), a product from canine hook worms that inhibits Mac-1 dependent adhesion, failed to reduce neutrophil emigration. Early studies

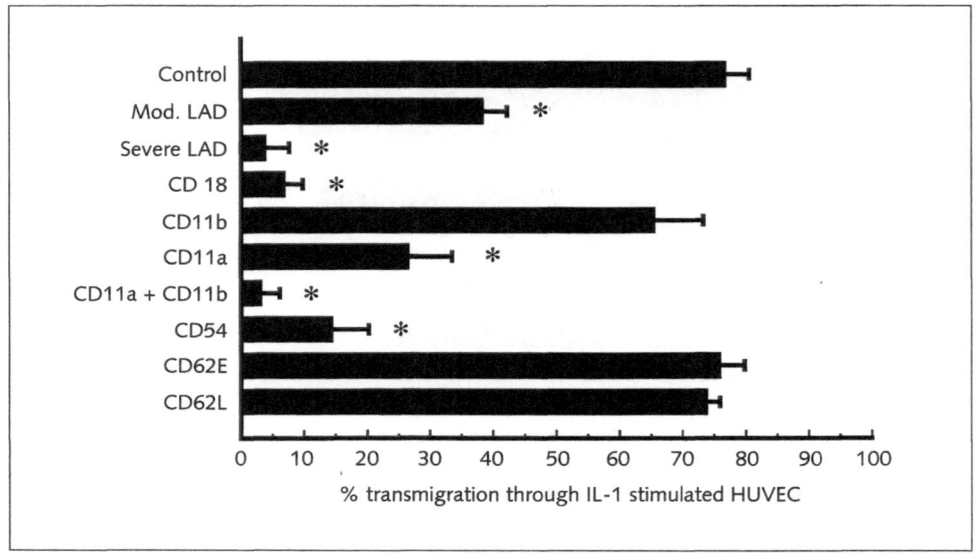

Figure 4

Transendothelial migration of neutrophils under static conditions. HUVEC monolayers were stimulated with IL-1 for 4 h and then placed in adhesion chambers. Isolated human neu-trophils were then injected into the chamber and allowed to settle onto the monolayer for a period of 500 seconds. The number of neutrophils in contact with the monolayer was counted on an inverted phase contrast microscope and the chamber was then inverted for an additional 500 seconds to allow unattached cells to fall away. At the end of this time the chamber was again examined to determine the percentage of the neutrophils originally con-tacting the monolayer that had transmigrated. Leukocytes were incubated either with or without known effective concentrations of blocking monoclonal antibodies to CD18, CD11b, CD11a, both CD11b and CD11a, or CD62L (L-selectin) prior to being injected into the chamber. The antibodies were retained through the period of adhesion and migration. The monolayers were incubated either with or without blocking concentrations of mono-clonal antibodies to CD54 (ICAM-1) or CD62E (E-selectin). With the exception of Mod. LAD and Severe LAD, all neutrophils were from healthy adult donors. *p < 0.01.

using blocking antibodies against CD11b gave the distinct impression that blocking Mac-1 would inhibit neutrophil emigration. In one study, Rosen and Gordon [70] found that monoclonal antibody 5C6 was inhibitory in a mouse peritoneal model, but this was only true if the antibody used was an IgG. If used as a F(ab′)$_2$ prepa-ration there was no inhibitory effect, raising questions regarding possible nonspe-cific effects (e.g., related to Fc interactions) of the IgG. We have analyzed peritoneal emigration of neutrophils in mice with a targeted deletion of CD11b [71]. These

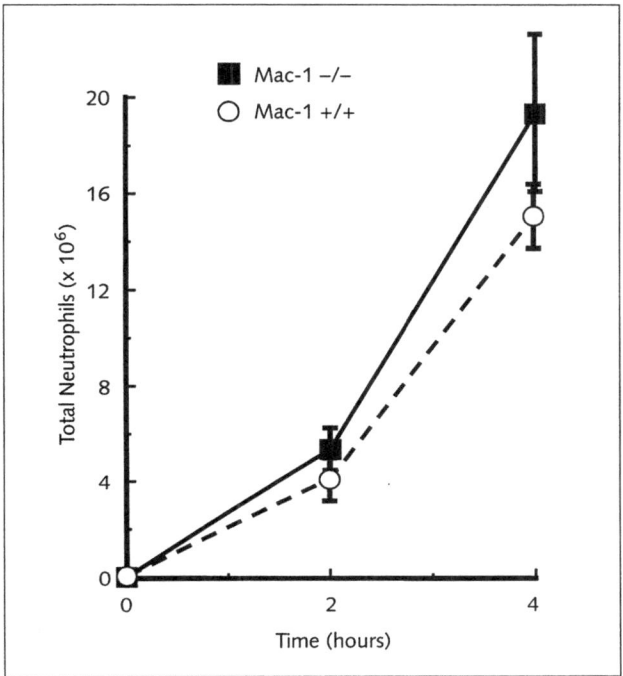

Figure 5
Neutrophil emigration in Mac-1-deficient mice. Mice with a targeted deletion of CD11b and wildtype mice were given intraperitoneal injections of thioglycollate [71]. Neutrophil emigration in the peritoneal cavity was determined in lavage fluid obtained either at 2 h or 4 h. No difference was found between Mac-1-deficient mice (Mac-1 −/−) and wildtype (Mac-1 +/+).

mice express no detectable Mac-1, and Mac-1-dependent functions *in vitro* were undetectable. However, the rate of neutrophil influx into the peritoneal cavity in the first 4 h of induced peritonitis was indistinguishable from that of wild type mice (Fig. 5), and was inhibited by monoclonal antibody to LFA-1. Additionally, in Mac-1 deficient mice, neutrophils in the peritoneal cavity were incapable of adhesion to fibrinogen-coated Mylar implants, a surface to which wild type neutrophils readily adhere [72]. Schmits et al. [73] found, in contrast to the study with CD11b deficient mice, that CD11a (LFA-1) deficient mice did exhibit a significant reduction in peritoneal influx of neutrophils.

Though the evidence just cited implicates a dominant role for LFA-1 in neutrophil emigration, Nolte et al. [74] found that F(ab′)$_2$ preparations of blocking monoclonal antibody to CD11b inhibited leukocyte sticking in an intravital model of ischemia/reperfusion in murine dorsal skin chambers. Similar intravital observations in rat and lapine models reveal similar contributions of Mac-1 to firm adhesion to venular endothelium [75,76]. Thus, it appears that different vascular beds may require different relative contributions of LFA-1 and Mac-1, and the differing studies *in vitro* reveal potential contributions of these integrins. It appears that Mac-1 and LFA-1 both contribute to the neutrophil's ability to stop rolling, and that LFA-1 may be dominant in the process of transendothelial migration.

The role of α_4 integrins in tethering and firm adhesion

The general model of leukocyte/endothelial interactions (rolling, stationary adhesion and transendothelial migration) covers all classes of leukocytes with such variations in the adhesion molecules and chemotactic stimuli that a high degree of specificity can be attained [77]. Selectins act as the dominant primary capture molecules for most if not all leukocytes. The interaction of VLA-4 ($\alpha_4\beta_1$, CD49d/CD29) with VCAM-1 (CD106) clearly functions as a secondary adhesion mechanism to stop rolling leukocytes. Luscinskas et al. [78] found that L-selectin, VLA-4 and CD18 integrins act in sequence to mediate the rolling, stable adhesion and spreading of monocytes on IL-4 stimulated HUVEC monolayers at venular shear rates. A similar behavior was seen for human eosinophils (which constitutively express VLA-4) on TNFα-stimulated HUVEC monolayers [79]. Jones et al. [80] found that T cells employ α_4 integrin/VCAM-1 and CD18 integrin/ICAM-1 for stable adhesion of IL-1-stimulated HUVEC.

As noted above, α_4 integrin is expressed on the leukocyte, concentrated at the tips of microvillus-like membranous projections where it may function as a primary tethering molecule [81, 82], and recent evidence indicates that it may serve such a function for some mononuclear leukocytes [80, 83], especially under circumstances were the endothelium expresses VCAM-1 and the wall shear stress is relatively low. The interaction between VLA-4 and VCAM-1 apparently permits rolling of leukocytes under flow, but most observers have found that the interaction between leukocytes and endothelial cells where this pair of adhesion molecules occurs involves little rolling. Jones et al. [80] observed that isolated T cells transiently roll, then stop on monolayers of L cells transfected with either the six or seven domain form of human VCAM-1. Recombinant or isolated native VCAM-1 immobilized on a foreign surface can support rolling and stable adhesion of lymphocytes [83]. Abe et al. [84] found that this adhesion molecule pair can function as a mechanism for primary capture of flowing leukocytes by endothelial cells. They also demonstrated that while both domains one and four of VCAM-1 can support VLA-4-dependent adhesion under static conditions, only domain one of VCAM-1 is involved in the primary tethering function of this molecule under conditions of flow.

Until recently, mature human neutrophils were thought not to express VLA-4. However, it is now clear that they can express this integrin under some conditions, and that α_4-dependent adhesion of these cells can occur. Early work revealed an intracellular storage pool of adhesion molecules for various matrix proteins [85], and stimuli such as chemotactic factors (e.g. C5a, platelet activating factor (PAF) or IL-8) have been shown to upregulate surface expression of α_4 integrin on mature neutrophils [86]. Demonstration of α_4 upregulation required treatment of the neutrophils with cytochalasin, possibly to promote extensive degranulation, or to prevent reinternalization of the integrin [86]. Reinhardt et al. [87] found that human neutrophils treated with dihydrocytochalasin B and a chemotactic stimulus to upregulate VLA-4 were able to tether and firmly adhere on VCAM-1 transfected L cell monolayers *in vitro* or TNFα-stimulated endothelial cells, and the adhesion was inhibited by anti-α_4 antibodies. Gao and Issekutz [88] found that C5a would induce the expression of VLA-4 on mature human neutrophils, resulting in α_4-dependent transmigration through monolayers of synovial and dermal fibroblasts. Thus, it is possible that neutrophils could utilize VLA-4 for firm adhesion to the luminal surface of endothelial cells if the appropriate stimulus conditions prevail.

The most likely function of neutrophil VLA-4 is after transendothelial migration. Such migration has been shown to upregulate VLA-4 expression on human and rat neutrophils [86, 89]. This increase in cell surface VLA-4 is not associated with increased adhesion unless the neutrophils are stimulated again with a chemotactic factor such as f-Met-Leu-Phe or a chemokine. The basis for the migration-induced VLA-4 expression remains to be determined, but it allows sustained expression and function much like the effects of cytochalasin described above. VLA-4 also binds to the extracellular matrix component fibronectin [90], and may function in the locomotion of neutrophils through extravascular connective tissue, a process apparently dependent on β_1 integrins but independent of CD18 integrins [91, 92]. The extravascular function of CD18 (β_2) integrins appears to be principally in the interaction of leukocytes with other cells such as fibroblasts [93] and parenchymal cells [94, 95].

Evidence for specific cellular localization of leukocyte arrest under flow

The topography of the adhesion molecules on leukocytes appears to play a significant role in the function of these adhesion molecules especially under conditions of shear stress. Burns was the first to show that L-selectin was not randomly distributed on the surface of neutrophils, but concentrated on the tips of membranous folds and microvillus-like projections from the cell surface [96, 97]. This distribution places L-selectin in a presumably favorable position for primary interaction with the endothelial surface. Other adhesion molecules that have been shown to function as primary tethers for flowing leukocytes also appear to colocalize with L-selectin at the tips of membranous surface projections. PSGL-1, a ligand for both E-selectin and P-selectin that mediates rolling of neutrophils [98], is found in this location [99], as are the α_4 integrins on lymphocytes [81, 82]. Von Andrian et al. [100] directly examined *in vitro* the functional consequences of microvillus localization of L-selectin on transfected lymphocytes in experiments involving domain exchanges between the ectodomain and transmembrane and intracellular domains of L-selectin and CD44. In contrast to the wild type L-selectin, the CD44 chimera was found predominately expressed on the cell body. In flow chamber assays, cells expressing the CD44 chimera were significantly less efficient in initiating tethering to isolated peripheral node addressin adsorbed to a planar surface, especially when shear rates were increased [100]. In addition, for those cells that tethered to the substratum under flow conditions, the rolling velocity for wild type L-selectin and the CD44 chimera was equivalent, and adhesion under static conditions was also equivalent. Thus, the advantage imparted by the microvillus presentation of L-selectin is in tethering efficiency under flow, but once rolling has been established the topography of L-selectin is without influence.

In contrast to the primary tethering molecules, the topography of the CD18 integrins appears to be random on the leukocyte surface, if not actually excluded from the membranous surface projections [97, 101, 102]. CD11b (Mac-1) is apparently excluded from the microvilli of neutrophils [97]. In addition to requiring an activation stimulus to augment the avidity of these integrins for adhesion, their surface distribution may be unfavorable to function as primary tethering molecules. However, as rolling proceeds, a combination of potentially important events occurs. The integrins are brought into proximity with the endothelial cell apical surface where there are ligands for the integrins, and chemotactic stimuli such as PAF and IL-8 that can rapidly activate the necessary avidity changes [26]. Rainger et al. [103] provided evidence in an *in vitro* model that IL-8 promotes conversion of rolling to stationary adhesion in a median of 240 ms, and PAF takes significantly longer to promote stationary adhesion (median of 720 ms). There is now evidence that the tethering process itself may contribute to integrin activation. Simon et al. [45] found that cross-linking L-selectin with antibodies results in significant activation of Mac-1-dependent adhesion, and that this response is synergistically enhanced when combined with low levels of PAF or IL-8 [59]. Several investigators have provided evidence for signaling through L-selectin [104–108].

The role of this signaling pathway in promoting stable adhesion of neutrophils on cytokine stimulated endothelial cells remains to be clearly shown. Evidence documenting a ligand for L-selectin on cytokine stimulated endothelial cells is critically lacking, so the basis for L-selectin-dependent signaling at sights of inflammation is yet to be defined. One possibility involves the interactions described earlier in this review; L-selectin-dependent tethering of neutrophils to each other through PSGL-1 on the opposing leukocyte. Another possibility involves the interaction of L-selectin and E-selectin. This potential mechanism is of interest regarding neutrophil adhesion since the difference in glycosylation of L-selectin by myeloid cells and lymphoid cells allows binding of E-selectin to myeloid derived L-selectin but not lymphoid derived L-selectin [96, 109]. In this situation, L-selectin would be functioning as a ligand presenting the carbohydrate recognized by E-selectin.

Once neutrophils arrest on the endothelial cells they promptly change shape and a high percentage begin to migrate. The following experiments *in vitro* provide evidence that transendothelial migration is strongly influenced by factors intrinsic to the monolayer. As noted above, cytokine-stimulated endothelial cells produce both PAF and IL-8, each contributing to the activation not only of adhesion, but of transmigration [26]. Endothelial cells appear to respond to neutrophil transmigation (in a transendothelial chemotactic gradient) as evidenced by a transient increase in cytosolic $[Ca^{2+}]_i$ that temporally corresponds to the transmigration of neutrophils [110]. Furthermore, these investigators found a corresponding myosin light chain phosphorylation in endothelial cells, and they demonstrated that when endothelial $[Ca^{2+}]_i$ was clamped at resting levels with a calcium buffer, neutrophil transmigration was inhibited [110, 111].

We have begun an evaluation of endothelial cell influence on the site of neutrophil firm adhesion and transmigration. Using HUVEC monolayers as an experimental model *in vitro*, we examined initially the site of neutrophil transmigration under static conditions [112]. In order to produce an endothelial monolayer with intercellular junctional characteristics (with particular reference to tight junctions, zonula occludens) similar to those found in postcapillary venules [113], we cultured the monolayers with astrocyte conditioned medium. Tight junctions appear to regulate macromolecular permeability, and they are situated in the interendothelial junctional complex closest to the luminal surface [114]. This position of tight junctions may regulate neutrophil transmigration, acting as the first barrier through which the neutrophil must pass. A model of transmigration should, therefore, include monolayers with tight junctions simulating those found *in vivo*. Exposing HUVEC to astrocyte conditioned medium was found to increase significantly both tight junctions (as revealed by transmission electron microscopy) and electrical resistance across the monolayer, without altering the upregulation of surface adhesion molecules following cytokine stimulation [112]. We found that the high level of transendothelial migration seen in Figure 4 was not reduced across monolayers with increased tight junctions. The site of transmigration was evaluated by fixing monolayers at the time of maximum neutrophil transmigration and staining endothelial junctions with silver nitrate to identify the positions of leukocyte migration. As shown in Figure 6, the dominate site of transmigration was at tricellular corners (i.e. the site where three endothelial cells meet). Quantitation of the site of migration revealed that $77.3 \pm 1.1\%$ of the neutrophils moved through the monolayer at tricellular corners, and the rest moved through at bicellular junctions. Morphometric analysis of the silver stained monolayers revealed that 6.4% of the perimeter of the endothelial cells is at the tricellular region, indicating that the apparent selection of

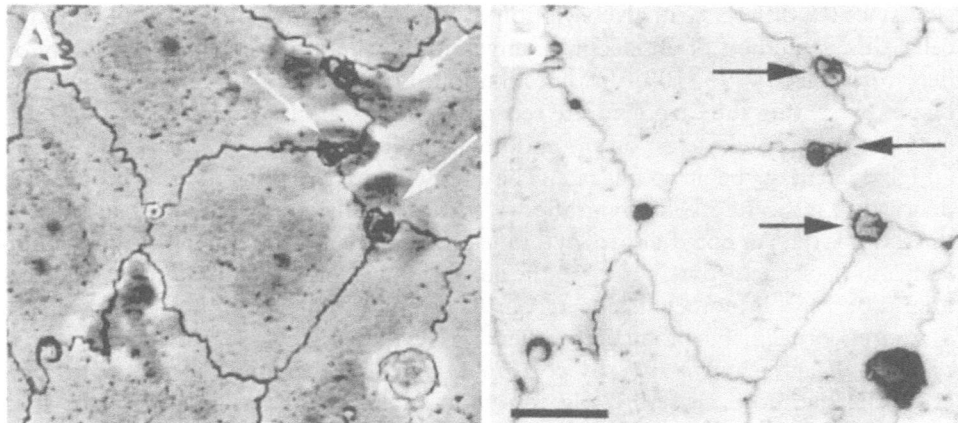

Figure 6

Transendothelial migration of human neutrophils at tricellular corners. HUVEC monolayers were stimulated with IL-1 for 4 h then placed in adhesion chambers. Isolated human neutrophils were injected into the chambers and allowed to settle onto the monolayer as described in Figure 4. At the time of maximum transendothelial migration the monolayers were fixed and silver stained to define the interendothelial borders. The phase contrast image of the monolayer is shown (A) and three neutrophils in the process of transmigation are identified (white arrows). The bright field image is shown (B) and the same three neutrophils are seen to be migrating at tricellular corners (the site where three endothelial cells meet). The scale bar is 10 μm.

this site for transmigration could not be a random process. Since Walker et al. [115] have shown ultrastructural discontinuities in tight junction strands at tricellular corners of endothelial cells *in vivo*, we investigated the distribution of occludin and ZO-1, tight junctional components, in these monolayers using immunofluorescence, and found consistent discontinuities in these components at tricellular junctions in monolayers that had not been exposed to neutrophils [112]. These observations raise the possibility that neutrophils may select intercellular regions of endothelial monolayers without tight junctions as sites for transmigration.

Since the above experiments were performed under static conditions, we also evaluated whether neutrophils would find tricellular corners for transmigration after firm arrest under conditions of flow. Using the model illustrated in Figure 2, we evaluated neutrophil locomotion after coming to firm arrest in the presence of a wall shear stress of 2 dynes/cm^2. We measured the distance the leukocyte moved from the site of arrest to the site of transmigration (illustrated in Fig. 7). The average migration distance for 30 randomly selected neutrophils was 5.9 ± 0.7 μm, and the median time from arrest to complete transmigration was 83.8 s. Since it was not

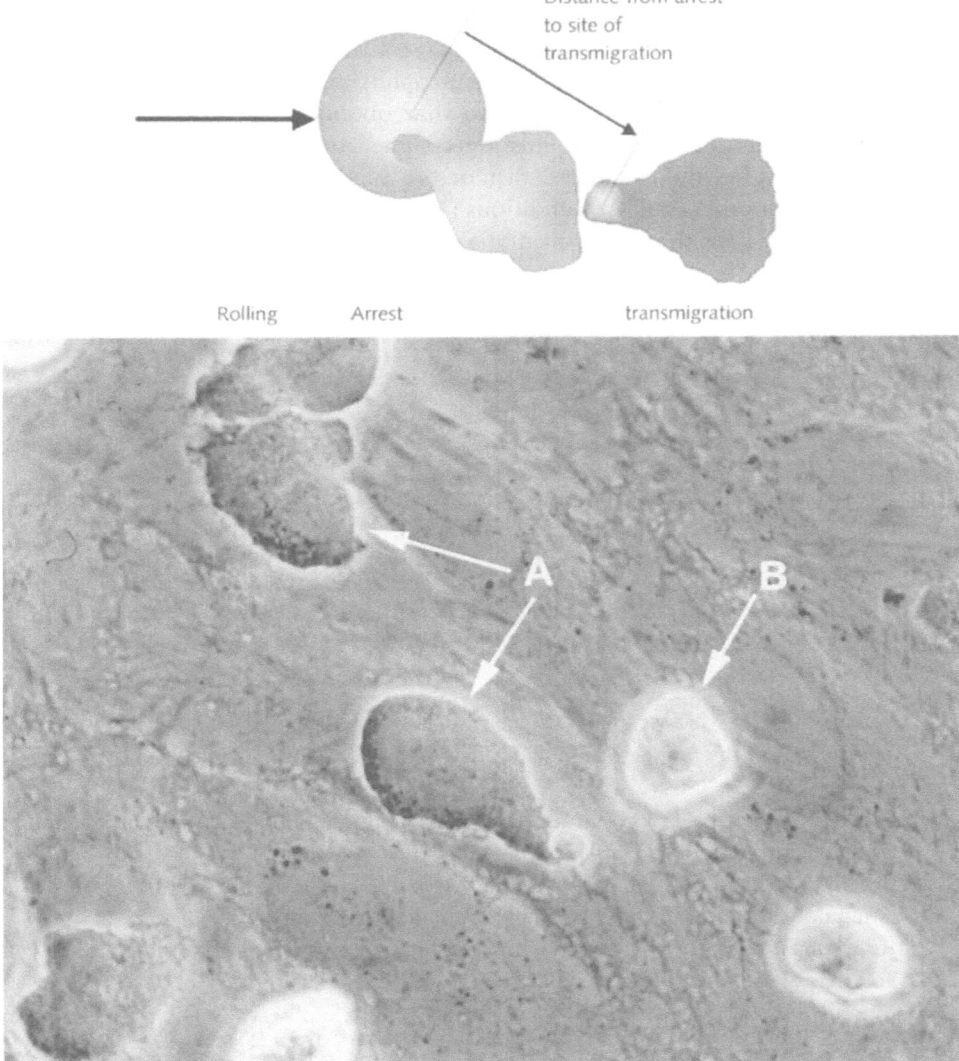

Figure 7

Transendothelial migration of human neutrophils. The upper figure illustrates the procedure used to measure the distance from the position a neutrophil arrested under flow conditions to the site where it transmigrated. The lower figure shows images of cells similar to those measured. The rounded, out of focus neutrophil (B) is on the apical surface of the HUVEC monolayer, and illustrates the appearance of cells firmly adherent under flow before they begin to change shape and migrate. The cells in shape focus (A) are beneath the endothelial monolayer. Notice the tip of the uropod still protruding through the monolayer as the cell transmigrates.

possible to visualize endothelial junctions using phase contrast microscopy, these flow experiments were repeated, the monolayers fixed and junctions stained with silver nitrate [112]. The percentage of neutrophils migrating at tricellular corners was $69.9 \pm 1.7\%$, a value very similar to that obtained for neutrophil migration under static conditions. If neutrophils are assumed to firmly arrest randomly over the monolayer, then the calculated distance of migration to tricellular corners in monolayers under these culture conditions [112] would be an average of 11 μm, significantly longer than that experimentally determined. This finding is not inconsistent with the idea that neutrophils arrest from the flow stream near the site of transmigration (i.e. near tricellular corners). A molecular or biophysical basis for this apparent localization of transmigration and adhesion under flow remains to be determined.

Acknowledgements

This work was supported in part by an Established Investigators Award of the American Heart Association (S.I.S.), NIH Grants HL42550, and AI19031 (C.W.S.).

References

1   Waller A (1846) Microscopic examination of some principal tissues of the animal frame as observed in the tongue of the living frog, toad, etc. *Lond Edinb Dubl Phil Mag* 29: 271–287

2   Clark ER, Clark EL (1935) Observations on changes in blood vascular endothelium in the living animal. *Am J Anat* 57: 385–438

3   Atherton A, Born GVR (1972) Quantitative investigations of the adhesiveness of circulating polymorphonuclear leukocytes to blood vessel walls. *J Physiol* 222: 447–474

4   Atherton A, Born GVR (1973) Relationship between the velocity of rolling granulocytes and that of the blood flow in venules. *J Physiol* 233: 157–165

5   Marchesi V, Florey HW (1960) Electron micrographic observations on the emigration of leucocytes. *Q J Exp Physiol* 45: 343–347

6   Anderson DC, Schmalstieg FC, Kohl S, Arnaout MA, Hughes BJ, Tosi MF, Buffone GJ, Brinkley BR, Dickey WD, Abramson JS et al (1984) Abnormalities of polymorphonuclear leukocyte function associated with a heritable deficiency of high molecular weight surface glycoproteins (GP138): Common relationship to diminished cell adherence. *J Clin Invest* 74: 536–551

7   Smith CW, Marlin SD, Rothlein R, Toman C, Anderson DC (1989) Cooperative interactions of LFA-1 and Mac-1 with intercellular adhesion molecule-1 in facilitating adherence and transendothelial migration of human neutrophils *in vitro*. *J Clin Invest* 83: 2008–2017

8   Smith CW, Rothlein R, Hughes BJ, Mariscalco MM, Schmalstieg FC, Anderson DC (1988) Recognition of an endothelial determinant for CD18-dependent human neutrophil adherence and transendothelial migration. *J Clin Invest* 82: 1746–1756

9   Diamond MS, Staunton DE, de Fougerolles AR, Stacker SA, Garcia-Aguilar J, Hibbs ML, Springer TA (1990) ICAM-1 (CD54): A counter-receptor for Mac-1 (CD11b/CD18). *J Cell Biol* 111: 3129–3139

10   Anderson DC, Kishimoto TK, Smith CW (1995) Leukocyte adhesion deficiency and other disorders of leukocyte adherence and motility. In: CR Scriver, AL Beaudet, WS Sly, D Valle (eds): *The metabolic and molecular bases of inherited disease*. McGraw-Hill, 3955–3994

11   Lawrence MB, McIntire LV, Eskin SG (1987) Effect of flow on polymorphonuclear leukocyte/endothelial cell adhesion. *Blood* 70: 1284–1290

12   Lawrence MB, Smith CW, Eskin SG, McIntire LV (1990) Effect of venous shear stress on CD18-mediated neutrophil adhesion to cultured endothelium. *Blood* 75: 227–237

13   Smith CW, Kishimoto TK, Abbassi O, Hughes BJ, Rothlein R, McIntire LV, Butcher E, Anderson DC (1991) Chemotactic factors regulate lectin adhesion molecule 1 (LECAM-1)-dependent neutrophil adhesion to cytokine-stimulated endothelial cells *in vitro*. *J Clin Invest* 87: 609–618

14   Abbassi O, Lane CL, Krater SS, Kishimoto TK, Anderson DC, McIntire LV, Smith CW (1991) Canine neutrophil margination mediated by lectin adhesion molecule-1 (LECAM-1) *in vitro*. *J Immunol* 147: 2107–2115

15   Bevilacqua MP, Stengelin S, Gimbrone MA Jr, Seed B (1989) Endothelial leukocyte adhesion molecule 1: An inducible receptor for neutrophils related to complement regulatory proteins and lectins. *Science* 243: 1160–1165

16   Abbassi O, Kishimoto TK, McIntire LV, Anderson DC, Smith CW (1993) E-Selectin supports neutrophil rolling *in vitro* under conditions of flow. *J Clin Invest* 92: 2719–2730

17   McEver RP (1991) Selectins: Novel receptors that mediate leukocyte adhesion during inflammation. *Thromb Haemostas* 65: 223–228

18   Jones DA, Abbassi O, McIntire LV, McEver RP, Smith CW (1993) P-selectin mediates neutrophil rolling on histamine-stimulated endothelial cells. *Biophys J* 65: 1560–1569

19   Smith CW (1993) Endothelial adhesion molecules and their role in inflammation. *Can J Physiol Pharmacol* 71: 76–87

20   Springer TA (1995) Traffic signals on endothelium for lymphocyte recirculation and leukocyte emigration. *Annu Rev Physiol* 57: 827–872

21   Ley K (1995) Gene-targeted mice in leukocyte adhesion research. *Microcirculation* 2: 141–150

22   Kishimoto TK, Jutila MA, Berg EL, Butcher EC (1989) Neutrophil Mac-1 and MEL-14 adhesion proteins inversely regulated by chemotactic factors. *Science* 245: 1238–1241

23   Simon SI, Chambers JD, Butcher E, Sklar LA (1992) Neutrophil aggregation is β_2-integrin- and L-selectin-dependent in blood and isolated cells. *J Immunol* 149: 2765–2771

24   Zimmerman GA, McIntyre TM, Mehra M, Prescott SM (1990) Endothelial cell-associ-

ated platelet-activating factor: A novel mechanism for signaling intercellular adhesion. *J Cell Biol* 110: 529–540

25 Webb LMC, Ehrengruber MU, Clark-Lewis I, Baggiolini M, Rot A (1993) Binding to heparan sulfate or heparin enhances neutrophil responses to interleukin 8. *Proc Natl Acad Sci USA* 90: 7158–7162

26 Kuijpers TW, Hakkert BC, Hart MHL, Roos D (1992) Neutrophil migration across monolayers of cytokine-prestimulated endothelial cells: A role for platelet-activating factor and IL-8. *J Cell Biol* 117: 565–572

27 Rainger GE, Fisher A, Shearman C, Nash GB (1995) Adhesion of flowing neutrophils to cultured endothelial cells after hypoxia and reoxygenation *in vitro. Am J Physiol* 269: H1398–H1406

28 Von Andrian UH, Hansell P, Chambers JD, Berger EM, Filho IT, Butcher EC, Arfors K-E (1992) L-selectin function is required for beta-2 integrin-mediated neutrophil adhesion at physiologic shear rates *in vivo. Am J Physiol* 263: H1034–H1044

29 Bongrand P, Capo C, Mege J-L, Benoliel A-M (1988) Use of hydrodynamic flows to study cell adhesion. In: P Bongrand (ed): *Physical basis of cell-cell adhesion.* CRC Press, Boca Raton, 125–156

30 Hammerschmidt PE, Bowers TK, Kammi-Kepfe CJ, Jacob HS, Craddock PR (1980) Granulocyte aggregometry: a sensitive technique for the detection of C5a and complement activation. *Blood* 55: 898–902

31 Craddock PR, Fehr J, Brigham KL, Broenerberg RS, Jacob HS (1977) Complement and leukocyte-mediated pulmonary dysfunction in hemodialysis. *N Eng J Med* 296: 769–774

32 Craddock PR, Hammerschmidt DE, White JG, Dalmasso AP, Jacob HS (1977) Complement (C5a)-induced granulocyte aggregation *in vitro*: A possible mechanism of complement-mediated leukostasis and leukopenia. *J Clin Invest* 60: 260–274

33 Craddock PR, Hammerschmidt DE, Moldow CF, Yamada O, Jacob HS (1979) Granulocyte aggregation as a manifestation of membrane interactions with complement. Possible role in leukocyte margination, microvascular occlusion, and endothelial damage. *Seminars in Hematology* 16: 140

34 McDonagh PF, Wilson DS, Iwamura H, Smith CW, Williams SK, Copeland JG (1996) CD18 Antibody treatment limits early myocardial reperfusion injury after initial leukocyte deposition. *J Surg Res* 64: 139–149

35 Lehr H-A, Weyrich AS, Saetzler RK, Jurek A, Arfors KE, Zimmerman GA, Prescott SM, McIntyre TM (1997) Vitamin C blocks inflammatory platelet-activating factor mimetics created by cigarette smoking. *J Clin Invest* 99: 2358–2364

36 Engler RL, Dahlgren MD, Morris DD, Peterson MA, Schmid-Schonbein GW (1986) Role of leukocytes in response to acute myocardial ischemia and reflow in dogs. *Am J Physiol* 251: H314–323

37 Alon R, Fuhlbrigge RC, Finger EB, Springer TA (1996) Interactions through L-selectin between leukocytes and adherent leukocytes nucleate rolling adhesions on selectins and VCAM-1 in shear flow. *J Cell Biol* 135: 849–865

38   Walcheck B, Moore KL, McEver RP, Kishimoto TK (1996) Neutrophil-neutrophil inter-
      actions under hydrodynamic shear stress involve L-selectin and PSGL-1. A mechanism
      that amplifies initial leukocyte accumulation on P-selectin *in vitro*. *J Clin Invest* 98:
      1081–1087

39   Walcheck B, Kahn J, Fisher JM, Wang BB, Fisk RS, Payan DG, Feehan C, Betageri R,
      Darlak K, Spatola AF et al (1996) Neutrophil rolling altered by inhibition of L-Selectin
      shedding *in vitro*. *Nature* 380: 720–723

40   Fuhlbrigge RC, Alon R, Puri KD, Lowe JB, Springer TA (1996) Sialylated, fucosylated
      ligands for L-selectin expressed on leukocytes mediate tethering and rolling adhesions in
      physiologic flow conditions. *J Cell Biol* 135: 837–848

41   Butcher EC (1991) Leukocyte-endothelial cell recognition: Three (or more) steps to
      specificity and diversity. *Cell* 67: 1033–1036

42   Kuijpers TW, Koenderman L, Weening RS, Verhoeven AJ, Roos D (1990) Continuous
      cell activation is necessary for stable interaction of complement receptor type 3 with its
      counter-structure in the aggregation response of human neutrophils. *Eur J Immunol* 20:
      501–508

43   Rochon YP, Frojmovic MM, Mills EL (1993) Comparative studies of microscopically
      determined aggregation degranulation, and light transmission after chemotactic activa-
      tion of adult and newborn neutrophils. *Blood* 75: 2053–2060

44   Smoluchowski MV (1917) Versuch einer mathematischen theorie der koagulationsk-
      inetik kolloider losungen. *Zeitschrift für Physikalische Chemie* 92: 129–168

45   Simon SI, Burns AR, Taylor AD, Gopalan PK, Lynam EB, Sklar LA, Smith CW (1995)
      L-Selectin (CD62L) crosslinking signals neutrophil adhesive functions via the Mac-1
      (CD11b/CD18) β_2-integrin. *J Immunol* 155: 1502–1514

46   Taylor AD, Neelamegham S, Hellums JD, Smith CW, Simon SI (1996) Molecular
      dynamics of of the transition from L-selectin- to β_2-integrin-dependent neutrophil adhe-
      sion under defined hydrodynamic shear. *Biophys J* 71: 3488–3500

47   Neelamegham S, Taylor AD, Hellums JD, Dembo M, Smith CW, Simon SI (1997) Mod-
      eling the reversible kinetics of neutrophil aggregation under hydrodynamic shear. *Bio-
      phys J* 72: 1527–1540

48   Hoffstein ST, Friedman RS, Weissmann G (1982) Degranulation, membrane addition,
      and shape change during chemotactic factor-induced aggregation of human neutrophils.
      J Cell Biol 95: 234–241

49   Sklar LA, Omann GM, Painter RG (1985) Relationship of actin polymerization and
      depolymerization to light scattering in human neutrophils: Dependence on receptor
      occupancy and intracellular Ca^{++}. *J Cell Biol* 101: 1161–1166

50   Arnaout MA, Hakim RM, Todd III RF, Dana N, Colten HR (1985) Increased expres-
      sion of an adhesion-promoting surface glycoprotein in the granulocytopenia of
      hemodialysis. *N Eng J Med* 312: 457–462

51   Schwartz BR, Ochs HD, Beatty PG, Harlan JM (1985) A monoclonal antibody-defined
      membrane antigen complex is required for neutrophil-neutrophil aggregation. *Blood* 65:
      1553–1556

52   Simon SI, Chambers JD, Sklar LA (1990) Flow cytometric analysis and modeling of cell-cell adhesive interactions: The neutrophil as a model. *J Cell Biol* 111: 2747–2756

53   Guyer DA, Moore KL, Lynam EB, Schammel CMG, Rogelj S, McEver RP, Sklar LA (1996) P-selectin glycoprotein ligand-1 (PSGL-1) is a ligand for L-selectin in neutrophil aggregation. *Blood* 88: 2415–2421

54   Puri KD, Chen S, Springer TA (1998) Modifying the mechanical property and shear threshold of L-Selectin adhesion independently of equilibrium properties. *Nature* 392: 930–933

55   Finger EB, Purl K, Alon R, Lawrence MB, von Andrian UH, Springer TA (1996) Adhesion through L-selectin requires a threshold hydrodynamic shear. *Nature* 379: 266–269

56   Lawrence MB, Kansas GS, Kunkel EJ, Ley K (1997) Threshold levels of fluid shear promote leukocyte adhesion through selectins (CD62L,P,E). *J Cell Biol* 136: 717–727

57   Simon SI, Taylor A, Neelamegham S, Hellums JD, Smith CW (1997) Neutrophil aggregation mediated by β_2-integrin and ICAM-3 at low hydrodynamic shear. *FASEB J* 11: A102

58   Campanero MR, del Pozo MA, Arroyo AG, Sanchez-Mateos P, Hernandez-Caselles T, Craig A, Pulido R, Sanchez-Madrid F (1993) ICAM-3 interacts with LFA-1 and regulates the LFA-1/ICAM-1 cell adhesion pathway. *J Cell Biol* 123: 1007–1016

59   Tsang YTM, Neelamegham S, Hu Y, Berg EL, Burns AR, Smith CW, Simon SI (1997) Synergy between L-selectin signaling and chemotactic activation during neutrophil adhesion and transmigration. *J Immunol* 159: 4566–4577

60   Gopalan PK, Smith CW, Lu H, Berg EL, McIntire LV, Simon SI (1997) Neutrophil CD18-dependent arrest on ICAM-1 in shear flow can be activated through L-selectin. *J Immunol* 158: 367–375

61   Wong J, Johnston B, Lee SS, Bullard DC, Smith CW, Beaudet AL, Kubes P (1997) A minimal role for selectins in the recruitment of leukocytes into the inflamed liver microvasculature. *J Clin Invest* 99: 2782–2790

62   Gaboury JP, Kubes P (1994) Reductions in physiologic shear rates lead to CD11/CD18-dependent, selectin-independent leukocyte rolling *in vivo*. *Blood* 83: 345–350

63   Lo SK, Detmer PA, Levin SM, Wright SD (1989) Transient adhesion of neutrophils to endothelium. *J Exp Med* 169: 1779–1793

64   Furie MB, Tancinco MCA, Smith CW (1991) Monoclonal antibodies to leukocyte integrins CD11a/CD18 and CD11b/CD18 or intercellular adhesion molecule-1 (ICAM-1) inhibit chemoattractant-stimulated neutrophil transendothelial migration *in vitro*. *Blood* 78: 2089–2097

65   Anderson DC, Springer TA (1987) Leukocyte adhesion deficiency: An inherited defect in the Mac-1, LFA-1 and p150,95 glycoproteins. *Ann Rev Med* 38: 175–194

66   Issekutz AC, Issekutz TB (1992) The contribution of LFA-1 (CD11a/CD18) and Mac-1 (CD11b/CD18) to the *in vivo* migration of polymorphonuclear leucocytes to inflammatory reactions in the rat. *Immunol* 76: 655–661

67   Rutter J, James TJ, Howat D, Shock A, Andrew D, De Baetselier P, Blackford J, Wilkin-

son JM, Higgs G, Hughes B, et al (1994) The *in vivo* and *in vitro* effects of antibodies against rabbit β$_2$-integrins. *J Immunol* 153: 3724–3733

68 Graf JM, Smith CW, Mariscalco MM (1996) Contribution of LFA-1 and Mac-1 to CD18-dependent neutrophil emigration in a neonatal rabbit model. *J Appl Physiol* 80: 1984–1992

69 Tang L, Eaton JW (1993) Fibrin(ogen) mediates acute inflammatory response to biomaterials. *J Exp Med* 178: 2147–2156

70 Rosen H, Gordon S (1987) Monoclonal antibody to the murine type 3 complement receptor inhibits adhesion of myelomonocytic cells *in vitro* and inflammatory cell recruitment *in vivo*. *J Exp Med* 166: 1685–1701

71 Lu H, Smith CW, Perrard J, Bullard D, Tang L, Shappell SB, Entman ML, Beaudet AL, Ballantyne CM (1997) LFA-1 is sufficient in mediating neutrophil emigration in Mac-1 deficient mice. *J Clin Invest* 99: 1340–1350

72 Tang L, Ugarova TP, Plow EF, Eaton JW (1996) Molecular determinants of acute inflammatory responses to biomaterials. *J Clin Invest* 97: 1329–1334

73 Schmits R, Kundig TM, Baker DM, Shumaker G, Simard JJL, Duncan G, Wakeham A, Shahinian A, van der Heiden A, Bachmann MF et al (1996) LFA-1-deficient mice show normal CTL responses to virus but fail to reject immunogenic tumor. *J Exp Med* 183: 1415–1426

74 Nolte D, Hecht R, Schmid P, Botzlar A, Menger MD, Neumueller C, Sinowatz F, Vestweber D, Messmer K (1994) Role of Mac-1 and ICAM-1 in ischemia-reperfusion injury in a microcirculation model of BALB/C mice. *Am J Physiol* 267: H1320–H1328

75 Kurose I, Anderson DC, Miyasaka M, Tamatani T, Paulson JC, Todd III RF, Rusche JR, Granger DN (1994) Molecular determinants of reperfusion-induced leukocyte adhesion and vascular protein leakage. *Cir Res* 74: 336–343

76 Zimmerman BJ, Holt JW, Paulson JC, Anderson DC, Miyasaka M, Tamatani T, Todd III RF, Rusche JR, Granger DN (1994) Molecular determinants of lipid mediator-induced leukocyte adherence and emigration in rat mesenteric venules. *Am J Physiol* 266: H847–H853

77 Alon R, Feizi T, Yuen CT, Fuhlbrigge RC, Springer TA (1995) Glycolipid ligands for selectins support leukocyte tethering and rolling under physiologic flow conditions. *J Immunol* 154: 5356–5366

78 Luscinskas FW, Kansas GS, Ding H, Pizcueta P, Schleiffenbaum BE, Tedder TF, Gimbrone MA Jr (1994) Monocyte rolling, arrest and spreading on IL-4-activated vascular endothelium under flow is mediated via sequential action of L-Selectin, β$_1$-integrins, and β$_2$-integrins. *J Cell Biol* 125: 1417–1427

79 Kitayama J, Fuhlbrigge RC, Puri KD, Springer TA (1997) P-selectin, L-selectin, and α$_4$ integrin have distinct roles in eosinophil tethering and arrest on vascular endothelial cells under physiological flow conditions. *J Immunol* 159: 3929–3939

80 Jones DA, McIntire LV, Smith CW, Picker LJ (1994) A two-step adhesion cascade for T cell/endothelial cell interactions under flow conditions. *J Clin Invest* 94: 2443–2450

81 Berlin C, Bargatze RF, Campbell JJ, von Andrian UH, Szabo MC, Hasslen SR, Nelson

RD, Berg EL, Erlandsen SL, Butcher EC (1995) Alpha-4 integrins mediate lymphocyte attachment and rolling under physiologic flow. *Cell* 80: 413–422

82 Abitorabi MA, Pachynski RK, Ferrando RE, Tidswell M, Erle DJ (1997) Presentation of integrins on leukocyte microvilli: a role for the extracellular domain in determining membrane localization. *J Cell Biol* 139: 563–571

83 Alon R, Kassner PD, Carr MW, Finger EB, Hemler ME, Springer TA (1995) The integrin VLA-4 supports tethering and rolling in flow on VCAM-1. *J Cell Biol* 128: 1243–1253

84 Abe Y, Ballantyne CM, Smith CW (1996) Functions of domain 1 and 4 of vascular cell adhesion molecule-1 in α_4 integrin-dependent adhesion under static and flow conditions are differentially regulated. *J Immunol* 157: 5061–5069

85 Singer II, Scott S, Kawka DW, Kazazis DM (1989) Adhesomes: Specific granules containing receptors for laminin, C3bi/fibrinogen, fibronectin, and vitronectin in human polymorphonuclear leukocytes and monocytes. *J Cell Biol* 109: 3169-3182

86 Kubes P, Niu X-F, Smith CW, Kehrli ME, Jr., Reinhardt PH, Woodman RC (1995) A novel β_1-dependent adhesion pathway on neutrophils: A mechanism invoked by dihydrocytochalasin B or endothelial transmigration. *FASEB J* 9: 1103–1111

87 Reinhardt PH, Elliott JF, Kubes P (1997) Neutrophils can adhere via $\alpha_4\beta_1$-integrin under flow conditions. *Blood* 89: 3837–3846

88 Gao JX, Issekutz AC (1997) The β_1 integrin, very late activation antigen-4 on human neutrophils can contribute to neutrophil migration through connective tissue fibroblast barriers. *Immunology* 90: 448–454

89 Reinhardt PH, Ward CA, Giles WA, Kubes P (1997) Emigrated rat neutrophils adhere to cardiac myocytes via α_4 integrin. Circ Res 81: 196–201

90 Elices MJ, Osborn L, Takada Y, Crouse C, Luhowskyj S, Hemler ME, Lobb RR (1990) VCAM-1 on activated endothelium interacts with the leukocyte integrin VLA-4 at a site distinct from the VLA-4/fibronecin binding site. *Cell* 60: 577–584

91 Bienvenu K, Harris N, Granger DN (1994) Modulation of leukocyte migration in mesenteric interstitium. *Am J Physiol* 267: H1573–H1577

92 Werr J, Xie X, Hedqvist P, Ruoslahti E, Lindbom L (1998) β_1 integrins are critically involved in neutrophil locomotion in extravascular tissue *in vivo. J Exp Med* 187: 2091–2096

93 Burns AR, Simon SI, Kukielka GL, Rowen JL, Mendoza LH, Brown ES, Entman ML, Smith CW (1996) Chemotactic factors stimulate CD18-dependent canine neutrophil adherence and motility on lung fibroblasts. *J Immunol* 156: 3389–3401

94 Nagendra AR, Mickelson JK, Smith CW (1997) CD18 integrin and CD54-dependent neutrophil adhesion to cytokine-stimulated human hepatocytes. *Am J Physiol* 272: G408–G416

95 Smith CW, Entman ML, Lane CL, Beaudet AL, Ty TI, Youker KA, Hawkins HK, Anderson DC (1991) Adherence of neutrophils to canine cardiac myocytes *in vitro* is dependent on intercellular adhesion molecule-1. *J Clin Invest* 88: 1216–1223

96 Picker LJ, Warnock RA, Burns AR, Doerschuk CM, Berg EL, Butcher EC (1991) The

neutrophil selectin LECAM-1 presents carbohydrate ligands to the vascular selectins ELAM-1 and GMP-140. *Cell* 66: 921–933

97 Erlandsen SL, Hasslen SR, Nelson RD (1993) Detection and spatial distribution of the beta-2 integrin (Mac-1) and L-selectin (LECAM-1) adherence receptors on human neutrophils by high-resolution field emission SEM. *J Histochem Cytochem* 41: 327–333

98 Patel KD, Moore KL, Nollert MU, McEver RP (1995) Neutrophils use both shared and distinct mechanisms to adhere to selectins under static and flow conditions. *J Clin Invest* 96: 1887–1896

99 Moore KL, Patel KD, Bruehl RE, Fugang L, Johnson DA, Lichenstein HS, Cummings RD, Bainton DF, McEver RP (1995) P-selectin glycoprotein ligand-1 mediates rolling of human neutrophils on P-selectin. *J Cell Biol* 128: 661–671

100 Von Andrian UH, Hasslen SR, Nelson RD, Erlandsen SL, Butcher EC (1995) A central role for microvillous receptor presentation in leukocyte adhesion under flow. *Cell* 82: 989–999

101 Thornhill MH, Kyan-Aung U, Haskard DO (1990) IL-4 increases human endothelial cell adhesiveness for T cells but not for neutrophils. *J Immunol* 144: 3060–3065

102 Hasslen SR, Burns AR, Simon SI, Smith CW, Starr K, Barclay AN, Michie SA, Nelson RD, Erlandsen SL (1996) Preservation of spatial organization and antigenicity of leukocyte surface molecules by aldehyde fixation: Flow cytometry and high-resolution FESEM studies of CD62L, CD11b, and Thy-1. *J Histochem Cytochem* 44: 1115–1122

103 Rainger GE, Fisher AC, Nash GB (1997) Endothelial-borne platelet-activating factor and interleukin-8 rapidly immobilize rolling neutrophils. *Am J Physiol* 272: H114–H122

104 Brenner B, Gulbins E, Schlottman K, Koppenhoefer U, Busch GL, Walzog B, Steinhausen M, Coggeshall KM, Linderkamp O, Lang F (1996) L-selectin activates the Ras pathway via the tyrosine kinase p56^{lck}. *Proc Natl Acad Sci USA* 93: 15376–15381

105 Brenner B, Gulbins E, Busch GL, Koppenhoefer U, Lang F, Linderkamp O (1997) L-selectin regulates actin polymerisation via activation of the small G-protein Rac2. *Biochem Biophys Res Commun* 231: 802–807

106 Waddell TK, Kialkow L, Chan CK, Kishimoto TK, Downey GP (1995) Signaling functions of L-selectin. *J Biol Chem* 270: 15403–15411

107 Gopalan PK, Smith CW, Lu H, Berg EL, McIntyre LV, Simon SI (1997) Neutrophil CD18-dependent arrest on ICAM-1 in shear flow can be activated through L-selectin. *J Immunol* 158: 367–375

108 Crockett-Torabi E (1998) Selectins and mechanisms of signal transduction. *J Leuk Biol* 63: 1–14

109 Zöllner O, Lenter MC, Blanks JE, Borges E, Steegmaier M, Zerwes HG, Vestweber D (1997) L-selectin from human, but not from mouse neutrophils binds directly to E-selectin. *J Cell Biol* 136: 707–716

110 Huang AJ, Manning JE, Bandak TM, Ratau MC, Hanser KR, Silverstein SC (1993) Endothelial cell cytosolic free calcium regulates neutrophil migration across monolayers of endothelial cells. *J Cell Biol* 120: 1371–1380

111 Hixenbaugh EA, Goeckeler ZM, Papaiya NN, Wysolmerski RB, Silverstein SC, Huang AJ (1997) Stimulated neutrophils induce myosin light chain phosphorylation and isometric tension in endothelial cells. *Am J Physiol* 272: H981–H988

112 Burns AR, Walker DC, Brown ES, Thurmon LT, Bowden RA, Keese CR, Simon SI, Entman ML, Smith CW (1997) Neutrophil transendothelial migration is independent of tight junctions and occurs preferentially at tricellular corners. *J Immunol* 159: 2893–2903

113 Simionescu M, Simionescu N, Palade GE (1976) Segmental differentiations of cell junctions in the vascular endothelium. Arteries and veins. *J Cell Biol* 68: 705–723

114 Staehelin LA (1975) A new occludens-like junction linking endothelial cells of small capillaries (probably venules) of rat jejunum. *J Cell Sci* 18: 545–551

115 Walker DC, MacKenzie A, Hosford S (1994) The structure of the tricellular region of endothelial tight junctions of pulmonary capillaries analyzed by freeze-fracture. *Microvasc Res* 48: 259–281

Production and presentation of chemokines by endothelial cells

Martha B. Furie

Department of Pathology, School of Medicine, State University of New York at Stony Brook, Stony Brook, NY 11794-8691, USA

Introduction

Recruitment of leukocytes at sites of tissue injury is governed by a complex network of cellular adhesion molecules, cytokines, and other inflammatory mediators. Chemokines (a contraction of *chemotactic cytokines*) play a prominent role in this process by attracting specific subsets of leukocytes [1–4]. Members of the chemokine family share common structural motifs, most notably conserved cysteine residues that form characteristic intramolecular disulfide bridges. There are at least four subfamilies of chemokines, defined by the presence and positioning of the two most amino-proximal cysteine residues. In the CXC subfamily, these two residues are separated by an intervening amino acid; in CC chemokines, the cysteine moieties are located immediately adjacent to one another. More recently, chemokine-like molecules have been cloned in which the cysteine residues are separated by three amino acids (CX_3C subfamily) [5] or in which only one of the two amino-proximal cysteine residues is present (C subfamily) [6]. More than 40 human chemokines have been identified so far, and searches of expressed sequence tag databases are rapidly adding to this number. An up-to-date listing of chemokines is available through the Cytokine Family cDNA Database web site (http://cytokine.medic. kumamoto-u.ac.jp/CFC/CK/Chemokine.html).

Many different cell types produce chemokines [1], and it is likely that any inflammatory reaction will involve chemokines from a number of cellular sources. However, the vascular endothelium, by virtue of its position at the interface between bloodstream and tissues, is uniquely situated to provide the chemokines that initially interact with an emigrating leukocyte. This chapter will briefly review the evidence that implicates chemokines in recruitment of leukocytes. The potential participation of the endothelium in generating chemokines and in displaying them to leukocytes as surface-bound molecules will then be considered in detail.

Vascular Adhesion Molecules and Inflammation, edited by J. D. Pearson
© 1999 Birkhäuser Verlag Basel/Switzerland

Chemokines and recruitment of leukocytes

Extravasation of leukocytes at sites of inflammation involves a precisely orchestrated sequence of events, as reviewed in the chapters by Ley and Smith et al. in this volume, and chemokines are thought to be involved at several points [3, 7]. The first step is transient adhesion of the leukocytes to the endothelium of postcapillary venules in the affected area, which is mediated in large part by the selectin family of adhesion molecules. This loose association, which results in rolling of the white cells along the vessels, allows the leukocytes to interact with chemoattractants that are generated in the area of damage. Chemokines, like other chemotactic agents, activate leukocytic integrins to render them competent to bind to ligands on endothelium [8, 9], thus establishing a firm adhesion between the two cell types.

Although the binding of integrins to their ligands results in a tight contact between leukocyte and endothelium, it is not a permanent one. Eventually, the leukocytes crawl across the vessel wall via endothelial junctional spaces and travel through the tissues until they reach their ultimate destination. The leukocytes are guided in this journey by chemoattractants. *In vitro*, chemoattractants cue leukocytes to move to the area of highest concentration when presented to the cells as a gradient. It is difficult to demonstrate the existence of such gradients *in vivo*; nonetheless, there is ample evidence that chemoattractants participate in recruitment of leukocytes in animal models of inflammation [3, 4, 7].

Chemoattractants such as bacterial formylated peptides, complement component C5a, and the arachidonic acid derivative leukotriene B_4 are rather nonspecific in their actions, in that they attract multiple types of leukocytes. In contrast, individual chemokines act on limited subsets of white cells. This unique property of the chemokines may explain the varying compositions of leukocytic infiltrates in different inflammatory settings. A frequently cited generalization is that CXC chemokines attract neutrophils, whereas CC chemokines exert their effects on other leukocytic subtypes. However, so many exceptions to this rule have been uncovered that it has lost much of its usefulness. Members of the CXC family that contain a glutamic acid-leucine-arginine (ELR) sequence located close to the amino terminus attract neutrophils, whereas those that lack it do not [1, 3, 4]. Moreover, members of both the CXC and CC subfamilies attract T lymphocytes, eosinophils, and basophils [2–4, 7]. The C chemokine lymphotactin, as its name suggests, acts on lymphocytes [6]. The CX_3C chemokine fractalkine predominantly attracts natural killer cells and a subset of T lymphocytes, with only a weak activity towards monocytes [10].

Once a leukocyte has arrived at a site of injury, chemokines and other chemoattractants may serve yet a third function by switching on antimicrobial functions of the white cell. Members of both CXC and CC subfamilies induce production of reactive oxygen intermediates and/or exocytosis of granules in their target cells *in vitro* [1, 7]. Although these functions are critical to host defense, they may also contribute to tissue damage in inflammatory foci. In a rabbit model of glomerulonephritis, an antibody to IL-8 reduces the influx of neutrophils by only 40% but completely reverses damage to the kidney, as measured by secretion of urinary protein [11]. In this instance, then, IL-8 may play a greater role in activation of neutrophils than in their recruitment. In contrast, localized overexpression of monocyte chemoattractan protein-1 (MCP-1) in transgenic mice can result in infiltration of mononuclear leukocytes without accompanying injury to the surrounding tissue [12]. The relative importance of chemokines in attracting versus activating leukocytes *in vivo* thus may vary among individual family members.

Production of chemokines by endothelial cells

As mentioned, chemokines made by endothelial cells are likely to be the first ones that a leukocyte encounters as it begins to roll along a venule at a site of inflammation. Like most other cells, cultured human endothelial cells produce low to undetectable levels of chemokines in the absence of a stimulus. Endothelium can be induced, however, to express at least 14 different chemokines (listed, with their abbreviations, in Tab. 1). For all of these chemokines, expression of mRNA in cultured endothelial cells has been verified; for most, production of protein also has been documented. The majority of studies that have examined synthesis of chemokines by cultured endothelium have used human umbilical vein endothelial cells (HUVEC), but human arterial [5, 13, 14] and microvascular [15, 16] endothelial cells also make these attractants. When compared in the same laboratory, HUVEC and microvascular endothelial cells from foreskins produce similar, but not completely identical, spectra of chemokines in response to a variety of stimuli [16].

Bacterial lipopolysaccharide (LPS) and the proinflammatory cytokines interleukin (IL)-1 and tumor necrosis factor α (TNFα) individually promote endothelial synthesis of most of the chemokines listed in Table 1 [5, 13–25]. The ability of these agents to induce endothelial expression of several chemokines of different subfamilies runs counter to the notion that these attractants are responsible for selective recruitment of leukocytes *in vivo*. However, it may be that other factors present in inflammatory lesions work in concert with IL-1, TNFα, or LPS to enhance or diminish expression of specific chemokines. For example, endothelial cells secrete little RANTES in response to either TNFα or interferon γ (IFNγ). However, a combination of the two cytokines strongly induces production [16, 26], which, in turn, is lessened by IL-4 or IL-13 [26]. In addition, the temporal expressions of various chemokines may differ even when endothelium is stimulated with a single agent [15, 23]. Lastly, IL-1, TNFα, and LPS may elicit production of chemokines in different proportions: TNFα is a stronger stimulus than IL-1 for secretion of IL-8 by pulmonary microvascular endothelium, whereas the opposite holds true for MCP-1 [15].

Table 1 - Chemokines produced by cultured human endothelial cells

	Chemokine	Selected references
CXC	ENA-78	[14, 23]
	GROα, GROβ, GROγ[1]	[13, 16, 17, 22]
	IL-8	[14-16, 18, 21, 22, 25, 28–30, 32]
	IP-10	[16, 22]
	mig	[22]
CC	Eotaxin	[20]
	MCP-1	[15, 16, 19, 20, 22, 27, 30, 31]
	MCP-3	[24]
	MCP-4	[19]
	MPIF-1 (MIP-3)	[80]
	MPIF-2	[80]
	RANTES	[16, 22, 26, 40]
CX$_3$C	Fractalkine	[5, 10]

[1]*The three GRO proteins are grouped together, since some of the studies of their expression used reagents that do not distinguish among them.*
Abbreviations: ENA, epithelial-derived neutrophil attractant; IL, interleukin; IP, IFNγ-inducible protein; mig, monokine induced by IFNγ; MCP, monocyte chemoattractant protein; MPIF, myeloid progenitor inhibitory factor; MIP, macrophage inflammatory protein; RANTES, regulated on activation, normal T expressed and secreted.

Endothelial cells also produce various chemokines in response to a diverse array of agents other than IL-1, TNFα, and LPS, including IFNγ [15, 16, 19, 20, 24], IL-4 [19, 20, 27], IL-13 [27], bacteria [21, 22, 28], oxidized low-density lipoproteins [13], histamine [18], thrombin [29], fibrin [25], complement [30], oxidants [31], and hypoxia followed by reoxygenation [32]. The degree to which these stimuli selectively upregulate expression of individual chemokines is largely unexplored. However, at least some may prove more restricted in their actions than are IL-1, TNFα, and LPS. For instance, IFNγ increases endothelial synthesis of IP-10 [16], eotaxin [20], MCP-1 [15, 16, 19, 20], and MCP-3 [24], but not IL-8 [14, 15] or ENA-78 [14]. IL-4 and IL-13 induce expression of MCP-1 by endothelium [19, 20, 27], but do not upregulate several other chemokines [14, 19, 20, 24, 27]. IL-4 also has different effects depending on the target endothelium, as it induces secretion of MCP-1 by HUVEC, but not by human dermal microvascular endothelial cells [16].

Many studies have documented increased expression of chemokines in animal models of disease and human illnesses that are characterized by leukocytic infiltrates [1, 3, 4, 7]. Several of these have demonstrated that chemokines are specifically associated with endothelium in human disorders, including osteoarthritis and rheumatoid arthritis [33], systemic sclerosis [34], aortic aneurysm [35], atherosclerosis [36, 37], idiopathic pulmonary fibrosis [38], inflammatory bowel disease [39], delayed-type hypersensitivity granulomas [40], and transplanted kidneys undergoing cell-mediated rejection [41]. As is the case for cultured endothelial cells, constitutive production of chemokines by endothelium *in vivo* is low. Although a few exceptions have been noted [34, 35, 38], chemokines generally are not detected in endothelium of healthy tissues [36, 37, 39–41].

The majority of studies that have examined expression of chemokines by endothelium *in vivo* used immunohistochemistry to detect the proteins themselves. If endothelial cells have the capacity to bind chemokines and present them to leukocytes, as discussed below, it is possible that the proteins so observed were synthesized by cells other than endothelium. That such a scenario may occur is supported by the finding that RANTES protein is associated with endothelial cells in transplanted kidneys undergoing cell-mediated rejection, but the corresponding mRNA cannot be detected [41]. However, most studies that looked for mRNA and protein found both [37, 39, 40], confirming that endothelium *in vivo* can indeed synthesize at least some chemokines. This result, of course, does not rule out the possibility that endothelial cells may also bind exogenously produced chemokines.

Presentation of chemokines by endothelium

The idea that endothelial cells or their surrounding matrix bind chemokines and "present" them to leukocytes was independently espoused by Rot in 1992 [42] and Tanaka et al. in 1993 [43, 44]. Presentation in this manner makes sense from a teleological point of view, since gradients of immobilized chemokines would not be subject to dilution by flowing blood. Furthermore, anchoring of chemokines would serve to confine their actions to the appropriate sites. The appeal of this hypothesis is such that it has gained widespread acceptance as fact, even though evidence to support it is largely indirect.

Binding of chemokines to endothelium

One important line of supportive evidence comes from studies that have demonstrated binding of chemokines to endothelium, either *in vivo*, *in situ*, or *in vitro*. Indeed, such a study was the origin for Rot's hypothesis [45]. Rot incubated small pieces of skin from humans and a variety of animal species with radiolabeled IL-8. Autoradiography was then used to demonstrate that the IL-8 becomes associated with endothelium of postcapillary venules (which are the primary sites of leukocytic trafficking) and small veins, but not with that of capillaries or arterioles. A similar distribution is seen 30 minutes to one hour after injection of IL-8 into the skin of living rabbits or rats [45]. Recently, these results have been extended to show that RANTES, MCP-1, and MCP-3 bind to the vasculature of skin with the same distribution as IL-8, whereas endothelial binding of MIP-1α is not detectable. RANTES, MCP-1, and MCP-3 also bind to the endothelium of dermal afferent lymphatic vessels, but IL-8 and MIP-1α do not [46]. In contrast, results of a kinetic study of the uptake of intravenously injected MIP-1α and MIP-1β by the brains of mice are most consistent with the interpretation that these chemokines associate reversibly with the luminal surface of the endothelium [47]. Whether the CXC chemokine platelet factor 4 (PF4) attracts leukocytes is a matter of debate [7], but it has been implicated in suppression of angiogenesis [48]. Consistent with a role in regulation of vessel growth, PF4 binds preferentially to endothelium of newly formed vasculature [49] and, in established vessels, to discrete regions that may represent foci of cellular replication [50].

PF4 also binds to cultured endothelium, including HUVEC [50, 51] and human arterial endothelial cells [50]. Whether other chemokines bind to endothelial cells *in vitro* has been a matter of controversy. Binding of IL-8 [32, 52, 53], MCP-1, RANTES, MIP-1α [53] and one or more of the GRO proteins [13] to HUVEC and additional types of cultured human endothelial cells has been reported. However, other investigators have been unable to demonstrate that either IL-8 or MCP-1 binds to HUVEC [54–56]. Subtle differences in the ways that endothelial cells are isolated or cultured might explain these discrepancies, as seems to be the case for discordant reports concerning the ability of IL-8 to stimulate proliferation of endothelium [54, 57]. This proliferation appears to depend on culture conditions that favor survival of a small, atypical population of IL-8-responsive cells, of either endothelial or non-endothelial origin, that indirectly mediates the replication of the rest of the culture [58].

Possible endothelial receptors for chemokines

If endothelial cells bind chemokines, what is the identity of the receptor? One possibility is that endothelial cells bear the same type of specific signaling receptors for chemokines as do leukocytes. There are at least 13 such receptors, all of which are members of the seven-transmembrane domain (7TM), G-protein-coupled receptor family. Most 7TM chemokine receptors bind more than one chemokine, and, conversely, many chemokines can bind to more than one such receptor. However, receptors for CC chemokines (CCR) do not bind CXC chemokines, and receptors for CXC chemokines (CXCR) do not bind CC chemokines [4]. Whether cultured endothelial cells express any of these receptors is as controversial as whether they bind the chemokines themselves. It has been reported that human large vein endothelial cells contain mRNA for CXCR1 [52], but others, using much the same experimental approaches, have failed to detect mRNA for CXCR1, CXCR2 [53, 54], or CCRs 1 through 5 [53]. Positive immunostaining for CXCR1 and, to a greater extent, CXCR2 is seen in microvascular endothelial cells of normal tissues and carcinomas of the head and neck [59], and Hub and Rot [46] have mentioned, as an unpublished observation, that endothelial cells of postcapillary venules and lymphatic vessels express CCR5.

If endothelial cells use 7TM receptors as a vehicle to present chemokines, how might a chemokine already bound to such a receptor interact with a second receptor on a leukocyte? Chemokines at high concentrations form dimers [2, 3], which theoretically would permit interaction of the multimeric molecules with two receptors. Alternatively, the ability of most chemokines to interact with more than one type of 7TM receptor raises the possibility that a monomeric chemokine molecule might interact simultaneously with two dissimilar receptors, one on an endothelial cell and the other on a leukocyte. The occurrence of such interactions, however, is purely speculative.

Another possible receptor for presentation of chemokines by endothelium is the so-called Duffy antigen receptor for chemokines (DARC). In 1993, it was recognized that red blood cells possess a promiscuous receptor that binds both CC and CXC chemokines [60]. The receptor is not completely without specificity, since it interacts weakly or not at all with the C chemokine lymphotactin [61], the CC chemokines MIP-1α and MIP-1β [60, 62, 63], and CXC chemokines that lack the ELR motif [61]. Cloning proved this receptor to be identical to the Duffy antigen, which also serves as a receptor for the malarial parasite *Plasmodium vivax* [62, 64]. Structurally, DARC is homologous to the 7TM receptors for chemokines, with the important difference that it does not appear to be associated with a G-protein and has not been shown to transduce a signal [64, 65]. The distribution of DARC *in vivo* is compatible with the view that it might serve to present chemokines, since it is constitutively expressed by endothelial cells of postcapillary venules in most tissues [63, 66].

Nearly all individuals in West Africa, as well as ~ 70% of African-Americans, lack DARC on their erythrocytes [65]. Absence of DARC prevents infection with *P. vivax* and has no obvious adverse consequences, which certainly provoked questions as to how DARC could serve any essential role relating to the function of chemokines. This apparent dilemma was resolved by Peiper et al. [66], who showed that people lacking DARC on their erythrocytes still express the molecule on endothelium. Specific repression in the erythrocytes of these individuals is due to a mutation in the *DARC* promoter [67]. However, there is a report of an apparently healthy woman with a mutant *DARC* gene that encodes a truncated protein. Presumably, none of the tissues of this woman expresses DARC, although lack of antigen has been confirmed only for her erythrocytes [68]. If DARC serves an essential function, then, it seems that there must be redundant mechanisms that operate in its absence.

Another unresolved question is whether chemokines that are bound to DARC retain activity for leukocytes. GROα binds to DARC and CXCR2 through distinct regions, raising the possibility that the DARC-bound chemokine might be capable of interacting with a target leukocyte [69]. However, IL-8 immobilized on erythrocytes does not stimulate neutrophils [70]. This observation led to the conclusion that DARC, rather than presenting chemokines, acts as a "sink" for their clearance from the circulation [70]. Whether chemokines other than IL-8 are rendered nonfunctional when bound to DARC is not known, nor is it known whether DARC on endothelium might function differently from DARC on erythrocytes, although both are products of the same gene [71].

Chemokines in general bind to heparin [72], and endothelial cells bear abundant amounts of heparan sulfate-containing proteoglycans on their surfaces [73]. It has therefore been proposed that heparan sulfate or other glycosaminoglycans (GAGs) are likely to be the binding sites for endothelial presentation of chemokines [44]. Chemokines immobilized on GAGs *in vitro* retain their ability to interact with 7TM receptors on leukocytes. MIP-1β adsorbed to a conjugate of heparin and albumin or to the proteoglycan CD44 promotes adhesion of CD8$^+$ T lymphocytes to substrates coated with vascular cell adhesion molecule-1 [43]. Similarly, MIP-1β or RANTES bound to extracellular matrix stimulates adhesion of resting CD4$^+$ T lymphocytes to the matrix [74]. GAGs may even enhance the efficacy of chemokines. Soluble heparan sulfate amplifies the response of neutrophils to IL-8, with respect to both chemotaxis and fluxes of cytosolic free calcium [75]. Competitive binding studies indicate that GAGs on cultured endothelial cells promote the oligomerization of IL-8, RANTES, and MCP-1, and it has been proposed that such aggregation may be important in increasing local concentrations of chemokines [53]. In addition, enzymatic removal of GAGs from Chinese hamster ovary cells transfected with CXCR1, CCR1, or CCR2 reduces binding of chemokines to the 7TM receptors by 40 to 70%. Low-affinity binding of chemokines to GAGs may thus facilitate their subsequent, high-affinity interactions with specific signaling receptors [53].

Evidence, then, is largely in favor of the view that chemokines bound to GAGs retain activity, and, in some instances, activity may be enhanced. Whether binding of chemokines to GAGs is required for their function is less certain. A mutant of MIP-1α that fails to bind to heparin still binds to CCR1 and elicits a transient increase in intracellular free calcium as efficiently as the wild-type molecule [76]. Likewise, a mutated PF4 that cannot bind heparin retains the ability to inhibit angiogenesis *in vivo* [77].

A number of *in vitro* and *in vivo* studies have attempted to identify the endothelial binding site for chemokines, but there is no clear consensus. Little evidence indicates that specific 7TM chemokine receptors on endothelium play a role. In fact, the patterns with which RANTES, MCP-1, MCP-3, MIP-1α and IL-8 compete with one another for binding to venular or lymphatic endothelium *in situ* are inconsistent with the binding properties of any known 7TM chemokine receptor [46]. The pattern of binding to venules is compatible with DARC being the endothelial receptor [46], but whether chemokines bound to DARC retain biological activity is unproven. Perhaps the most likely candidates for ligands that present chemokines are GAGs, since, as discussed, chemokines immobilized on GAGs can interact with specific signaling receptors on leukocytes. That GAGs are endothelial ligands for chemokines is supported by the observation that heparin displaces endothelial-bound GRO [13] and PF4 [51] *in vitro*, as well as PF4 *in vivo* [49, 50]. Treatment of cultured endothelial cells or their underlying matrix with various glycosidases also partially reduces binding of PF4 [51], MIP-1β [74], IL-8, RANTES, and MCP-1 [53, 74]. Likewise, digestion with heparitinase of frozen sections of skin previously injected with IL-8 removes much of the chemokine from the venular endothelium [56].

MIP-1α binds to heparin [76] but not to dermal microvascular or lymphatic endothelium [46], which argues against a role for GAGs as endothelial ligands for chemokines. However, it may be that MIP-1α interacts with only a specific subset of GAGs that is not expressed by vessels in the skin. The affinities of different chemokines for heparan sulfate and subspecies of heparin vary, suggesting that the types of GAGs that endothelial cells display at different anatomic locations may determine the particular chemokines that are bound [72]. Moreover, individual chemokines may employ different strategies to bind to endothelium. A case in point is the recently discovered CX_3C chemokine, fractalkine. Fractalkine is comprised of a chemokine domain attached to a mucin-like stalk, a transmembrane region, and a cytoplasmic tail [5]. Fractalkine is found on the surface of cytokine-stimulated, but not resting, endothelial cells *in vitro* [5, 10], and the membrane-bound molecule can interact with a 7TM receptor on leukocytes [10]. Fractalkine, then, may be a chemokine that can be presented by endothelium to circulating leukocytes without the need for an intermediary receptor.

Participation of immobilized chemokines in recruitment of leukocytes

Only a few studies have investigated whether chemokines mediate extravasation of leukocytes as soluble or tethered molecules. IL-8 [78] and RANTES [41] dried on microporous filters induce haptotaxis (i.e., directed migration along a substrate-bound gradient) of neutrophils and monocytes, respectively. In a more physiologically relevant setting, IL-8 produced by epithelial cells in response to *Salmonella typhimurium* forms an immobilized gradient on the subcellular extracellular matrix, and this gradient induces the directed movement of neutrophils [79]. IL-8 added to cultured HUVEC promotes the adhesion of neutrophils under conditions of flow, even if the endothelium is vigorously washed prior to addition of the leukocytes [32]. Cultured aortic endothelial cells that are exposed to minimally modified low-density lipoprotein express elevated amounts of one or more of the GRO chemokines on their surfaces. Although GRO is not chemotactic for monocytes, the surface-bound form nonetheless appears to mediate adhesion of monocytes to the stimulated endothelial cells. The aortic endothelial cells also synthesize increased amounts of MCP-1 when activated by these same agents, but nearly all of this MCP-1 is found in the culture medium rather than bound to the cells [13]. MCP-1 also fails to associate with cultures of HUVEC grown on acellular connective tissue substrates prepared from human amnion. In such cultures, endogenous MCP-1 that is constitutively produced by the HUVEC promotes migration of monocytes across the endothelium. Extensive washing of the cultures removes nearly all of the MCP-1 and greatly suppresses transmigration of monocytes, confirming that the MCP-1 functions predominantly in a soluble form in this model system [55].

Whether MCP-1 or other chemokines can act as strictly soluble molecules to recruit leukocytes in the complex *in vivo* milieu is still an open question. The most compelling evidence that chemokines must be anchored to function comes from a recent study by Middleton et al. [56], who used electron microscopy to follow the fate of IL-8 and RANTES injected intradermally into rabbits or into pieces of human skin. The injected chemokines are internalized by endothelium of small veins at the abluminal surface, transported in vesicles across the cells, and displayed on the luminal surface. Quantitative analysis of the luminal distribution of IL-8 showed that it is particularly concentrated on microvilli, where it is presumably more available to interact with circulating leukocytes. When a truncated version of IL-8 with reduced ability to bind to heparin is injected into skin *ex vivo*, little accumulates within or on the apical surface of endothelium. When injected into peritoneal cavities of mice or skin of monkeys *in vivo*, the truncated IL-8 is substantially poorer at eliciting accumulation of neutrophils than is the native molecule. In contrast, the truncated and native forms of IL-8 stimulate release of elastase by neutrophils to a similar degree. Taken together, these results are consistent with the conclusion that the truncated IL-8 fails to recruit neutrophils normally due to its inability to become immobilized, rather than to an inability to interact with signaling receptors on the leukocytes.

At present, there is no direct proof that chemokines produced by endothelial cells themselves must be surface-bound to function in extravasation of leukocytes. The hypothesis that endothelial cells present chemokines, whether self-derived or exogenous, to leukocytes in an immobilized form makes a great deal of sense, and it has nearly attained the status of dogma on that basis alone. However, it should be appreciated that evidence in support of this concept is, for the most part, circumstantial. Presentation of chemokines by endothelium or its underlying matrix may well prove to be essential for recruitment of leukocytes, but it is premature to rule out the possibility that chemokines are targeted to where they are needed by other, less obvious mechanisms.

Acknowledgments
I regret that limitations on the length of this review prevented me from citing a great many excellent and relevant publications. I thank Antal Rot for providing a preprint

of Reference 46 and for insightful discussion of issues in the field, Margaret Burns and Howard Fleit for critiquing the manuscript, and Lori Horb and Jennifer Raffanello for clerical assistance.

References

1   Baggiolini M, Dewald B, Moser B (1994) Interleukin-8 and related chemotactic cytokines – CXC and CC chemokines. *Adv Immunol* 55: 97–179

2   Baggiolini M, Dewald B, Moser B (1997) Human chemokines: an update. *Annu Rev Immunol* 15: 675–705

3   Rollins BJ (1997) Chemokines. *Blood* 90: 909–928

4   Luster AD (1998) Chemokines – chemotactic cytokines that mediate inflammation. *N Engl J Med* 338: 436–445

5   Bazan JF, Bacon KB, Hardiman G, Wang W, Soo K, Rossi D, Greaves DR, Zlotnik A, Schall TJ (1997) A new class of membrane-bound chemokine with a CX_3C motif. *Nature* 385: 640–644

6   Kelner GS, Kennedy J, Bacon KB, Kleyensteuber S, Largaespada DA, Jenkins NA, Copeland NG, Bazan JF, Moore KW, Schall TJ et al (1994) Lymphotactin: a cytokine that represents a new class of chemokine. *Science* 266: 1395–1399

7   Furie MB, Randolph GJ (1995) Chemokines and tissue injury. *Am J Pathol* 146: 1287–1301

8   Detmers PA, Lo SK, Olsen-Egbert E, Walz A, Baggiolini M, Cohn ZA (1990) Neutrophil-activating protein 1/interleukin 8 stimulates the binding activity of the leukocyte adhesion receptor CD11b/CD18 on human neutrophils. *J Exp Med* 171: 1155–1162

9   Weber C, Alon R, Moser B, Springer TA (1996) Sequential regulation of $\alpha 4\beta 1$ and $\alpha 5\beta 1$ integrin avidity by CC chemokines in monocytes: implications for transendothelial chemotaxis. *J Cell Biol* 134: 1063–1073

10 Imai T, Hieshima K, Haskell C, Baba M, Nagira M, Nishimura M, Kakizaki M, Takagi S, Nomiyama H, Schall TJ et al (1997) Identification and molecular characterization of fractalkine receptor CX_3CR1, which mediates both leukocyte migration and adhesion. *Cell* 91: 521–530

11 Wada T, Tomosugi N, Naito T, Yokoyama H, Kobayashi K, Harada A, Mukaida N, Matsushima K (1994) Prevention of proteinuria by the administration of anti-interleukin 8 antibody in experimental acute immune complex-induced glomerulonephritis. *J Exp Med* 180: 1135–1140

12 Gunn MD, Nelken NA, Liao X, Williams LT (1997) Monocyte chemoattractant protein-1 is sufficient for the chemotaxis of monocytes and lymphocytes in transgenic mice but requires an additional stimulus for inflammatory activation. *J Immunol* 158: 376–383

13 Schwartz D, Andalibi A, Chaverri-Almada L, Berliner JA, Kirchgessner T, Fang Z-T, Tekamp-Olson P, Lusis AJ, Gallegos C, Fogelman AM et al (1994) Role of the GRO

family of chemokines in monocyte adhesion to MM-LDL-stimulated endothelium. *J Clin Invest* 94: 1968–1973

14 Lukacs NW, Kunkel SL, Allen R, Evanoff HL, Shaklee CL, Sherman JS, Burdick MD, Strieter RM (1995) Stimulus and cell-specific expression of C-X-C and C-C chemokines by pulmonary stromal cell populations. *Am J Physiol* 268: L856–L861

15 Brown Z, Gerritsen ME, Carley WW, Strieter RM, Kunkel SL, Westwick J (1994) Chemokine gene expression and secretion by cytokine-activated human microvascular endothelial cells: differential regulation of monocyte chemoattractant protein-1 and interleukin-8 in response to interferon-γ. *Am J Pathol* 145: 913–921

16 Goebeler M, Yoshimura T, Toksoy A, Ritter U, Bröcker E-B, Gillitzer R (1997) The chemokine repertoire of human dermal microvascular endothelial cells and its regulation by inflammatory cytokines. *J Invest Dermatol* 108: 445–451

17 Haskill S, Peace A, Morris J, Sporn SA, Anisowicz A, Lee SW, Smith T, Martin G, Ralph P, Sager R (1990) Identification of three related human *GRO* genes encoding cytokine functions. *Proc Natl Acad Sci USA* 87: 7732–7736

18 Jeannin P, Delneste Y, Gosset P, Molet S, Lassalle P, Hamid Q, Tsicopoulos A, Tonnel AB (1994) Histamine induces interleukin-8 secretion by endothelial cells. *Blood* 84: 2229–2233

19 Garcia-Zepeda EA, Combadiere C, Rothenberg ME, Sarafi MN, Lavigne F, Hamid Q, Murphy PM, Luster AD (1996) Human monocyte chemoattractant protein (MCP)-4 is a novel CC chemokine with activities on monocytes, eosinophils, and basophils induced in allergic and nonallergic inflammation that signals through the CC chemokine receptors (CCR)-2 and -3. *J Immunol* 157: 5613–5626

20 Garcia-Zepeda EA, Rothenberg ME, Ownbey RT, Celestin J, Leder P, Luster AD (1996) Human eotaxin is a specific chemoattractant for eosinophil cells and provides a new mechanism to explain tissue eosinophilia. *Nature Med* 2: 449–456

21 Burns MJ, Sellati TJ, Teng EI, Furie MB (1997) Production of interleukin-8 (IL-8) by cultured endothelial cells in response to *Borrelia burgdorferi* occurs independently of secreted IL-1 and tumor necrosis factor alpha and is required for subsequent trans-endothelial migration of neutrophils. *Infect Immun* 65: 1217–1222

22 Ebnet K, Brown KD, Siebenlist UK, Simon MM, Shaw S (1997) *Borrelia burgdorferi* activates nuclear factor-κB and is a potent inducer of chemokine and adhesion molecule gene expression in endothelial cells and fibroblasts. *J Immunol* 158: 3285–3292

23 Imaizumi T, Albertine KH, Jicha DL, McIntyre TM, Prescott SM, Zimmerman GA (1997) Human endothelial cells synthesize ENA-78: relationship to IL-8 and to signaling of PMN adhesion. *Am J Respir Cell Mol Biol* 17: 181–192

24 Polentarutti N, Introna M, Sozzani S, Mancinelli R, Mantovani G, Mantovani A (1997) Expression of monocyte chemotactic protein-3 in human monocytes and endothelial cells. *Eur Cytokine Netw* 8: 271–274

25 Qi J, Goralnick S, Kreutzer DL (1997) Fibrin regulation of interleukin-8 gene expression in human vascular endothelial cells. *Blood* 90: 3595–3602

26 Marfaing-Koka A, Devergne O, Gorgone G, Portier A, Schall TJ, Galanaud P, Emilie D

(1995) Regulation of the production of the RANTES chemokine by endothelial cells: synergistic induction by IFN-γ plus TNF-α and inhibition by IL-4 and IL-13. *J Immunol* 154: 1870–1878

27   Goebeler M, Schnarr B, Toksoy A, Kunz M, Bröcker EB, Duschl A, Gillitzer R (1997) Interleukin-13 selectively induces monocyte chemoattractant protein-1 synthesis and secretion by human endothelial cells: involvement of IL-4Rα and Stat6 phosphorylation. *Immunology* 91: 450–457

28   Vernier A, Diab M, Soell M, Haan-Archipoff G, Beretz A, Wachsmann D, Klein J-P (1996) Cytokine production by human epithelial and endothelial cells following exposure to oral viridans streptococci involves lectin interactions between bacteria and cell surface receptors. *Infect Immun* 64: 3016–3022

29   Kaplanski G, Fabrigoule M, Boulay V, Dinarello CA, Bongrand P, Kaplanski S, Farnarier C (1997) Thrombin induces endothelial type II activation *in vitro*: IL-1 and TNF-α-independent IL-8 secretion and E-selectin expression. *J Immunol* 158: 5435–5441

30   Kilgore KS, Schmid E, Shanley TP, Flory CM, Maheswari V, Tramontini NL, Cohen H, Ward PA, Friedl HP, Warren JS (1997) Sublytic concentrations of the membrane attack complex of complement induce endothelial interleukin-8 and monocyte chemoattractant protein-1 through nuclear factor-κB activation. *Am J Pathol* 150: 2019–2031

31   Kilgore KS, Imlay MM, Szaflarski JP, Silverstein FS, Malani AN, Evans VM, Warren JS (1997) Neutrophils and reactive oxygen intermediates mediate glucan-induced pulmonary granuloma formation through the local induction of monocyte chemoattractant protein-1. *Lab Invest* 76: 191–201

32   Rainger GE, Fisher AC, Nash GB (1997) Endothelial-borne platelet-activating factor and interleukin-8 rapidly immobilize rolling neutrophils. *Am J Physiol* 272: H114–H122

33   Koch AE, Kunkel SL, Shah MR, Fu R, Mazarakis DD, Haines GK, Burdick MD, Pope RM, Strieter RM (1995) Macrophage inflammatory protein-1β: a C-C chemokine in osteoarthritis. *Clin Immunol Immunopathol* 77: 307–314

34   Koch AE, Kronfeld-Harrington LB, Szekanecz Z, Cho MM, Haines GK, Harlow LA, Strieter RM, Kunkel SL, Massa MC, Barr WG et al (1993) In situ expression of cytokines and cellular adhesion molecules in the skin of patients with systemic sclerosis: their role in early and late disease. *Pathobiology* 61: 239–246

35   Koch AE, Kunkel SL, Pearce WH, Shah MR, Parikh D, Evanoff HL, Haines GK, Burdick MD, Strieter RM (1993) Enhanced production of the chemotactic cytokines interleukin-8 and monocyte chemoattractant protein-1 in human abdominal aortic aneurysms. *Am J Pathol* 142: 1423–1431

36   Takeya M, Yoshimura T, Leonard EJ, Takahashi K (1993) Detection of monocyte chemoattractant protein-1 in human atherosclerotic lesions by an anti-monocyte chemoattractant protein-1 monoclonal antibody. *Hum Pathol* 24: 534–539

37   Pattison JM, Nelson PJ, Huie P, Sibley RK, Krensky AM (1996) RANTES chemokine expression in transplant-associated accelerated atherosclerosis. *J Heart Lung Transplant* 15: 1194–1199

38   Antoniades HN, Neville-Golden J, Galanopoulos T, Kradin RL, Valente AJ, Graves DT (1992) Expression of monocyte chemoattractant protein 1 mRNA in human idiopathic pulmonary fibrosis. *Proc Natl Acad Sci USA* 89: 5371–5375

39   Grimm MC, Doe WF (1996) Chemokines in inflammatory bowel disease mucosa: expression of RANTES, macrophage inflammatory protein (MIP)-1α, MIP-1β, and γ-interferon-inducible protein-10 by macrophages, lymphocytes, endothelial cells, and granulomas. *Infl Bowel Dis* 2: 88–96

40   Devergne O, Marfaing-Koka A, Schall TJ, Leger-Ravet M-B, Sadick M, Peuchmaur M, Crevon M-C, Kim T, Galanaud P, Emilie D (1994) Production of the RANTES chemokine in delayed-type hypersensitivity reactions: involvement of macrophages and endothelial cells. *J Exp Med* 179: 1689–1694

41   Wiedermann CJ, Kowald E, Reinisch N, Kaehler CM, von Luettichau I, Pattison JM, Huie P, Sibley RK, Nelson PJ, Krensky AM (1993) Monocyte haptotaxis induced by the RANTES chemokine. *Curr Biol* 3: 735–739

42   Rot A (1992) Endothelial cell binding of NAP-1/IL-8: role in neutrophil emigration. *Immunol Today* 13: 291–294

43   Tanaka Y, Adams DH, Hubscher S, Hirano H, Siebenlist U, Shaw S (1993) T-cell adhesion induced by proteoglycan-immobilized cytokine MIP-1β. *Nature* 361: 79–82

44   Tanaka Y, Adams DH, Shaw S (1993) Proteoglycans on endothelial cells present adhesion-inducing cytokines to leukocytes. *Immunol Today* 14: 111–115

45   Rot A (1992) Binding of neutrophil attractant/activation protein-1 (interleukin 8) to resident dermal cells. *Cytokine* 4: 347–352

46   Hub E, Rot A (1998) Binding of RANTES, MCP-1, MCP-3 and MIP-1α to cells in human skin. *Am J Pathol* 152: 749–757

47   Banks WA, Kastin AJ (1996) Reversible association of the cytokines MIP-1α and MIP-1β with the endothelia of the blood-brain barrier. *Neurosci Lett* 205: 202–206

48   Maione TE, Gray GS, Petro J, Hunt AJ, Donner AL, Bauer SI, Carson HF, Sharpe RJ (1990) Inhibition of angiogenesis by recombinant human platelet factor-4 and related peptides. *Science* 247: 77–79

49   Hansell P, Maione TE, Borgström P (1995) Selective binding of platelet factor 4 to regions of active angiogenesis *in vivo*. *Am J Physiol* 269: H829–H836

50   Hansell P, Olofsson M, Maione TE, Arfors K-E, Borgström P (1995) Differences in binding of platelet factor 4 to vascular endothelium *in vivo* and endothelial cells *in vitro*. *Acta Physiol Scand* 154: 449–459

51   Busch C, Dawes J, Pepper DS, Wasteson A (1980) Binding of platelet factor 4 to cultured human umbilical vein endothelial cells. *Thromb Res* 19: 129–137

52   Schönbeck U, Brandt E, Petersen F, Flad H-D, Loppnow H (1995) IL-8 specifically binds to endothelial but not to smooth muscle cells. *J Immunol* 154: 2375–2383

53   Hoogewerf AJ, Kuschert GSV, Proudfoot AEI, Borlat F, Clark-Lewis I, Power CA, Wells TNC (1997) Glycosaminoglycans mediate cell surface oligomerization of chemokines. *Biochemistry* 36: 13570–13578

54   Petzelbauer P, Watson CA, Pfau SE, Pober JS (1995) IL-8 and angiogenesis: evidence that

human endothelial cells lack receptors and do not respond to IL-8 *in vitro*. *Cytokine* 7: 267–272

55   Randolph GJ, Furie MB (1995) A soluble gradient of endogenous monocyte chemoattractant protein-1 promotes the transendothelial migration of monocytes *in vitro*. *J Immunol* 155: 3610–3618

56   Middleton J, Neil S, Wintle J, Clark-Lewis I, Moore H, Lam C, Auer M, Hub E, Rot A (1997) Transcytosis and surface presentation of IL-8 by venular endothelial cells. *Cell* 91: 385–395

57   Koch AE, Polverini PJ, Kunkel SL, Harlow LA, DiPietro LA, Elner VM, Elner SG, Strieter RM (1992) Interleukin-8 as a macrophage-derived mediator of angiogenesis. *Science* 258: 1798–1801

58   Watson CA, Camera-Benson L, Palmer-Crocker R, Pober JS (1995) Variability among human umbilical vein endothelial cultures. *Science* 268: 447–448

59   Richards BL, Eisma RJ, Spiro JD, Lindquist RL, Kreutzer DL (1997) Coexpression of interleukin-8 receptors in head and neck squamous cell carcinoma. *Am J Surg* 174: 507–512

60   Neote K, Darbonne W, Ogez J, Horuk R, Schall TJ (1993) Identification of a promiscuous inflammatory peptide receptor on the surface of red blood cells. *J Biol Chem* 268: 12247–12249

61   Szabo MC, Soo KS, Zlotnik A, Schall TJ (1995) Chemokine class differences in binding to the Duffy antigen-erythrocyte chemokine receptor. *J Biol Chem* 270: 25348–25351

62   Chaudhuri A, Zbrzezna V, Polyakova J, Pogo AO, Hesselgesser J, Horuk R (1994) Expression of the Duffy antigen in K562 cells: evidence that it is the human erythrocyte chemokine receptor. *J Biol Chem* 269: 7835–7838

63   Hadley TJ, Lu Z, Wasniowska K, Martin AW, Peiper SC, Hesselgesser J, Horuk R (1994) Postcapillary venule endothelial cells in kidney express a multispecific chemokine receptor that is structurally and functionally identical to the erythroid isoform, which is the Duffy blood group antigen. *J Clin Invest* 94: 985–991

64   Neote K, Mak JY, Kolakowski LF, Jr., Schall TJ (1994) Functional and biochemical analysis of the cloned Duffy antigen: identity with the red blood cell chemokine receptor. *Blood* 84: 44–52

65   Hadley TJ, Peiper SC (1997) From malaria to chemokine receptor: the emerging physiologic role of the Duffy blood group antigen. *Blood* 89: 3077–3091

66   Peiper SC, Wang Z, Neote K, Martin AW, Showell HJ, Conklyn MJ, Ogborne K, Hadley TJ, Lu Z, Hesselgesser J et al (1995) The Duffy antigen/receptor for chemokines (DARC) is expressed in endothelial cells of Duffy negative individuals who lack the erythrocyte receptor. *J Exp Med* 181: 1311–1317

67   Tournamille C, Colin Y, Cartron JP, Le Van Kim C (1995) Disruption of a GATA motif in the Duffy gene promoter abolishes erythroid gene expression in Duffy-negative individuals. *Nature Genet* 10: 224–228

68   Mallinson G, Soo KS, Schall TJ, Pisacka M, Anstee DJ (1995) Mutations in the erythrocyte chemokine receptor (Duffy) gene: the molecular basis of the Fy^a/Fy^b antigens

and identification of a deletion in the Duffy gene of an apparently healthy individual with the Fy(a-b-) phenotype. *Br J Haematol* 90: 823–829

69 Hesselgesser J, Chitnis CE, Miller LH, Yansura DG, Simmons LC, Fairbrother WJ, Kotts C, Wirth C, Gillece-Castro BL, Horuk R (1995) A mutant of melanoma growth stimulating activity does not activate neutrophils but blocks erythrocyte invasion by malaria. *J Biol Chem* 270: 11472–11476

70 Darbonne WC, Rice GC, Mohler MA, Apple T, Hébert CA, Valente AJ, Baker JB (1991) Red blood cells are a sink for interleukin 8, a leukocyte chemotaxin. *J Clin Invest* 88: 1362–1369

71 Chaudhuri A, Polyakova J, Zbrzezna V, Williams K, Gulati S, Pogo AO (1993) Cloning of glycoprotein D cDNA, which encodes the major subunit of the Duffy blood group system and the receptor for the *Plasmodium vivax* malaria parasite. *Proc Natl Acad Sci USA* 90: 10793–10797

72 Witt DP, Lander AD (1994) Differential binding of chemokines to glycosaminoglycan subpopulations. *Curr Biol* 4: 394–400

73 Rosenberg RD, Shworak NW, Liu J, Schwartz JJ, Zhang L (1997) Heparan sulfate proteoglycans of the cardiovascular system: specific structures emerge but how is synthesis regulated? *J Clin Invest* 99: 2062–2070

74 Gilat D, Hershkoviz R, Mekori YA, Vlodavsky I, Lider O (1994) Regulation of adhesion of CD4+ T lymphocytes to intact or heparinase-treated subendothelial matrix by diffusible or anchored RANTES and MIP-1β. *J Immunol* 153: 4899–4906

75 Webb LMC, Ehrengruber MU, Clark-Lewis I, Baggiolini M, Rot A (1993) Binding to heparan sulfate or heparin enhances neutrophil responses to interleukin 8. *Proc Natl Acad Sci USA* 90: 7158–7162

76 Koopmann W, Krangel MS (1997) Identification of a glycosaminoglycan-binding site in chemokine macrophage inflammatory protein-1α. *J Biol Chem* 272: 10103–10109

77 Maione TE, Gray GS, Hunt AJ, Sharpe RJ (1991) Inhibition of tumor growth in mice by an analogue of platelet factor 4 that lacks affinity for heparin and retains potent angiostatic activity. *Cancer Res* 51: 2077–2083

78 Rot A (1993) Neutrophil attractant/activation protein-1 (interleukin-8) induces *in vitro* neutrophil migration by haptotactic mechanism. *Eur J Immunol* 23: 303–306

79 McCormick BA, Hofman PM, Kim J, Carnes DK, Miller SI, Madara JL (1995) Surface attachment of *Salmonella typhimurium* to intestinal epithelia imprints the subepithelial matrix with gradients chemotactic for neutrophils. *J Cell Biol* 131: 1599–1608

80 Patel VP, Kreider BL, Li Y, Li H, Leung K, Salcedo T, Nardelli B, Pippalla V, Gentz S, Thotakura R et al (1997) Molecular and functional characterization of two novel human C-C chemokines as inhibitors of two distinct classes of myeloid progenitors. *J Exp Med* 185: 1163–1172

Platelet-activating factor: A signaling molecule for leukocyte adhesion

Diane E. Lorant[1,6], Thomas M. McIntyre[1,2,4,5], Stephen M. Prescott[2,3,4] and Guy A. Zimmerman[1,2,4]

[1]The Nora Eccles Harrison Cardiovascular Research and Training Institute; [2]The Eccles Program in Human Molecular Biology and Genetics, and the [3]Departments of Biochemistry, [4]Internal Medicine, [5]Pathology, and [6]Pediatrics at the University of Utah Health Sciences Center, 95 South 2000 East, Salt Lake City, UT 84112, USA

Overview

Platelet-activating factor (PAF) is a phospholipid signaling molecule that mediates intercellular interactions [1–3]. Many of the most precisely-characterized signaling effects of PAF occur in the inflammatory and vascular systems, where it transmits information between endothelial cells, leukocytes, and other cell types in both physiological and pathological conditions [3–6]. In this chapter we focus on signaling of adhesion of polymorphonuclear leukocytes (PMNs; neutrophils) by PAF when it is synthesized by human endothelial cells or platelets, and on additional functional consequences of this intercellular signaling.

When PAF is synthesized by vascular or inflammatory cells [2] it can bind to receptors (see below) on the plasma membranes of PMNs or other cell types, inducing their activation and changes in their phenotypes. Thus, it transmits signals between the signaling cells and the target cell [3]. When PMNs are the target cells, signaling from the outside to intracellular transduction pathways (outside-in signaling) via the PAF receptor induces activation of β_2 integrins (leukocyte integrins; CD11/CD18 integrins), making them competent to recognize intercellular adhesion molecule-1 (ICAM-1), ICAM-2 and other ligands on adjacent cells as well as fibrinogen, fibronectin and other proteins in extracellular matrix structures (see below and [2–6]). We focus much of this review on this action of PAF when it is presented to neutrophils by stimulated human endothelial cells, where it functions as a juxtacrine signaling molecule for PMN adhesion (tethering) [3, 6, 7]. Since the PAF receptor can transmit outside-in signals leading to activation of leukocyte integrins (the latter process is also termed inside-out signaling [8]), it can induce the critical triggering step [9] in the sequential events that lead to regulated targeting, activation and transmigration of PMNs and other myeloid leukocytes [4, 5, 10]. The individual components of this multistep process are discussed in detail in the chapters by Ley, Smith et al. and Muller in this volume. PAF also induces leukocyte responses besides integrin-mediated adhesion, including shape change, motility, priming for granular secretion, altered distribution of selectin ligands, and expression of genes that encode mediators that amplify inflammatory responses (see below and [2, 11]. Studies with isolated human cells in static interactions, in *in vitro* models of leukocytes interacting with endothelial cells or platelets under conditions of flow, and in *in vivo* animal models, establish that PAF has signaling functions in adhesive interactions. While it has the potential to act as an endocrine, paracrine and/or autocrine signal [1,2], its juxtacrine actions at the surfaces of stimulated endothelial cells and platelets are critical aspects of its signaling portfolio.

Platelet-activating factor (PAF) is a phospholipid signaling molecule that mediates regulated interactions between cells

PAF is a phospholipid, 1-alkyl-2-acetyl-*sn*-glycero-3-phosphocholine [1]. While there is structural heterogeneity in the molecular species of PAF that are synthesized by human endothelial cells and other signaling cells [12], there are well-defined requirements for recognition of these homologs by the receptor [1, 12–14]. The receptor for PAF spans the plasma membrane seven times and is linked via G proteins to intracellular signal transduction pathways [14]. Messenger RNA for the receptor is present in human neutrophils and monocytes and certain other cell types [5, 14–18]. The receptor for PAF on PMNs and other leukocytes undergoes homologous and heterologous desensitization under the appropriate conditions [19–21]. This provides a mechanism for regulation of biological responses to PAF by rapid modulation of the receptor. Manipulation of the PAF receptor on leukocytes by desensitization with specific agonists and, more recently, with specific competitive receptor antagonists has been an important approach in dissecting its signaling functions (see below). There is evidence that there is transcriptional and post-transcriptional regulation of expression of the PAF receptor in monocytes [15, 17] but it is unknown if this occurs in PMNs. It is also unknown how the receptor for PAF is developmentally regulated in embryonic and/or neonatal animals or humans.

An additional mechanism for regulating the signaling actions of PAF is its rapid degradation by a family of lipases, the PAF acetylhydrolases [22]. There are both intracellular and extracellular forms of PAF acetylhydrolase; the extracellular or "plasma" enzyme is constitutively present in human blood where it is associated with low density and high density lipoproteins and limits the half life of exogenous PAF in physiologically-relevant concentrations to a few minutes. Both the naturally-occurring and recombinant forms of plasma PAF acetylhydrolase have restricted substrate specificities that allow them to degrade PAF, and oxidatively-modified phospholipids that have similar structures (also called PAF-like lipids) [23–26], without attacking the "building-block" phospholipids in cellular membranes [22]. By degrading PAF, the naturally-occurring and recombinant forms of plasma PAF acetylhydrolase prevent activation of the receptors expressed on polymorphonuclear leukocytes or on transfected cells [27, 28]. Because of this property the enzyme has been called a "signal terminator" [29]. Hereditary, developmental, and acquired deficiencies of PAF acetylhydrolase have been described, and there is evidence that deficient activity of the enzyme is associated with increased frequency and severity of inflammatory syndromes [22].

The features of the PAF signaling system briefly outlined above indicate specialization of function and several levels of regulation that appear to have evolved to control precisely its biological actions. Restriction of PAF synthesis to certain signaling cells, and tight control of the synthetic enzymes, are additional regulatory features [1, 13, 14] (see below). Early studies demonstrated that human endothelial cells have the capacity to synthesize PAF [30, 31]. Since there was evidence in initial experiments that both the accumulation and distribution of PAF are regulated in human endothelium [31–33], its functions in this cell type were carefully explored leading to the discovery that PAF is an endothelial signaling molecule that induces spatially-localized activation and adhesion of PMNs. These points are reviewed in the following sections.

PAF is synthesized and displayed by stimulated endothelial cells

PAF is not constitutively present in endothelial cells but is rapidly synthesized in a regulated fashion in response to specific stimuli. Its distribution and the duration of its accumulation in endothelial cells are tightly controlled [5, 13]. The majority of the studies characterizing the synthesis and distribution of PAF have been done using cultured human umbilical vein endothelial cells [34], an extremely useful model of post-capillary venular endothelium, but its regulated synthesis has also been demonstrated in human endothelial cells from other sources [35]. Furthermore, stimulated synthesis with features similar to those in cultured endothelial cells occurs in endothelium *in situ* [13, 34].

The major route of PAF synthesis by stimulated endothelial cells has been called the "remodeling pathway" [1, 5, 13]. The first step is the activation of a phospholipase A_2 that catalyses the hydrolysis of *sn*-2 fatty acyl residues of membrane phospholipids yielding an intermediate, 1-O-alkyl-*sn*-glycero-3-phosphocholine (lyso-PAF), and a free fatty acid. Endothelial cells also produce an analog of PAF that has a fatty acid at the *sn*-1 position; this compound has similar properties to PAF but is less potent [12]. A major fatty acid released by activation of the phospholipase(s) A_2 in endothelial cells is arachidonic acid, because the enzyme prefers a phospholipid that has arachidonate at the *sn*-2 position [1, 13]. Endothelial cells predominantly synthesize prostacyclin (PGI_2) from the released arachidonic acid; PGI_2 is a potent inhibitor of platelet aggregation and secretion of platelet granule contents and can also inhibit granulocyte adhesiveness [20]. At first glance it is paradoxical that

endothelial cells simultaneously produce both PGI_2 and PAF, since they have opposite effects on platelet and leukocyte functions. However, the simultaneous production of the two signaling molecules with opposing actions provides a mechanism for
tight regulation of responses of these blood cells at the endothelial surface [36]. Furthermore, PGI_2 is released into solution and acts as a paracrine signal, with the
potential to inhibit platelet and leukocyte aggregation in flowing blood, whereas
PAF is retained by the endothelial cells and acts as a juxtacrine signal (see below).
An additional potential function of PGI_2 is to inhibit PAF production by endothelial cells, providing a negative feedback mechanism [37].

The second step in PAF synthesis in endothelial cells is the acetylation of lyso-
PAF by the enzyme acetyl-coenzyme A:lyso-PAF acetyl transferase [1, 5, 13]. Both
the initial phospholipase A_2-catalyzed reaction and the acetyltransferase are regulated in human endothelial cells [38]. Regulation at both steps of the synthetic pathway is unusual and indicates that precise control of the pathway is required. The
phospholipase A_2 is regulated by the concentration of intracellular calcium and by
G proteins [13], whereas activation of the acetyltransferase is via phosphorylation-
dependent events [38]. There is evidence that key regulatory features of the PAF synthetic pathway that have been demonstrated using cultured human endothelial cells
also occur in endothelium *in situ* [13, 34]. The site of PAF synthesis in endothelial
cells is likely the endoplasmic reticulum based on the location of phospholipid synthesis in mammalian cells and the locations of phospholipases A_2 and the acetyltransferase in other cell types [5, 13].

The synthesis of PAF in human endothelial cells is induced by inflammatory and
prothrombotic agonists including thrombin, histamine, bradykinin, and sulfidopeptide leukotrienes that bind to plasma membrane receptors [5]. It is also induced by
certain pathological agonists that do not utilize surface receptors on the endothelial
cells and, therefore, are not subject to their regulatory constraints. These stimuli
include oxidants and bacterial toxins [39-43]. TNFα and IL-1α are also reported to
promote the synthesis of PAF in endothelial cells [5, 44]. A proposed mechanism
involves the synthesis of a serine protease in endothelial cells that then activates
acetyl-coenzyme A:lyso-PAF acetyl transferase [45]. This issue has been controversial, however, because other investigators did not find PAF synthesis in human
endothelial monolayers stimulated with IL-1 [46]. More recently, in experiments
using incorporation of radiolabeled acetate into PAF we found that its synthesis was
trivial in IL-1-stimulated human endothelial cells compared to monolayers stimulated with thrombin in parallel [47], similar to earlier results with TNFα-stimulated endothelial cells [48]. Thus the role of PAF in neutrophil adhesion to IL-1- or
TNFα-stimulated endothelial cells (see below) remains incompletely defined. Under
some conditions PAF that is synthesized by PMNs in response to signals delivered
by the cytokine-activated endothelial monolayers may be involved [49].

PAF produced by stimulated endothelial cells is not released into solution but
instead remains associated with the cell. This distribution is maintained even when

human endothelial monolayers are stimulated to produce PAF in the presence of a high concentration of an acceptor protein such as albumin, which binds hydrophobic PAF [31, 32, 36]. However, a portion of the newly synthesized PAF in stimulated human endothelial cells is rapidly translocated to the plasma membrane, where it is transiently available to interact with target leukocytes. Thus PAF is "displayed" by stimulated endothelial cells in a spatially-restricted fashion rather than diffusing into solution – a key feature that controls its mode of signaling in interactions of endothelial cells with PMNs (see below). The mechanism of PAF's intracellular transport to the plasma membrane and its orientation at the endothelial cell surface are unknown. Two potential mechanisms of transport are flow of vesicles containing PAF to the plasma membrane with subsequent membrane fusion, and translocation of PAF in association with a transport protein with subsequent transfer to the outer leaflet of the plasma membrane via a "flippase" [5, 36]. Once at the surface of the endothelial cell, PAF may be intercalated into the outer leaflet of the lipid bilayer, potentially localized in patches at high surface density, and/or noncovalently associated with one or more surface proteins. Neither of these possibilities has been rigorously explored. After transient display at the endothelial surface PAF is rapidly reinternalized and degraded by an intracellular acetylhydrolase [31–33].

Initial experiments revealed that PAF purified from stimulated human endothelial cells triggers adhesiveness of isolated human PMNs, using cellular aggregation, which is mediated by β_2 integrins [50], as the reporting assay [31]. This observation established a potential mechanism by which endothelial cells can directly signal activation and tethering of leukocytes in a spatially-localized fashion in inflammatory responses, rather than simply being a passive surface that only presents counterligands for leukocyte integrins as was largely believed at the time the studies were reported. Additional detailed *in vitro* experiments documented that PAF acts as a signaling molecule for neutrophil adhesion at the endothelial surface, functioning as a juxtacrine signaling molecule.

PAF is a juxtacrine signal for neutrophil adhesion

PAF induces not only aggregation of isolated neutrophils in suspension but also adhesion of PMNs to endothelial surfaces. Experimental findings using exogenous synthetic PAF and isolated human PMNs established this proadhesive property. PAF triggers PMN adhesion to proteins immobilized on planar surfaces [51, 52]. More importantly, exogenous synthetic PAF causes isolated PMNs to adhere to unstimulated endothelial monolayers (i.e. endothelial cells that have not been treated with thrombin or another agonist, so no endogenous PAF is present) [20]. Adhesion of PMNs stimulated with exogenous PAF to endothelial cells occurs within minutes and is modulated so that the leukocytes do not remain irreversibly attached to the endothelial surfaces but, instead, can polarize and release. The rapidity and reversib-

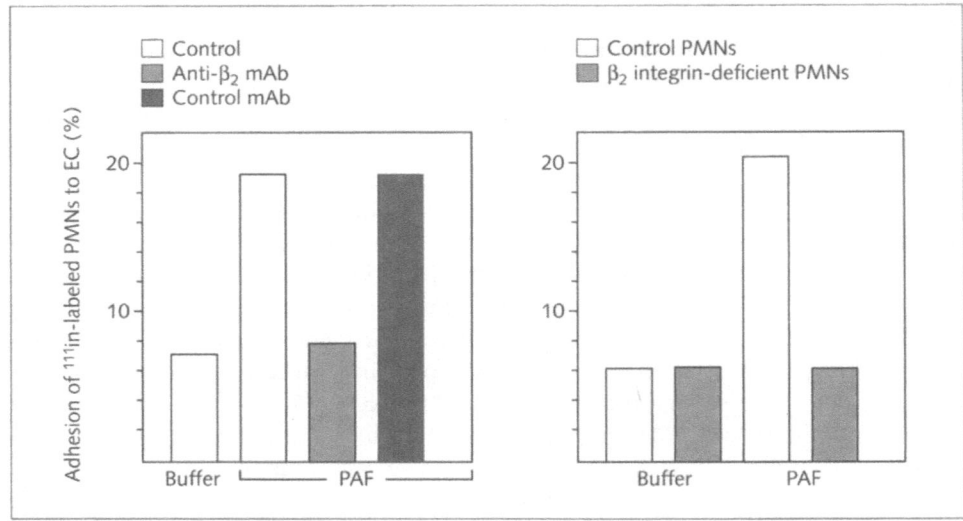

Figure 1
PAF triggers inside-out signaling of β_2 integrins and adhesion of PMNs to endothelial cells. Isolated radiolabeled human PMNs were layered over unstimulated human endothelial monolayers, PAF or control buffer was added, and adhesion was measured after a 5 min incubation period. In the left panel, PMNs were preincubated with a blocking anti-β_2 integrin monoclonal antibody (mAb) or with a control mAb. In the right panel, PMNs from a control subject or a subject with leukocyte adhesion deficiency type I were compared. Both strategies demonstrated that β_2 integrins mediate adhesion of PMNs to resting endothelial cells in response to PAF. See text and [54] for details.

ility of PMN adhesion triggered by PAF are consistent with key features of neutrophil targeting and directional migration in acute inflammation *in vivo* [6]. The ability of PAF to rapidly signal adhesion of PMNs to endothelial cells, first demonstrated in static incubations [20], has also been examined under conditions of flow. In an *in vitro* perfusion system in which PMN adhesion was examined under conditions of shear, exogenously-added PAF triggered stationary arrest of neutrophils rolling on P-selectin (see below) expressed on endothelial surfaces within one second [53].

PAF-stimulated adhesion of neutrophils to endothelial cells requires the β_2 integrins on the leukocyte surface. The tethering interaction is inhibited by blocking monoclonal antibodies directed against the β_2 (CD18) chain of the α/β heterodimers or by antibodies against α subunits (α_a or CD11a, and α_M or CD11b) [52, 54] (Fig. 1). This finding has been consistent in studies in several laboratories in which a variety of different blocking antibodies were used to interrupt adhesion of PAF-

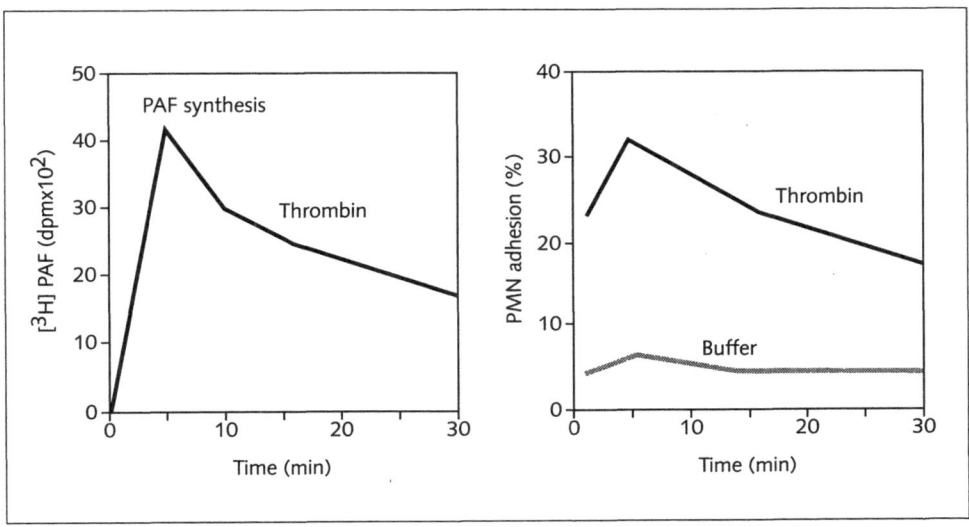

Figure 2
Human endothelial cells stimulated with thrombin synthesize PAF, which signals PMN adhesion. See text and [5, 20, 31] for details.

stimulated human PMNs to human endothelial cells [52, 55, 56], as well as in studies in which exogenous PAF triggered PMN adhesion and transmigration in the vessels of experimental animals [57]. In addition, the requirement for β_2 integrins was directly demonstrated using mutant PMNs from a subject with leukocyte adhesion deficiency type I (LAD I) (Fig. 1), which lack these adhesion molecules on their surfaces [50]. Thus, the receptor for PAF on PMNs is linked to cytoplasmic pathways that trigger inside-out signaling of β_2 integrin heterodimers [58], and this mechanism accounts for its ability to stimulate neutrophil tethering to endothelial cells. The experiments with exogenous PAF and resting endothelial monolayers (Fig. 1) also demonstrate that counterligands for the activated β_2 integrins on PAF-triggered neutrophils are constitutively present on the surfaces of human endothelial cells. Studies using blocking monoclonal antibodies indicate that intercellular adhesion molecule 1 (ICAM-1) and at least one other counterligand are involved [54].

While studies with exogenous PAF were useful as proof of principle, establishing that PAF endogenously synthesized by stimulated endothelial cells signals PMN adhesion was considerably more difficult and posed several technical challenges. As noted above, a critical feature of the handling of PAF by cultured endothelial cells is that it is not released into solution. Thus, if it signals target leukocytes it must do so when expressed at the endothelial surface and strategies to confirm this membrane-anchored mode of action were required. Also, its accumulation is rapid and

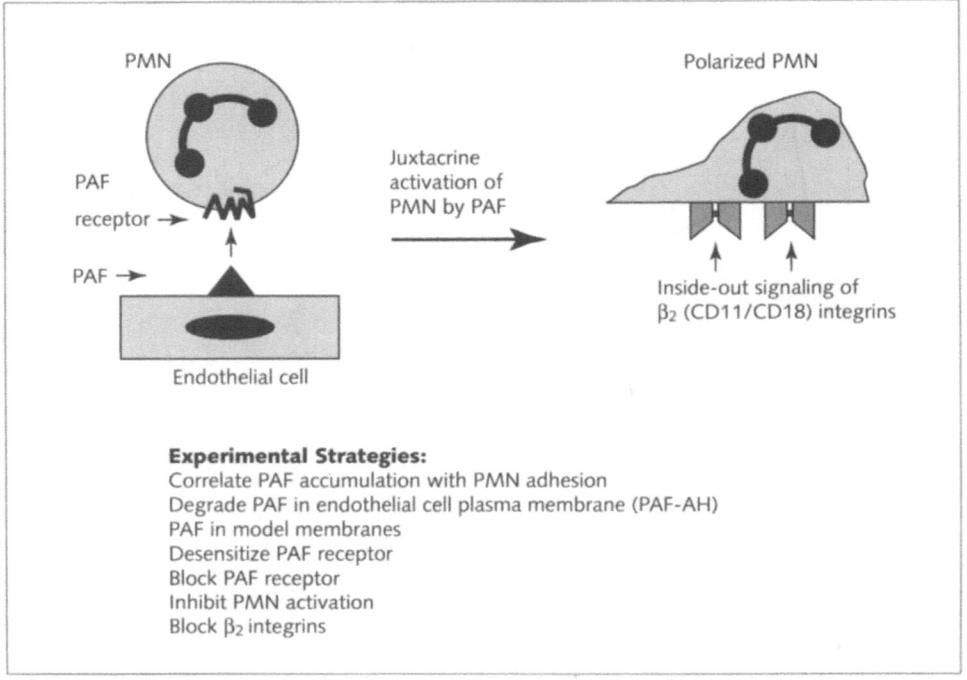

PMN

Polarized PMN

PAF receptor →

Juxtacrine activation of PMN by PAF

PAF →

Inside-out signaling of β_2 (CD11/CD18) integrins

Endothelial cell

Experimental Strategies:
Correlate PAF accumulation with PMN adhesion
Degrade PAF in endothelial cell plasma membrane (PAF-AH)
PAF in model membranes
Desensitize PAF receptor
Block PAF receptor
Inhibit PMN activation
Block β_2 integrins

Figure 3
PAF synthesized by stimulated human endothelial cells is a juxtacrine signaling molecule for PMNs.
PAF displayed and retained on the plasma membranes of stimulated endothelial cells binds to its receptor on PMNs, triggering inside-out signaling of β_2 integrins and adhesion of the leukocytes to the endothelial surface. See text and [59, 60] for details. β_2 integrins are not shown on the surface of the PMN in the left part of the figure for convenience.

transient in cultured human endothelial monolayers, peaking at 5–10 min in response to thrombin or histamine, with degradation complete by 20–30 min [31, 32] (Fig. 2). Reporting assays aimed at dissecting actions of cell-associated PAF in signaling of PMNs and their adhesion needed to be fast enough to measure events within this time frame. Finally, because PAF is a phospholipid, no specific blocking monoclonal antibodies exist that could be used as experimental tools. In addition, no specific inhibitors of the synthetic pathway for PAF exist. Furthermore, the key synthetic enzymes (see above) and the receptor for PAF had not been cloned; thus, genetic manipulation was not an option. To deal with these hurdles a variety of experimental strategies, largely involving cell biological approaches, were devised

[59, 60]. Together they demonstrated that PAF is a juxtacrine signaling molecule for PMN adhesion when it is synthesized by human endothelial cells (Fig. 3). Key evidence for this conclusion follows.

The accumulation of PAF and PMN adhesion are temporally coupled when human endothelial cells are activated

Tethering of PMNs to stimulated endothelial monolayers follows the same time course as accumulation and degradation of PAF when the two events are measured by microscopy and quantitative assay of adhesion of radiolabeled neutrophils, and by metabolic labeling of newly-synthesized PAF, respectively [20, 31] (Fig. 2). This temporal coupling is seen when receptor-mediated agonists that induce different time courses of transient PAF accumulation and neutrophil adhesion are studied [33, 54] or when oxidants or bacterial toxins induce prolonged PAF synthesis [39, 41, 43]. The concentration dependencies of agonists such as thrombin that induce both PAF synthesis and endothelial cell-dependent PMN adhesion, and other biological features of the responses, are also closely correlated [20, 35].

Degradation of endogenous PAF at the surfaces of stimulated human endothelial cells inhibits PMN adhesion

Treatment of stimulated endothelial monolayers with partially-purified PAF acetylhydrolase, an enzyme that specifically cleaves and inactivates the phospholipid (see above), accelerated the degradation of endogenously-synthesized radiolabeled PAF and inhibited neutrophil adhesion to human endothelial monolayers stimulated to synthesize PAF with thrombin [35, 59]. Catalytically-inactivated preparations of the enzyme did not have these effects. The conditions of the experiments were set to exclude the possibility of internalization of the degrading enzyme and thus provided additional evidence that cell-associated PAF is displayed on the plasma membranes of the endothelial cells. More recently a similar strategy, employing recombinant PAF acetylhydrolase, was used to examine signaling of PMN adhesion by PAF at the surfaces of stimulated human platelets [61].

PAF in model membranes and exogenous PAF bound to the endothelial cell surface signal PMN adhesion

We found that PAF incorporated into liposomal model membranes induces activation of PMNs and their adhesion [59]. The enhanced adhesion was blocked by competitive inhibitors of the PAF receptor on the neutrophils. This experimental result supported the hypothesis that PAF localized to the plasma membranes of endothelial cells can interact with its receptor on target leukocytes. We next asked if exogenous PAF added to resting endothelial cells binds to the endothelial plasma membrane and can signal in this position, and found that exogenous PAF associates with low affinity binding sites on the surfaces of unstimulated endothelial cells and can specifically induce PMN adhesion [59]. We found no evidence for activation of endothelial cells by PAF under these conditions. Whether the structures that exogenous PAF associates with are the same binding sites that are used when endothelial cells display endogenously-synthesized PAF at the cell surface is unknown. Regardless, the experiments established that PAF has the capacity to deliver intercellular signals to target leukocytes while localized at the plasma membrane of the signaling endothelial cell – a key requirement for a juxtacrine signaling molecule [7, 62, 63]. Others have also shown that exogenously-added PAF associates with the endothelial surface and can signal PMN adhesion from this location under conditions of flow [53].

Desensitizing the PAF receptor on PMNs prevents neutrophil adhesion to endothelial cells stimulated to synthesize and display PAF

Using protocols for homologous desensitization of the PAF receptor [19,21], we demonstrated that this manipulation blocks PMN adhesion to thrombin-stimulated endothelial monolayers [20]. Desensitization of the neutrophil PAF receptor with low concentrations of exogenous PAF also inhibits PMN adhesion to endothelial cells stimulated to synthesize PAF by other agonists [33, 39]. Thus, this strategy supported the hypothesis that PAF displayed at the endothelial cell surface is recognized by its receptor on the PMN and that signal transduction via the receptor is required to induce PMN adhesion to thrombin-stimulated endothelial cells (Fig. 3). A limitation of the strategy, however, is that pretreatment of PMNs with "desensitizing" concentrations of PAF might also have other effects – such as shedding of L-selectin [64] or modification of ligands for endothelial selectins [65] (see below) – that influence the adhesive interaction independent of desensitization of the PAF receptor. Direct inhibition of binding of PAF presented by stimulated endothelial cells to receptors on neutrophils using specific competitive antagonists resolved this issue and confirmed the interpretation of the desensitization experiments.

Blocking the PAF receptor on PMNs prevents neutrophil adhesion to human endothelial cells stimulated to display PAF

Treatment of PMNs with competitive antagonists of the PAF receptor inhibits neutrophil adhesion to human endothelial monolayers stimulated with thrombin or histamine under conditions in which the endothelial cells synthesize and display PAF [59, 60]. This result was consistent in experiments using three structurally-unrelated PAF receptor antagonists, and the potencies of the compounds in inhibiting PMN adhesion to stimulated endothelial cells were consistent with their relative affinities for the receptor [59]. The conditions of the experiments and concentrations of the receptor antagonists used were chosen based on rigorous characterization that demonstrated specific blockade of the PAF receptor without inhibition of signaling via other receptors on the neutrophil surface, such as that for the bacterial peptide fMLP. Competitive blockade of the PAF receptor on PMNs also inhibits their tethering to endothelial cells induced to synthesize PAF by treatment with bacterial toxins or oxidant peroxides in *in vitro* models of septic and ischemia/reperfusion vascular injury, respectively [41, 43]. In contrast, blocking the neutrophil PAF receptor did not inhibit their adhesion to human endothelial cells treated with TNFα which, as noted above, induced little or no accumulation of PAF in comparison to monolayers stimulated with thrombin or histamine [41, 59].

Juxtacrine signaling by PAF

Together the experimental strategies outlined above dissected the signaling actions of PAF at the surfaces of stimulated endothelial cells and the requirement for the signal-transducing receptor on PMNs, establishing a new mechanism for triggering neutrophil adhesion [59]. The bimolecular system consisting of PAF localized to the endothelial plasma membrane and its receptor on the PMN fulfill key requirements for juxtacrine intercellular signaling as originally proposed by Anklesaria, Massagué et al. [62, 63], in which a "nondiffusible" ligand on the surface of a signaling cell engages a receptor on a target cell leading to activation and functional alterations of the target. Signaling of PMN adhesion by endothelial cell-associated PAF (Fig. 3) is one of the best-characterized juxtacrine mechanisms to date, and is the only one involving a lipid signaling molecule yet to be described. All other established or putative juxtacrine signaling molecules are membrane-anchored polypeptides or proteins. A difference in juxtacrine signaling by PAF and the original juxtacrine mechanism is that in the latter case binding of the signaling molecule (pro-TGFα on bone marrow stromal cells) to its receptor (the EGF receptor on hematopoietic stem cells) both tethers the target cell (i.e. directly mediates intercellular adhesion) and activates it [62, 63]. In contrast, binding of PAF on endothelial cells to its receptor on PMNs activates the leukocytes but does not directly tether the two cells together; if activation of the target neutrophil is prevented adhesion is also prevented [59]. As noted above, PAF induces activation-dependent inside-out signaling of β_2 integrins that then bind to counterligands on the endothelial surface, providing the adhesive component [59, 60] (Fig. 3). This variation on the theme of juxtacrine cellular interactions [7], involving different molecular pairs for signaling and adhesion, provides the potential for additional points of regulation over and above those inherent to a single membrane-anchored signaling molecule and its receptor. Such precise regulation of intercellular interactions has biological advantages [54, 60] and appears to be particularly important in the tightly-controlled and dynamic targeting and activation of PMNs at endothelial surfaces in physiological inflammation *in vivo* [6]. Spatial control of adhesion and signaling of PMNs in inflamed vessels is a characteristic of physiological defensive inflammation, one that may be disrupted in pathological injurious inflammatory syndromes [6]. The juxtacrine mechanism exhibited by endothelial cells stimulated to synthesize PAF and tether neutrophils establishes a molecular mechanism for such spatial regulation. Coordinate expression of PAF with P-selectin at the surfaces of stimulated endothelial cells as components of a juxtacrine signaling system (see below) adds a further increment of precision and regulatory potential [60].

Additional observations confirm that PAF acts as a juxtacrine signal for PMNs when it is synthesized and expressed by endothelial cells. Experiments done under shear conditions in a parallel plate flow chamber [66] indicated that endothelial-associated PAF induces PMN adhesion that is inhibited by blocking the leukocyte PAF receptor. This was demonstrated using cultured human endothelial cells stimulated with thrombin or with TNFα. The latter result is different from our earlier studies [41, 59] in which we found no evidence that blocking the PAF receptor inhibits PMN adhesion to TNF-stimulated endothelial cells under static conditions (see above). The reason for this difference is unknown but, regardless, the central findings [66] support the concept that PAF can signal PMN adhesion while localized at the endothelial surface. In a second model, Rainger et al. examined adhesive interactions between PMNs and endothelial cells subjected to hypoxia and reoxygenation under flow conditions. Experiments that again utilized receptor blockade demonstrated that PAF presented by endothelial cells induces adhesion and immobilizes rolling neutrophils and acts in parallel with IL-8, which is also generated under the conditions of the studies [53, 56]. Previous studies had indicated that PAF is a signal for PMN activation and adhesion after hypoxia/reoxygenation or ischemia/reperfusion [55, 67]. The apparent kinetics of signaling by PAF in the hypoxia/reoxygenation model under flow conditions were measured in milliseconds, and were calculated to induce stationary adhesion of PMNs within short distances of their initial rolling interaction with activated endothelial cells [53]. Experiments with blocking monoclonal antibodies demonstrated that β_2 integrins mediate immobilization of the PMNs. Thus these experiments indicate that PAF expressed by endothelial cells can engage its receptor and trigger inside-out signaling of β_2 integrins when PMNs are subjected to shear, supporting predictions from studies using static assays [59, 60] (Fig. 3). The ability of endothelial cell-associated PAF to operate under conditions of flow is consistent with a key requirement for signaling in post-capillary venules and other vessels *in vivo* [6, 9].

PAF also acts as a juxtacrine signal in interactions of platelets with neutrophils. Platelets express the receptor for PAF and undergo inside-out signaling of integrin $\alpha_{IIb}\beta_3$ and aggregation when it is engaged [37]. PAF retained on the surfaces of stimulated PMNs induces activation and aggregation of target platelets [68, 69], indicating juxtacrine signaling. More recent studies have utilized experimental systems involving neutrophils rolling on immobilized human platelets to explore signaling in the other direction, from platelets to neutrophils. In one report, signaling of rolling PMNs by PAF synthesized by immobilized thrombin-stimulated platelets induced tight adhesion of the neutrophils by activating their β_2 integrins. This required the neutrophil PAF receptor and was blocked by receptor antagonists [70]. Thus, this is a juxtacrine mechanism analogous to that exhibited by thrombin- or histamine-stimulated endothelial cells (see [59, 60] and below). In a different approach, tight adhesion of neutrophils rolling on platelets immobilized on collagen was inhibited by treatment of the platelets with recombinant PAF acetylhydrolase, the signal-terminating regulatory enzyme (see above), as well as by blocking the neutrophil PAF receptor [61]. These experiments also documented the requirement for β_2 integrins for PMN arrest.

In addition to supporting a juxtacrine action of PAF, studies in flowing systems utilizing endothelial cells and platelets stimulated to display PAF and signal PMNs also examined its cooperative action with P-selectin at the surfaces of the signaling cells [53, 56, 61, 70]. This signaling complex was first worked out in static assays using cultured human endothelial cells [60] and is discussed in detail in the next section.

While we have focused on triggering of adhesion when endothelial cells signal neutrophils using surface-bound PAF (Fig. 3), there are other functional consequences as well. Signaling via the PAF receptor under these conditions induces an increase in intracellular Ca^{2+}, polarization, and priming for enhanced granular secretion [71] (Fig. 4). Each of these responses is important in the migration of PMNs to extravascular sites after their initial targeting in inflamed vessels, and/or for antimicrobial and wound repair functions of the leukocytes. Thus, juxtacrine signaling by PAF can trigger neutrophil responses besides tight adhesion that are required for effective defense of the host. Under some conditions, however, priming of PMNs for release of granular enzymes and generation of oxygen radicals by endothelial-bound PAF may contribute to vascular injury [72].

PAF and P-selectin: An adhesion and signaling system at cellular surfaces

While signaling functions of endothelial PAF were being characterized, it also became clear that a component of the endothelial cell-dependent adhesion of neutrophils induced by thrombin, histamine, or other rapidly-acting agonists is independent of the β_2 integrin adhesive mechanism [52]. This finding, although contrary

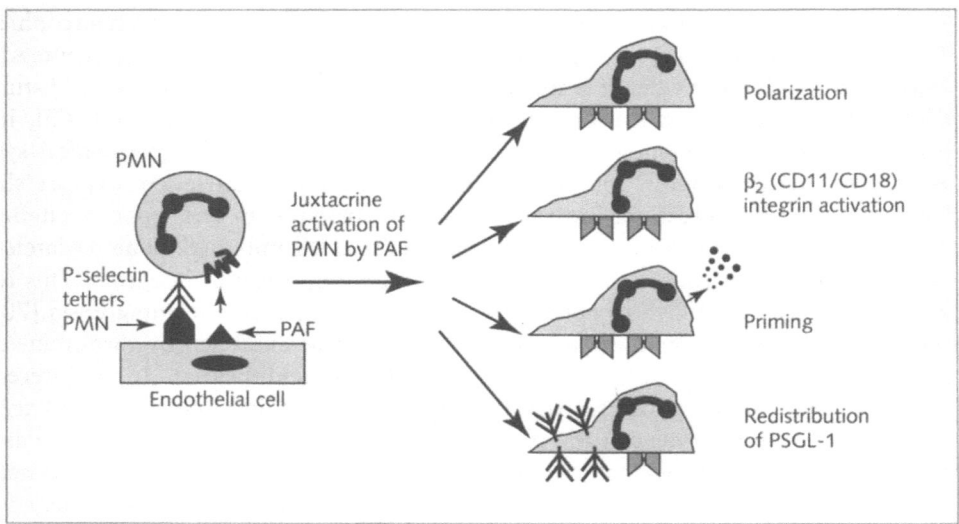

Figure 4

PAF and P-selectin are components of a juxtacrine signaling system at the endothelial sur-face.

PAF and P-selectin are coordinately displayed on the plasma membranes of stimulated human endothelial cells and, together with the PAF receptor and PSGL-1 on the neutrophil, form an adhesion and juxtacrine signaling system. PAF and P-selectin each have specific actions that lead to localized activation and adhesion of PMNs. See text and [5, 6, 60] for details. β_2 integrins are not shown on the PMN at the left of the figure for convenience.

to earlier dogma in the field that β_2 integrin-dependent adhesion is the dominant or only mechanism of leukocyte targeting, indicated that a parallel tethering mecha-nism operates at the surfaces of endothelial cells stimulated with these agonists. The β_2 integrin-independent tethering mechanism at the surfaces of thrombin- or hista-mine-stimulated endothelial cells is provided by P-selectin (previously called GMP-140) [73, 74], an integral membrane glycoprotein that is constitutively present in Weibel-Palade bodies of endothelial cells and alpha granules of platelets [75]. After initial cloning and molecular characterization of P-selectin by McEver and co-work-ers, it was shown to be rapidly translocated from these subcellular storage granules to the plasma membranes of endothelial cells and platelets in response to cellular stimulation and to be transiently localized at their surfaces before rapid reinternal-ization [75, 76]. In the case of human endothelial cells, the agonists that induce this event – thrombin, histamine, sulfidopeptide leukotrienes, oxidant peroxides – are the same as those that induce PAF synthesis and surface translocation [5, 75]. In addition, the time courses of surface expression of P-selectin and accumulation and degradation of PAF coincide, paralleling the time course of neutrophil adhesion [54, 60] (Fig. 2). P-selectin was shown to directly tether human neutrophils to the surfaces of stimulated endothelial cells and to transfected cells [73], establishing its adhesive function. A large number of studies from many laboratories have confirmed and further characterized this adhesive function of P-selectin, demonstrating that it is specialized to "capture" and loosely tether PMNs under conditions of flow [reviewed in 10,75]. P-selectin is thus one of the key adhesion molecules that mediates rolling of PMNs on the endothelial surfaces of inflamed post-capillary venules ([75]; see also the chapter by Ley, this volume). Several studies have demonstrated the tethering functions of P-selectin *in vivo* using thrombin, histamine, and sulfidopeptide leukotrienes as the agonists for its expression at the endothelial surface [77–79]. These reports are consistent with earlier experiments utilizing cultured human endothelial cells under static conditions (see above), and underscore the utility of the latter system.

P-selectin on the plasma membranes of stimulated endothelial cells or platelets is recognized by a glycoprotein ligand on the PMN plasma membrane, P-selectin glycoprotein ligand 1 (PSGL-1). PSGL-1 was characterized by Moore et al. [80, 81] and was recently cloned [82]. PSGL-1 is constitutively present on microvilli of resting PMNs, a position that favors interaction with P-selectin [75, 81], and is randomly distributed over the surfaces of spherical non-activated neutrophils with a topography consistent with its participation in an initial rolling interaction [65]. Cellular activation is not required for PSGL-1 to recognize P-selectin [65, 73, 81] and it is neither stored in subcellular granules nor translocated to the surface from other sites in stimulated human leukocytes [83]. These features indicate specialization of PSGL-1 for initial tethering events, since cellular activation is not required for its adhesive function. While it is possible that other ligands for P-selectin are expressed by PMNs or other leukocytes [81, 84], blockade of PSGL-1 on human neutrophils completely inhibits their interaction with P-selectin presented in purified form immobilized on microspheres [65] and at cellular surfaces under static or shear conditions [85].

PAF and P-selectin displayed on the endothelial surface together with their corresponding counterstructures on neutrophil plasma membranes, the PAF receptor and PSGL-1, constitute a multi-molecular juxtacrine signaling system for spatially-localized activation and adhesion of the leukocytes (Fig. 4). Parallel adhesion and signaling by endothelial cell-associated P-selectin and PAF was dissected by individual or combined blockade of each molecular "axis" using monoclonal antibodies and competitive receptor antagonists [60]. Under these conditions blocking either the P-selectin/PSGL-1 axis or the PAF/PAF receptor component blocks adhesion of PMNs by greater than 50%, indicating that the two molecular pairs act in a cooperative rather than additive fashion; blocking P-selectin completely inhibited neutrophil adhesion whereas blocking the PAF receptor inhibited by ~70% [60].

This finding suggests that engagement of the PMNs by P-selectin is required for the PAF-dependent component to act efficiently and to induce maximal adhesion. Binding of P-selectin to PSGL-1 may be required to bring the neutrophils close to the endothelial plasma membrane so that PAF at the surface can engage and trigger its receptor.

As a consequence of the outside-in signals delivered by PAF through its receptor, activation of β_2 integrins on the leukocytes and their binding to counterligands on the endothelial cells recruits an additional molecular interaction to the juxtacrine system (Fig. 4). In thrombin- or histamine-stimulated endothelial cells (Fig. 4), the specific requirements for PAF-stimulated activation of the PMNs and inside-out signaling of β_2 integrins (Fig. 3) were demonstrated using metabolic blockade, blocking monoclonal antibodies against β_2 integrins, and mutant neutrophils from a subject with leukocyte adhesion deficiency type I lacking surface β_2 heterodimers [60]. The latter experiments also demonstrated that P-selectin and β_2 integrins are each required for maximal adhesion. Analogous observations of initial tethering of PMNs by P-selectin and subsequent β_2 integrin-dependent "tight" adhesion triggered by cellular activation were reported using purified selectins and signaling molecules under conditions of flow [86]. Similar events have also been observed in a variety of other endothelial models (see the chapters by Ley and Smith et al., this volume). As noted above, a juxtacrine signaling system consisting of P-selectin and PAF also operates at the surfaces of stimulated human platelets [61, 70].

Experiments using purified P-selectin and PAF [71] further demonstrated that each molecule contributes specific functions to the juxtacrine system (Fig. 4). Separate but integrated actions of PAF and P-selectin establish the potential for control, or "editing", of the neutrophil responses [6] that would not be available if a single molecular pair mediated both adhesion and juxtacrine signaling [63] (see above). The specific question of whether engagement of PSGL-1 by P-selectin triggers activation of β_2 integrins on PMNs was explored using P-selectin in purified immobilized form and in model membranes. Under these conditions it neither triggered inside-out signaling of $\alpha_L\beta_2$ integrin (CD11a/CD18) or $\alpha_M\beta_2$ integrin (CD11b/CD18) nor induced translocation of integrin heterodimers from subcellular granules to the surface [71]. In contrast, PAF in purified form triggers both events [2, 71]. Lawrence and Springer also reported evidence that P-selectin alone does not induce β_2 integrin activation [86]. Although P-selectin does not directly trigger inside-out signaling of β_2 integrins on PMNs, its binding to their surfaces enhances this response when it is stimulated by PAF or by other neutrophil agonists [60]. This indicates that engagement of PSGL-1 on the PMN integrates signals delivered through the PAF receptor, a variation on the theme of adhesion-dependent signaling [6]. Integration of intracellular signals generated by engagement of PSGL-1 and binding of PAF to its receptor also occurs in human monocytes, leading to nuclear translocation of Rel (NF-κB) transcription factors and induction of genes for chemokines [87]. In neutrophils, PSGL-1 is linked to p42 and p44 mitogen-activated protein kinases [88] but it is unknown if these kinases are the critical points of integration between the intracellular signaling via PSGL-1 and the transduction cascade triggered through the PAF receptor [89].

An additional interplay between the PAF receptor and PSGL-1 on PMNs may indicate how stable "tight" adhesion of PMNs at endothelial surfaces is modified so that the leukocytes can loosen their tethers and move from initial points of attachment to extravascular sites of tissue damage or microbial invasion. When PMNs are activated by PAF the tightness of their binding to P-selectin expressed on the surfaces of transfected cells is reduced, and the leukocytes release from the monolayer [65]. This reduction in adhesiveness, which suggests modification of the affinity of the interaction of PSGL-1 with P-selectin, requires several minutes to develop rather than seconds. Thus it is rapid, but slower than the time required for PAF to trigger β_2 integrin-dependent adhesion of PMNs to endothelial cells [20, 53]. Furthermore, it requires blocking the neutrophil β_2 integrins to be fully seen [65]. The time course and other aspects of the "loosening" response suggest that juxtacrine signals delivered by PAF at the endothelial surface first trigger activation of β_2 integrins, which amplifies the initial tethering by P-selectin and arrests the rolling neutrophils (see above), and then within minutes induce loosening of the PSGL-1/P-selectin bond. The latter event may be a component of the complex sequence that allows the leukocytes to release from their initial tethers and transmigrate. In addition to this modification, activation of PMNs by PAF causes PSGL-1 to redistribute from its dispersed pattern over the plasma membranes of resting leukocytes (see above) so that it becomes localized at the uropods of activated, polarized PMNs and monocytes [65,83] (Fig. 5). The specific relationship between the apparent affinity modulation of PSGL-1 (Fig. 5) and the alteration in its topography has not been clearly worked out. Other signaling molecules for PMNs share with PAF the ability to induce these changes, including IL-8 and FMLP [65]. Triggering of neutrophil activation by PAF may also induce "cross-talk" between PSGL-1 and PECAM-1 (CD-31) that influences the migratory behavior of the leukocytes [90].

Signaling of neutrophil adhesion by PAF: Prototypes and paradigms

PAF is the first signaling molecule for neutrophils to be identified as a regulated product of stimulated human endothelial cells. It is also the first signaling molecule to be shown to act in a juxtacrine fashion at the surfaces of endothelial cells stimulated with inflammatory agonists. In this regard it has been a prototype for other signaling molecules that are synthesized by endothelial cells and/or that can be primarily or secondarily tethered to the endothelial cell surface and signal in a spatially-restricted and localized fashion [4, 6]. IL-8, a chemokine that is produced by inflamed endothelial cells and by adjacent cells in extravascular tissues, can associ-

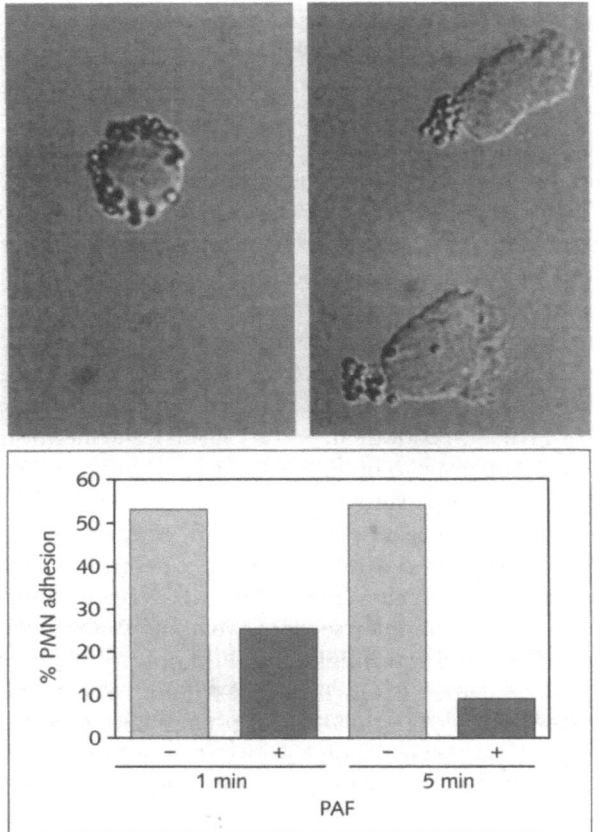

Figure 5

Activation of PMNs induces redistribution of PSGL-1 and reduces their adhesion to P-selectin.

In the upper panel, latex beads were coated with P-selectin and the distribution of their binding to resting and activated PMNs was examined by Normarski interference contrast microscopy. Binding of beads was uniform over the surfaces of resting unactivated PMNs (left) when many cells and focal planes were examined, indicating that PSGL-1 is randomly distributed on leukocyte plasma membrane (a single focal plane is shown). In contrast, when PMNs are activated by PAF or certain other agonists, PSGL-1 redistributes to the uropods of polarized cells as indicated by specific binding of P-selectin-coated beads in this region (right). In the lower panel, radiolabeled PMNs were added to transfected CHO cells that express P-selectin on their plasma membranes, PAF (closed bars) or control buffer (stippled bars) was added, and adhesion was measured at the indicated times. The β_2 integrins on the PMNs were blocked with a monoclonal antibody. Under these conditions activation of the PMNs by PAF induced release of the leukocytes from the P-selectin tethers. See text and [65] for details.

ate with the endothelial plasma membrane and signal in this fashion [4, 53, 91, 92]. It is unknown if ENA-78, another CXC chemokine that activates PMNs and is synthesized by stimulated human endothelial cells [93], does the same. Fractalkine, a variant chemokine that is tethered in the plasma membrane and directly mediates both adhesion and activation in a fashion similar to the original concept of juxtacrine signaling [63], broadens the number of target leukocyte subtypes that may be subject to adhesion-dependent signaling [6] by virtue of the fact that its receptor is present on the surfaces of natural killer cells and monocytes ([94]; for more details see the chapter by Furie, this volume). For chemokines, as with PAF, spatially-restricted signaling of leukocyte adhesion and trafficking at the surfaces of endothelial cells has specific biological advantages [4, 6]. Thus, PAF has been useful as a prototype of inflammatory mediators of different classes that signal in a spatially-restricted fashion at cell surfaces.

Discovery that PAF operates as part of a juxtacrine system at the surfaces of stimulated human endothelial cells in cooperation with P-selectin established a paradigm for spatially-localized triggering by an endogenously-synthesized and transiently-expressed signaling molecule, with consequent amplification of adhesion by inside-out signaling of neutrophil β_2 integrins (Fig. 4). The sequence of initial tethering (resulting in rolling under flow), triggering, and tight adhesion can also be shown using purified selectins and exogenous signaling molecules, as described in the chapters by Ley and Smith et al., this volume. The endothelial cell juxtacrine system consisting of PAF and P-selectin demonstrates that these events can be accomplished by an endogenously-synthesized signaling molecule together with a constitutive selectin [60]. Thus, the stimulated or inflamed endothelial cell is sufficient, and no accessory cell is required as a source of the triggering factor. Because coordinate tethering and signaling by P-selectin and PAF also occurs *in vivo* in experimental models [78, 79, 95], perhaps induced in some cases by local generation of thrombin or plasmin in response to inflammatory stimuli [96], the paradigm may have practical as well as conceptual utility. Several reports indicate that PAF also acts in parallel with E-selectin and IL-8 at the surfaces of endothelial cells stimulated with TNFα or IL-1 [66, 97–101], although this system is not as clearly defined. Finally, the PAF/P-selectin juxtacrine signaling system also provides a framework on which to base understanding of how individual components of adhesion and signaling cascades become dysregulated, leading to inflammatory vascular injury [39, 41–43, 53, 55–57], rather than to the localized, controlled, and dynamic tethering and activation of leukocytes that is characteristic of homeostatic acute inflammation [6].

Acknowledgments
We thank Michelle Bills and Leona Montoya for help in preparing the manuscript, our technical associates, students, and fellows for their support and efforts, and

many colleagues for direct contributions to work cited. This work was supported by the Nora Eccles Treadwell Foundation, grants from the National Institutes of Health (HL-44525, HL-44513, HL-46022), a Special Center of Research in ARDS (HL-50153), an American Lung Association Asthma Research Center, and a Center of Excellence in Molecular Hematology (DK-49219).

References

1   Prescott SM, Zimmerman GA, McIntyre TM (1990) Platelet-activating factor (PAF). *J Biol Chem* 265: 17381–17384

2   Zimmerman GA, McIntyre TM, Prescott SM (1992) Platelet-activating factor: A fluid-phase and cell-associated mediator of inflammation. In: JI Gallin, IM Goldstein, R Snyderman (eds): Inflammation: *Basic principles and clinical correlates.* 2nd ed. Raven Press, New York, 149–176

3   Zimmerman GA, McIntyre TM, Prescott SM (1996) Cell-to-cell communication. In: RG Crystal, JB West, ER Weibel, PJ Barnes (eds): *The lung scientific foundations.* 2nd ed. Raven Press, New York, 289–304

4   Zimmerman GA, Prescott SM, McIntyre TM (1992) Endothelial cell interactions with granulocytes: tethering and signaling molecules. *Immunol Today* 13: 93–100

5   Lorant DE, Zimmerman GA, McIntyre TM, Prescott SM (1995) Platelet-activating factor mediates procoagulant activity on the surface of endothelial cells by promoting leukocyte adhesion. *Semin Cell Biol* 6: 295–303

6   Zimmerman GA, McIntyre TM, Prescott SM (1996) Adhesion and signaling in vascular cell-cell interactions. *J Clin Invest* 98: 1699–1702

7   Zimmerman GA, Lorant DE, McIntyre TM, Prescott SM (1993) Juxtacrine intercellular signaling: Another way to do it. *Am J Resp Cell Mol Biol* 9: 573–577

8   Hynes RO, Lander AD (1992) Contact and adhesive specificities in the associations, migrations and targeting of cells and axons. *Cell* 68: 303–322

9   Ebnet K, Kaldjian EP, Anderson AO, Shaw S (1996) Orchestrated information transfer underlying leukocyte endothelial interactions. *Annu Rev Immunol* 14: 155–177

10 McEver RP (1998) Interactions of leukocytes with the vessel wall. In: J Loscalzo, AI Schafer (eds): *Thrombosis and hemorrhage.* 2nd ed. Williams and Wilkins, Baltimore, 321–336

11 Zimmerman GA, Elstad MR, Lorant DE, McIntyre TM, Prescott SM, Topham MK, Weyrich AS, Whatley RE (1997) Platelet-activating factor (PAF): signaling and adhesion in cell-cell interactions. In: S Nigam, G Kunkel, SM Prescott (eds): *Platelet-activating factor and related lipid mediators 2. Roles in health and disease.* Advances in Experimental Medicine and Biology, vol. 416. Plenum Publishing Corporation, New York, 297–304

12 Whatley RE, Clay KL, Chilton FH, Triggiani M, Zimmerman GA, McIntyre TM,

Prescott SM (1992) Relative amounts of 1-O-alkyl- and 1-acyl-2-acetyl-*sn*-glycero-3-phosphocholine in stimulated endothelium cells. *Prostaglandins* 43: 21–29

13 Whatley RE, Zimmerman GA, Prescott SM, McIntyre TM (1996) Platelet-activating factor and PAF-like mimetics. In: RM Bell, JH Exton, SM Prescott (eds): *Handbook of lipid research, Chapter 7, Vol. 8: Lipid second messengers*. Plenum Press, New York, 239–276

14 Prescott SM, McIntyre TM, Zimmerman GA (1999) Platelet-activating factor (PAF): a phospholipid mediator of inflammation. In: JI Gallin, R Snyderman (eds): *Inflammation: Basic principles and clinical correlates*, 3rd ed. Raven Press, New York, 387–396

15 Müller E, Dagenais P, Alami N, Rola-Pleszczynski M (1993) Identification and functional characterization of platelet-activating factor receptors in human leukocyte population using polyclonal anti-peptide antibody. *Proc Natl Acad Sci USA* 90: 5818–5822

16 Thivierge M, Alami N, Müller E, de Brum-Fernandes AJ, Rola-Pleszczynski M (1993) Transcriptional modulation of platelet-activating factor receptor gene expression by cyclic AMP. *J Biol Chem* 268: 17457–17462

17 Simon HU, Tsao PW, Siminovitch KA, Mills GB, Blaser K (1994) Functional platelet-activating factor receptors are expressed by monocytes and granulocytes but not by resting or activated T-lymphocyte and B-lymphocyte from normal individuals or patients with asthma. *J Immunol* 153: 364–377

18 Thivierge M, Parent J-L, Stankova J, Rola-Pleszczynski M (1996) Modulation of human platelet-activating factor receptor gene expression by protein kinase C activation. *J Immunol* 157: 4681–4687

19 O'Flaherty JT, Lees CJ, Miller CH, McCall CE, Lewis JC, Love SH, Wykle RL (1981) Selective desensitization of neutrophils: further studies with 1-O-alkyl-sn-glycero-3-phosphocholine analogues. *J Immunol* 127: 731–737

20 Zimmerman GA, McIntyre TM, Prescott SM (1985) Thrombin stimulates the adherence of neutrophils to human endothelial cells *in vitro*. *J Clin Invest* 76: 2235–2246

21 Richardson RM, Haribabu B, Ali H, Snyderman R (1996) Cross-desensitization among receptors for platelet activating factor and peptide chemoattractants: evidence for independent regulatory pathways. *J Biol Chem* 271: 28717–28724

22 Stafforini DM, McIntyre TM, Zimmerman GA, Prescott SM (1997) Platelet-activating factor acetylhydrolases. *J Biol Chem* 272: 17895–17898

23 Smiley PL, Stremler KE, Prescott SM, Zimmerman GA, McIntyre TM (1991) Oxidatively-fragmented phosphatidylcholines activate human neutrophils through the receptor for platelet-activating factor. *J Biol Chem* 266: 11104–11110

24 Patel KD, Zimmerman GA, Prescott SM, McIntyre TM (1992) Novel leukocyte agonists are released by endothelial cells exposed to peroxide. *J Biol Chem* 267: 15168–15175

25 McIntyre TM, Patel KP, Zimmerman GA, Prescott SM (1995) Oxygen radical-mediated leukocyte adherence. In: G Schmid-Schonbein, DN Granger (eds): *Physiology and pathophysiology of leukocyte adhesion*. Oxford University Press, Oxford, 261–277

26 Lehr H-A, Weyrich AS, Saetzler RK, Jurek A, Arfors KE, Zimmerman GA, Prescott SM,

McIntyre TM (1997) Vitamin C blocks inflammatory platelet-activating factor mimetics created by cigarette smoking. *J Clin Invest* 99: 2358–2364

27 Tjoelker LW, Wilder C, Eberhardt C, Stafforini DM, Dietsch G, Schimpf B, Hooper S, Trong HL, Cousens LS, Zimmerman GA, Yamada Y, McIntyre TM, Prescott SM, Gray PW (1995) Anti-inflammatory properties of a platelet-activating factor acetylhydrolase. *Nature* 374: 549–552

28 Heery JM, Kozak M, Jones DA, Zimmerman GA, McIntyre TM, Prescott SM (1995) Oxidatively modified LDL contains phospholipids with PAF-like activity and stimulates the growth of smooth muscle cells. *J Clin Invest* 96: 2322–2330

29 Bazan N (1995) A signal terminator. *Nature* 374: 501–502

30 Camussi G, Aglietta M, Malavasi F et al (1983) The release of platelet-activating factor from human endothelial cells in culture. *J Immunol* 131: 2397–2403

31 Prescott SM, Zimmerman GA, McIntyre TM (1984) Human endothelial cells in culture produce platelet-activating factor (1-alkyl-2-acetyl-*sn*-glycero-3-phosphocholine) when stimulated with thrombin. *Proc Natl Acad Sci USA* 81: 3534–3538

32 McIntyre TM, Zimmerman GA, Satoh K, Prescott SM (1985) Cultured endothelial cells synthesize both platelet-activating factor and prostacyclin in response to histamine, bradykinin and ATP. *J Clin Invest* 76: 271–280

33 McIntyre TM, Zimmerman GA, Prescott SM (1986) Leukotrienes C_4 and D_4 stimulate human endothelial cells to synthesize platelet-activating factor and bind neutrophils. *Proc Natl Acad Sci USA* 83: 2204–2208

34 Zimmerman GA, Whatley RE, Benson DE, McIntyre TM, Prescott SM (1990) Endothelial cells for studies of platelet-activating factor and arachidonate metabolites. *Meth Enzymol* 187: 520–535

35 Carveth HJ, Shaddy RE, Whatley RE, McIntyre TM, Zimmerman GA, Prescott SM (1992) Regulation of platelet-activating factor (PAF) synthesis and PAF-mediated neutrophil adhesion to endothelial cells activated by thrombin. *Sem Thrombos Hemostas* 18: 126–134

36 Prescott SM, McIntyre TM, Zimmerman GA (1990) The role of platelet-activating factor in endothelial cells. *Thrombos Hemostas* 64: 99–103

37 Zimmerman GA, McIntyre TM, Prescott SM (1985) Human vascular endothelial cells produce platelet-activating factor (1-alkyl-2-acetyl-*sn*-glycero-3-phosphocholine): Evidence for a requirement for specific agonists and modulation by prostacyclin. *Circulation* 72: 718–727

38 Holland MR, Venable ME, Whatley RE, Zimmerman GA, McIntyre TM, Prescott SM (1992) Activation of the acetyl coenzyme A: lysoPAF acetyltransferase regulates PAF synthesis in human endothelial cells. *J Biol Chem* 267: 22883–22890

39 Lewis ML, Whatley RE, Cain P, McIntyre TM, Prescott SM, Zimmerman GA (1988) Hydrogen peroxide stimulates the synthesis of platelet-activating factor by endothelium and induces endothelial cell-dependent neutrophil adhesion. *J Clin Invest* 82: 2045–2055

40 Whatley RE, Nelson P, Zimmerman GA, Stevens DL, Parker CJ, McIntyre TM, Prescott

SM (1989) The regulation of platelet-activating factor synthesis in endothelial cells. The role of Calcium and Protein Kinase C. *J Biol Chem* 264: 6325–6333

41   Patel KD, Zimmerman GA, Prescott SM, McEver RP, McIntyre TM (1991) Oxygen radicals induce human endothelial cells to express GMP-140 and bind neutrophils. *J Cell Biol* 112: 749–759

42   Krüll M, Dold C, Hippenstiel S, Rosseau S, Lohmeyer J, Suttorp N (1996) Escherichia coli hemolysin and *Staphylococcus aureus* α-toxin potently induce neutrophil adhesion to cultured human endothelial cells. *J Immunol* 157: 4133–4140

43   Bunting M, Lorant DE, Bryant AE, Zimmerman GA, McIntyre TM, Stevens DL, Prescott SM (1997) Alpha toxin from Clostridium perfringens induces proinflammatory changes in endothelial cells. *J Clin Invest* 100: 565–574

44   Mantovani A, Bussolino F, Dejana E (1992) Cytokine regulation of endothelial cell function. *FASEB J* 6: 2591–2599

45   Bussolino F, Arese M, Silvestro L, Soldi R, Benfenati E, Sanavio F, Aglietta M, Bosia A, Camussi G (1994) Involvement of a serine protease in the synthesis of platelet-activating factor by endothelial cells stimulated by tumor necrosis factor-agr; or interleukin-1α. *Eur J Immunol* 24: 3131–3139

46   Zavoico GB, Ewenstein BM, Schafer AI, Pober JS (1989) IL-1 and related cytokines enhance thrombin-stimulated PGI_2 production in cultured endothelial cells without affecting thrombin-stimulated von Willebrand factor secretion or platelet-activating factor biosynthesis. *J Immunol* 142: 3993–3999

47   Topham MK, Carveth HJ, McIntyre TM, Prescott SM, Zimmerman GA (1998) Human endothelial cells regulate polymorphonuclear leukocyte degranulation. *FASEB J* 12: 733–746

48   Zimmerman GA, McIntyre TM, Prescott SM, Otsuka K (1990) Molecular mechanisms of neutrophil adhesion to endothelial cells involving platelet-activating factor and cytokines. *J Lipid Mediators* 2: S31–S43

49   Breviario F, Bertocchi F, Dejana E, Bussolino F (1988) IL-1-induced adhesion of polymorphonuclear leukocytes to cultured human endothelial cells. Role of platelet-activating factor. *J Immunol* 141: 3391–3397

50   Harlan JM (1993) Leukocyte adhesion deficiency syndrome: insights into the molecular basis of leukocyte emigration. Clin Immunol Immunopathol 67: S16–S24

51   Zimmerman GA, Prescott SM, McIntyre TM (1986) Thrombin stimulates neutrophil adherence by an endothelial cell-dependent mechanism: Characterization of the response and relationship to platelet-activating factor synthesis. *Ann New York Acad Sci* 485: 349–367

52   Zimmerman GA, McIntyre TM (1988) Neutrophil adherence to human endothelium *in vitro* occurs by CDw18 (Mo1, MAC-1/LFA-1/GP 150,95) glycoprotein-dependent and -independent mechanisms. *J Clin Invest* 81: 531–537

53   Rainger GE, Fisher AC, Nash GB (1997) Endothelial-borne platelet-activating factor and interleukin-8 rapidly immobilize rolling neutrophils. *Am J Physiol* 272: H114–H122

54 Patel KD, Lorant DE, Jones DA, Prescott SM, McIntyre TM, Zimmerman GA (1993) Juxtacrine interactions of endothelial cells with leukocytes: Tethering and signaling molecules. In: C Sorg, N Hogg, D Ruiter (eds): *The vascular endothelium in inflammation* (Symposium), *Behring Inst Mitt* 92: 144–164

55 Arnould T, Michiels C, Remacle R (1993) Increased PMN adherence on endothelial cells after hypoxia: involvement of PAF, CD18/CD11b, and ICAM-1. *Am J Physiol* 264: C1102–C1110

56 Rainger GE, Fisher A, Shearman C, Nash GB (1995) Adhesion of flowing neutrophils to cultured endothelial cells after hypoxia and reoxygenation *in vitro. Am J Physiol* 269: H1398–H1406

57 Kubes P, Suzuki M, Granger DN (1990) Platelet-activating factor-induced microvascular dysfunction: role of adherent leukocytes. *Am J Physiol* 258: G158–G163

58 Gahmberg CG (1997) Leukocyte adhesion: CD11/CD18 integrins and intercellular adhesion molecules. *Curr Opin Cell Biol* 9: 643–650

59 Zimmerman GA, McIntyre TM, Mehra M, Prescott SM (1990) Endothelial cell-associated platelet-activating factor: a novel mechanism for signaling intercellular adhesion. *J Cell Biol* 110: 529–540

60 Lorant DE, Patel KD, McIntyre TM, McEver RP, Prescott SM, Zimmerman GA (1991) Coexpression of GMP-140 and PAF by endothelium stimulated by histamine or thrombin: A juxtacrine system for adhesion and activation of neutrophils. *J Cell Biol* 115: 223–234

61 Ostrovsky L, King AJ, Bond S, Mitchell D, Lorant DE, Zimmerman GA, Larsen R, Niu XF, Kubes P (1998) A juxtacrine mechanism for neutrophil adhesion on platelets involves platelet-activating factor and a selectin-dependent activation process. *Blood* 91: 3028–3036

62 Anklesaria P, Teixidó J, Laiho M, Pierce JH, Greenberger JS, Massagué J (1990) Cell-cell adhesion mediated by binding of membrane-anchored transforming growth factor α to epidermal growth factor receptors promotes cell proliferation. *Proc Natl Acad Sci USA* 87: 3289–3293

63 Massagué J (1990) Transforming growth factor-α. A model for membrane-anchored growth factors. *J Biol Chem* 265: 21393–21396

64 Smith CW, Kishimoto TK, Abbass O, Hughes B, Rothlein R, McIntire LV, Butcher E, Anderson DC (1991) Chemotactic factors regulate lectin adhesion molecule 1 (LECAM-1)-dependent neutrophil adhesion to cytokine-stimulated endothelial cells *in vitro. J Clin Invest* 87: 609–618

65 Lorant DE, McEver RP, McIntyre TM, Moore KL, Prescott SM, Zimmerman GA (1995) Activation of polymorphonuclear leukocytes reduces their adhesion to P-selectin and causes redistribution of ligands for P-selectin on their surfaces. *J Clin Invest* 96: 171–182

66 Macconi D, Foppolo M, Paris S, Noris M, Aiello S, Remuzzi G, Remuzzi A (1995) PAF mediates neutrophil adhesion to thrombin or TNF-stimulated endothelial cells under shear stress. *Am J Physiol* 269: C42–C47

67 Kubes P, Ibbotson G, Russell J, Wallace JL, Granger DN (1990) Role of platelet acti-

vating factor in ischemia/reperfusion-induced leukocyte adherence. *Am J Physiol* 259: G300–G305

68 Ninio E, Leyravaud S, Bidault J, Jurgens P, Benveniste J (1991) Cell adhesion by membrane-bound paf-acether. *Int Immunol* 3: 1157–1163

69 Zhou W, Javors MA, Olson MS (1992) Platelet-activating factor as an intercellular signal in neutrophil-dependent platelet activation. *J Immunol* 149: 1763–1769

70 Weber C, Springer TA (1997) Neutrophil accumulation on activated, surface-adherent platelets in flow is mediated by interaction of Mac-1 with fibrinogen bound to αIIbβ3 and stimulated by platelet-activating factor. *J Clin Invest* 100: 2085–2093

71 Lorant DE, Topham MK, Whatley RE, McEver RP, McIntyre TM, Prescott SM, GA Zimmerman (1993) Inflammatory roles of P-selectin. *J Clin Invest* 92: 559–570

72 Vercellotti GM, Wickham NWR, Gustafson KS, Yin HQ, Hebert M, Jacob HS (1989) Thrombin-treated endothelium primes neutrophil functions: inhibition by platelet-activating factor receptor antagonists. *J Leuk Biol* 45: 483–490

73 Geng J-G, Bevilacqua MP, Moore KL, McIntyre TM, Prescott SM, Kim JM, Bliss GA, Zimmerman GA, McEver RP (1990) Rapid neutrophil adhesion to activated endothelium mediated by GMP-140. *Nature* 343: 757–760

74 Toothill VJ, Van Mourik JA, Niewenhuis HK, Metzelaar MJ, Pearson JD (1990) Characterization of the enhanced adhesion of neutrophil leukocytes to thrombin-stimulated endothelial cells. *J Immunol* 145: 283–291

75 McEver RP, Moore KL, Cummings RD (1995) Leukocyte trafficking mediated by selectin-carbohydrate interactions. *J Biol Chem* 270: 11025–11028

76 Hattori R, Hamilton KK, Fugate RD, McEver RP, Sims PJ (1989) Stimulated secretion of endothelial von Willebrand factor is accompanied by rapid redistribution to the cell surface of the intracellular granule membrane protein GMP-140. *J Biol Chem* 264: 7768–7771

77 Kubes P, Kanwar S (1994) Histamine induces leukocyte rolling in post-capillary venules. A P-selectin-mediated event. *J Immunol* 152: 3570–3577

78 Gaboury JP, Johnston B, Niu X-F, Kubes P (1995) Mechanisms underlying acute mast cell-induced leukocyte rolling and adhesion *in vivo*. *J Immunol* 154: 804–813

79 Kanwar S, Johnston B, Kubes P (1995) Leukotriene C4/D4 induces P-selectin and sialyl Lewis^x-dependent alterations in leukocyte kinetics *in vivo*. *Circ Res* 77: 879–887

80 Moore KL, Varki A, McEver RP (1991) GMP-140 binds to glycoprotein receptors on human neutrophils: evidence for a lectin-like interaction. *J Cell Biol* 112: 491–499

81 McEver RP, Cummings RD (1997) Role of PSGL-1 binding to selectins in leukocyte recruitment. *J Clin Invest* 100: 485–492

82 Sako D, Chang X-J, Barone KM, Vachino G, White HM, Shaw G, Veldman GM, Bean KM, Ahern TJ, Furie B et al (1993) Expression cloning of a functional glycoprotein ligand for P-selectin. *Cell* 75: 1179–1186

83 Bruehl RE, Moore KL, Lorant DE, Borregaard N, Zimmerman GA, McEver RP, Bainton DF (1997) Leukocyte activation induces surface redistribution of P-selectin glycoprotein ligand-1. *J Leuk Biol* 61: 489–499

84 Varki A (1997) Selectin ligands: will the real ones please stand up? *J Clin Invest* 99: 158–162

85 Patel KD, Moore KL, Nollert MU, McEver RP (1995) Neutrophils use both shared and distinct mechanisms to adhere to selectins under static and flow conditions. *J Clin Invest* 96: 1887–1896

86 Lawrence MB, Springer TA (1991) Leukocytes roll on a selectin at physiologic flow rates: distinction from and prerequisite for adhesion through integrins. *Cell* 65: 859–873

87 Weyrich AS, McIntyre TM, McEver RP, Prescott SM, Zimmerman GA (1995) Monocyte tethering by P-selectin regulates monocyte chemotactic protein-1 and tumor necrosis factor-α secretion: Signal integration and NF-κB translocation. *J Clin Invest* 95: 2297–2303

88 Hidari KIPJ, Weyrich AS, Zimmerman GA, McEver RP (1997) Engagement of PSGL-1 enhances tyrosine phosphorylation and activates MAP kinases in human neutrophils. *J Biol Chem* 272: 28750–28756

89 Nick JA, Avdi NJ, Young SK, Knall C, Gerwins P, Johnson GL, Worthen GS (1997) Common and distinct intracellular signaling pathways in human neutrophils utilized by platelet activating factor and FMLP. *J Clin Invest* 99: 975–986

90 Rainger GE, Buckley C, Simmons DL, Nash GB (1997) Cross-talk between cell adhesion molecules regulates the migration velocity of neutrophils. *Curr Biol* 7: 316–325

91 Rot A (1992) Endothelial cell binding of NAP-1/IL-8: role in neutrophil emigration. *Immunol Today* 13: 291–294

92 Middleton J, Neil S, Wintle J, Clark-Lewis I, Moore H, Lam C, Auer M, Hub E, Rot A (1997) Transcytosis and surface presentation of IL-8 by venular endothelial cells. *Cell* 91: 385–395

93 Imaizumi T, Albertine KH, Jicha DL, McIntyre TM, Prescott SM, Zimmerman GA (1997) Human endothelial cells synthesize ENA-78: Relationship to IL-8 and to signaling of PMN adhesion. *Am J Respir Cell Mol Biol* 17: 181–192

94 Imai T, Hieshima K, Haskell C, Baba M, Nagira M, Nishimura M, Kakizaki M, Takagi S, Nomiyama H, Schall TJ, Yoshie O (1997) Identification and molecular characterization of fractalkine receptor CX_3CR1, which mediates both leukocyte migration and adhesion. *Cell* 91: 521–530

95 Coughlan AF, Hau H, Dunlop LC, Berndt MC, Hancock WW (1994) P-selectin and platelet-activating factor mediate initial endotoxin-induced neutropenia. *J Exp Med* 179: 329–334

96 Montrucchio G, Lupia E, De Martino A, Silvestro L, Savu SR, Cacace G, De Filippi PG, Emanuelli G, Camussi G (1996) Plasmin promotes an endothelium-dependent adhesion of neutrophils: Involvement of platelet activating factor and P-selectin. *Circulation* 93: 2152–2160

97 Kuijpers TW, Hakkert BC, Hoogerwerf M, Leeuwenberg JFM, Roos D (1991) Role of endothelial leukocyte adhesion molecule-1 and platelet-activating factor in neutrophil adherence to IL-1-prestimulated endothelial cells. *J Immunol* 147: 1369–1376

98 Kuijpers TW, Hakkert BC, Hart MHL, Roos D (1992) Neutrophil migration across

monolayers of cytokine-prestimulated endothelial cells: a role for platelet-activating factor and IL-8. *J Cell Biol* 117: 565–572

99   Hill ME, Bird IN, Daniels RH, Elmore MA, Finnen MJ (1994) Endothelial cell-associated platelet-activating factor primes neutrophils for enhanced superoxide production and arachidonic acid release during adhesion to but not transmigration across IL-1β-treated endothelial monolayers. *J Immunol* 153: 3673–3683

100 Nourshargh S, Larkin SW, Das A, Williams TJ (1995) Interleukin-1-induced leukocyte extravasation across rat mesenteric microvessels is mediated by platelet-activating factor. *Blood* 85: 2553–2558

101 von Asmuth EJU, Buurman WA (1995) Endothelial cell associated platelet-activating factor (PAF), a costimulatory intermediate in TNF-α-induced H_2O_2 release by adherent neutrophil leukocytes. *J Immunol* 154: 1383–1390

Tight junctions and adherens junctions in endothelial cells: structure and regulation

James M. Staddon[1] and Tetsuaki Hirase[2]

[1]Eisai London Research Laboratories Ltd., Bernard Katz Building, University College London, Gower Street, London WC1E 6BT, UK; [2]1st Department of Internal Medicine, School of Medicine, Kobe University, 7-5-2 Kusunoki-cho, Chuo-ku, Kobe-city 650, Japan

Introduction

Endothelial cells lining the vasculature provide a crucial interface between plasma and tissue environments, separating the solute, macromolecular and cellular composition of the plasma from that of the interstitial fluid [1–3]. This chapter will focus on the role of endothelial cell-cell adhesion as relates to this function. In particular, the tight junction plays the most important role in the separation of plasma and tissue environments. The tight junction also plays a crucial role in the establishment and maintenance of cellular polarity, the separation of the plasma membrane into apical and basolateral compartments, important for the vectorial transport of essential nutrients and factors across endothelia with especially well developed tight junctions [4]. An example of such a differentiated endothelium is the blood-brain barrier, where tight junctions are so well developed that even ionic permeability is severely limited [5]. In epithelial cells [6] and endothelial cells [3, 7, 8], the establishment of tight junctions is dependent on the prior formation of intercellular adherens junctions. For this reason, the adherens junction will also be discussed. Both tight and adherens junctions are composed of transmembrane proteins with associated cytoplasmic components. Also, both junctions are linked to the actin-based cytoskeleton which in itself is subject to complex regulation.

To understand endothelial cell-cell adhesion, it is necessary to understand the molecular components of the intercellular junctions, and in this field much progress has recently been made. Furthermore, it is becoming increasingly clear that cell-cell junctions are not simply passive mechanical entities, rather they are targets for a variety of signalling processes that play a role in the regulation of endothelial biology in both normal physiology and pathology. In this respect, understanding such regulatory processes becomes important for the development of new therapeutic strategies where aberrant regulation of endothelial cell-cell junctions may occur.

Vascular Adhesion Molecules and Inflammation, edited by J. D. Pearson

Molecular architecture of tight junctions

Tight junctions were initially identified in epithelial cells, where a junctional complex consists of tight junctions, adherens junctions, desmosomes and gap junctions [9]. In this junctional complex the tight junction exists on the most apical side of the lateral membranes. The tight junction has been recognized for a long time as the barrier for solutes in both endothelia and epithelia [2, 10, 11]. Early on, a meshwork of fibrils called strands, a key structure of tight junctions, was observed by electron microscopy of freeze fracture replicas [12], and tight junctions were studied mainly by morphological and physiological approaches. In the last decade progress has been made in describing this intercellular coupling on a molecular level, enabling analysis of tight junctions in terms of the function of proteins. Recent key issues have been the identification of the proteins localized at tight junctions and progress towards an understanding of their functions [13–16].

Much has been learned from studies of epithelial cells, and these have generated tools, especially antibodies, to extend such work to endothelial cells. The flow of information has been in this direction because of the availability of excellent lines of epithelial cells with well developed tight junctions. A problem has been how to identify protein components of cell-cell junctions in the absence of any known biochemical properties. In this regard, the use of junctional preparations as immunogens with subsequent characterization of antibody epitopes has been a powerful approach [17].

The first tight junction associated protein to be identified was from mouse liver and was the 220 kDa protein ZO-1, for zonula occludens-1 [18]. ZO-1 is localized at tight junctions in epithelial cells [18] and in endothelial cells [19]. Interestingly, ZO-1 is also associated with the adherens junction complex in fibroblasts and cardiac muscle cells, which lack tight junction structure [20]. In immunoprecipitation experiments, anti-ZO-1 antibodies coprecipitated a 160 kDa protein termed ZO-2 [21] that turned out to be related to ZO-1 by cDNA sequence [20, 22–24]. Also ZO-1 has two isoforms, α^+ and α^-, where the α domain is alternatively spliced [25]. The function of the α domain is not fully understood, although the α^+ isoform may be related to maturation and plasticity of tight junctions [25–28]. Both ZO-1 and ZO-2 are cytoplasmic, peripherally associated tight junction proteins.

Thus the molecular analysis of tight junctions has been initiated and is making good progress. However, for a long time, the existence of integral membrane proteins at tight junctions was one of the most intriguing issues in this field [29]. In 1993 an exciting breakthrough was achieved: An integral membrane protein localized at tight junctions was identified, and it was termed occludin [30]. Occludin was initially identified in junctional preparations from chicken liver. cDNA sequence analysis of chicken occludin [30] and, subsequently, mammalian homologues [31] showed that the protein has two extracellular loops and four transmembrane domains with a comparatively long region at the carboxy terminus. *In vitro* binding assays using recombinant occludin and junctional preparations established that it binds to a complex of ZO-1 and ZO-2 via its C-terminal cytoplasmic tail [32]. p130 was also identified as a protein associating, somehow, with ZO-1 and ZO-2 [33]. Therefore, tight junctions seem to consist of at least one occludin: ZO-1: ZO-2: p130 complex. Since ZO-1 is known to be associated with spectrin [34], this complex appears to be linked to the cytoskeleton. Other studies have indicated that occludin plays a functional role in cell adhesion and barrier formation [35–37]. From these findings, the occludin: ZO-1: ZO-2: p130 complex appears to be a key player in the formation and maintenance of tight junctions.

Recent observations from the cDNA sequence of ZO-1 [20, 22] and ZO-2 [23, 24] revealed that ZO-1 and ZO-2 are comprised of three PDZ (PSD-95/DlgA/ZO-1 homology domain) domains, an SH3 domain and a domain homologous to guanylate kinase, and are therefore members of the MAGUK (membrane-associated guanylate kinase) protein family [38]. Since members of the MAGUK protein family are suggested to mediate protein-protein interactions, ZO-1 and ZO-2 might be involved in clustering of occludin (or unknown membrane proteins of tight junctions) and the docking of submembranous tight junction components to occludin.

Several other cytoplasmic components of tight junctions are known, and these include cingulin [39], the 7H6 antigen [40], the small GTPase rab13 [41] and symplekin [42]. However, symplekin seems not to be expressed in vascular endothelial cells. Information about the primary structures of some of these proteins has not yet been established. In addition, the mechanisms whereby these peripheral membrane components interact, if at all, with the occludin: ZO-1: ZO-2: p130 complex are not yet clear.

Molecular architecture of adherens junctions

Cadherins

The calcium dependence of tight junction permeability has been a long established fact for epithelial cells [43], and also holds true for endothelial cells [8]. Removal of extracellular calcium destroys the barrier properties of tight junctions. The basis for this calcium dependence was revealed by Gumbiner and Simons [6]. Their experiments demonstrated that the calcium-dependent establishment of tight junctions in epithelial cells was blocked by antibody to cadherin. It appears that initial intercellular contacts are mediated by cadherins, and tight junction formation follows. Established tight junctions in endothelial cells are still dependent on the adherens junction, because disruption of cadherin interaction leads to an increase in paracellular permeability [8, 44]. These observations have made it necessary to consider the molecular architecture and regulation of the adherens junction in the control of endothelial tight junction permeability.

The classical cadherins, such as E, P and N, are single-pass transmembrane glycoproteins that interact homotypically with cadherin on neighbouring cells [10, 45]. The basis for the calcium-dependence of cadherin adhesiveness has been recently established [46–48]. It appears that calcium stabilizes cadherin structure such that cadherin dimers form within the membrane of a cell, these then interact with similar dimers on neighbouring cells to form a zipper-like structure. Endothelial cells from peripheral tissues express a more recently described cadherin, termed VE-cadherin or cadherin-5, which appears to be the major cadherin at cell-cell contacts [49–53]. N-cadherin is also expressed in endothelial cells [54, 55] but its distribution appears to be extrajunctional [55]. The possibility that expression of a particular cadherin determines endothelial phenotype, such as that of brain endothelial cells, has not been fully explored.

Catenins

Essential for adhesiveness of these cadherins is their cytoplasmic tail which associates with a group of proteins termed catenins [see 10, 56, 57]. Initially, three catenins were identified: α, β and γ. β-catenin possesses twelve copies of a motif originally identified in the segment polarity gene product armadillo and binds directly to cadherin. Structural studies suggest that the repeats form a superhelix of helices, creating a positively charged groove that may interact with acidic regions in the cytoplasmic tail of cadherin [58]. α-catenin is a vinculin homologue binding to β-catenin and probably links cadherins to the actin-based cytoskeleton. γ-catenin is related to β and can substitute for it in the complex. All of these catenins are expressed and localized to junctions in endothelial cells [44, 59, 60]. The calcium-dependence of tight junction permeability is probably explained by the linkage of cadherins to the actin-based cytoskeleton. Removal of calcium simply reveals the cytoskeletal tension, allowing cell retraction and tight junction opening [7, 61].

More recently, another catenin was identified. p120, also termed p120[cas] and p120[ctn], is a 120 kDa protein that was initially identified as a substrate for the tyrosine kinase src, and tyrosine phosphorylation of p120 appeared to be necessary for cellular transformation [62]. Cloning and sequencing of p120 revealed that it had some structural relationship to β-catenin, i.e. the presence of armadillo repeats [63, 64]. Splice variants of p120 exist and the relative expression of these variants can vary amongst cell-types, although the functional significance of this is not yet clear [59, 65, 66]. A variety of approaches has shown p120 association with the cadherin/catenin complex in epithelial cells [59, 66–68]. Classically, the original catenins were observed as methionine-labelled proteins present in cadherin immunoprecipitates [56]. p120 was not identified by this approach because it does not possess as many methionines as the other catenins, and is also present in the complex in lower amounts [59]. p120 also exists as part of the cadherin/catenin complex in endothelial cells [59, 69], so it appears that, so far, the cytoplasmic components of adherens junctions in epithelial and endothelial cells are very similar.

Signalling and endothelial cell-cell adhesion

Another feature of endothelial cells is that their tight junction permeability, as established under certain conditions, can be rapidly altered, especially by modulators of signalling processes. This is especially clear in culture and plays a role *in vivo*, creating problems associated with oedema. In the case of the central nervous system, oedema following a stroke or head trauma is especially serious and severely exacerbates the clinical management of such problems. Another situation where signalling and endothelial cell-cell adhesion are important is during immune cell transmigration across endothelial cells, where endothelial signalling appears to be crucial ([70, 71]; see also the chapter by Muller, this volume).

Cyclic AMP

As shown for cultured brain endothelial cells, cyclic AMP-elevating agents or membrane-permeant analogues of cyclic AMP induce a decrease in tight junction permeability [19, 44, 72]. Peripheral endothelial cells respond similarly [73]. Associated with this decrease in permeability is a reorganized actin cytoskeleton [19, 44]. Untreated cultures contain actin stress fibres throughout their cytoplasm but after cyclic AMP treatment these become less abundant and the cortical belt of actin becomes well defined. Associated with the absence of stress fibres is the disappearance of focal contacts, as revealed by antibody staining of proteins such as paxillin and focal adhesion kinase [44].

The mode of action of cyclic AMP is probably related to inhibition of myosin light chain phosphorylation, which appears to be a key regulator of contractility in endothelial cells [74]. In this mechanical model, cyclic AMP causes relaxation of the actin-based cytoskeleton which, due to its linkage to the adherens and tight junctions, results in an improved development of cell-cell contacts, and therefore decreased tight junction permeability. This does not exclude the possibility of additional mechanisms; so far we have yet to observe any changes in localization or distribution of adherens or tight junction proteins, but this does not exclude the possibility of effects on phosphorylation of these proteins. The effect of cyclic AMP on endothelial cell permeability, however, opens up therapeutic possibilities to control oedema through phosphodiesterase inhibition [19, 75, 76].

Lysophosphatidic acid and rho proteins

Interestingly, although studies with peripheral endothelial cells have established histamine and thrombin as permeability increasing agents [see 61], these apparently have no effect on cultured brain endothelial cells, perhaps due to the absence of appropriate receptors (Staddon et al., unpublished observations). In our search for potential permeability altering agents for brain endothelial cells, lysophosphatidic acid emerged as a possible candidate [44]. This agent, released from platelets during clotting [77], increased tight junction permeability of brain endothelial cells in a reversible manner. Associated with this increase in permeability was an increase in stress fibre formation and the appearance of tyrosine phosphorylated protein at focal contacts. Lysophosphatidic acid reversed the effect of cyclic AMP on both permeability and the cytoskeleton [44].

In other systems such as fibroblasts, effectors of lysophosphatidic acid-triggered signalling are being identified. The small GTP-binding protein rho appears to be a key effector of lysophosphatidic acid signalling especially in the control of stress fibre formation and myosin light chain phosphorylation [78–80]. Mechanisms regulating rho activation may therefore also be vital in the control of endothelial tight junction permeability. However, the situation appears complex in that in epithelial cells, establishment of cadherin-dependent cell-cell adhesion requires rho activity [81]. As mentioned below, lysophosphatidic acid signalling also has effects on phosphorylation of proteins localized at cell-cell contacts.

Tyrosine phosphorylation

A variety of observations has indicated that tyrosine phosphorylation of proteins at cell-cell junctions may be involved in their regulation. In the late 1980s, Takata and Singer [82] suggested that decreased tyrosine phosphorylation of proteins at cell-cell contacts during development may correlate with the acquisition of barrier function in tissue. Tyrosine kinases of the src family are localized at adherens junctions in epithelial cells [83], and β-catenin appears to be a very significant src substrate since stoichiometry of phosphorylation is very high in src transfected cells [84, 85]. Furthermore, although controversial [86], receptor protein tyrosine phosphatases appear to be associated with the cadherin-catenin complex [87–90].

In studies using cultured epithelial and brain endothelial cells, treatment with tyrosine phosphatase inhibitors resulted in a rapid increase in tight junction permeability [91]. Furthermore, tyrosine phosphorylation of proteins associated with cell-cell junctions was increased. In the epithelial cells, these proteins included β-catenin and ZO-1 [91], suggesting that both adherens and tight junction proteins were targets for tyrosine kinases. However, although elicited by pharmacological agents, the physiological significance of tyrosine phosphorylation of junctional proteins remains to be determined. Ligands acting via cell surface receptors have yet to be identified especially for brain endothelial cells. Recently, evidence has been presented that tyrosine phosphorylation of junction proteins may be involved in contact inhibition in endothelial cells [69, 92]. Cell-cell contact may involve ligand and counter-receptor engagement, regulating processes such as direct activation of receptor protein tyrosine phosphatases, controlling tyrosine phosphorylation.

p120

Another set of observations linking signalling and the regulation of cell-cell adhesion derives from studies of p120. As mentioned, this 120 kDa protein was initially discovered as a src substrate [62]. p120 and the associated protein p100 in general migrate as broad bands on SDS polyacrylamide gels. Initially, the significance of this was not clear. However, these clusters of bands may represent differentially phosphorylated forms of protein. This was suggested by work on epithelial cells where pharmacological activation of protein kinase C triggered rapid and reversible serine/threonine dephosphorylation of p120 and p100, resulting in tighter, faster migrating bands [93]. p120 is thus a target for both tyrosine kinase- and serine/threonine-kinase-based signalling, providing further evidence that junctions are targets for signalling processes. In the epithelial cells, p120/p100 dephosphorylation correlated with increased tight junction permeability [93].

Brain endothelial cells also express p120 and p100 which migrate as broad bands [59] and, although unresponsive to protein kinase C activation, dephosphorylation can be triggered by exogenous lysophosphatidic acid in parallel with increased tight junction permeability (Ratcliffe and Staddon, unpublished observations). These data indicate that lysophosphatidic acid activates signalling connections with the adherens junctions, and so, plausibly, could be involved in permeability control. However, much remains to be established about p120 signalling pathways before this can be tested experimentally.

Occludin phosphorylation

The possibility that occludin function itself is regulated by phosphorylation and signalling pathways has also been suggested. In epithelial cells cultured in medium containing low concentrations of calcium, such that tight junctions cannot form, occludin migrates as a tight band on SDS polyacrylamide gels. Addition of calcium to the culture medium initiates tight junction formation and this correlates with retarded mobility of occludin on the gels. This retardation is due to phosphorylation of occludin on serine residues [94]. The identity of the kinase is not known.

115

Interestingly, in brain endothelial cells, when the gel mobility of occludin is compared with that from peripheral endothelial cells it appears as a more retarded protein, and its mobility is more like that from epithelial cells [27]. Thus there may be differential phosphorylation of occludin in brain endothelial cells and peripheral endothelial cells. However, agents such as cyclic AMP and lysophosphatidic acid, permeability modulators with opposite effects, do not have any apparent effect on occludin mobility suggesting that these agents do not regulate occludin phosphorylation [27]. It still remains possible that occludin phosphorylation is involved in the establishment of tight junctions but not in their subsequent regulation.

Protein expression and junctional phenotype

The absolute permeability of endothelial cells varies enormously, ranging from fully leaky to more epithelial-like, as in brain endothelial cells. The molecular basis for such differences is not yet established. So far, levels of ZO-1 [27] and ZO-2 (Hirase, Ratcliffe, Staddon, unpublished observations) appear to be very similar in peripheral and brain endothelial cells. Expression of the catenins is also very similar [27] but cadherin types in brain endothelial cells have not been characterized. Interestingly, however, occludin expression is much higher in brain endothelial cells than in peripheral endothelial cells [27], suggesting that it may be a key determinant of the permeability phenotype. This difference in expression was observed both in cultured cells and *in vivo*. It is also relevant to note that tight and adherens junctions in peripheral endothelial cells are discontinuous and fragmented, whereas those in brain endothelial cells are seamless, at least under the light microscope, suggesting a correlation between tightness of tight junctions and continuity of junctional structures at cell-cell contacts. The 7H6 tight junction-associated antigen may also be a regulator of permeability in endothelial cells [95].

Thus, occludin is a junctional component that differs in its expression in different types of endothelial cells and therefore could be a determinant of tight junction permeability. These observations raise several issues. One is that of stoichiometry. What is the binding partner of ZO-1 in tight junctions of peripheral endothelial cells? This concern only applies if ZO-1 and occludin are expressed in similar molar amounts in brain endothelial cells. However, because tight junction proteins need harsh detergent conditions to be solubilized, it is technically difficult to study the stoichiometry of these complexes. Another observation which indicates the possible existence of an occludin isoform or a binding partner of ZO-1 is that, in blots of mRNA isolated from brain endothelial cells, occludin cDNA hybridises with a fainter band in addition to the main band [27]. Since occludin expression in brain endothelial cells seems to be transcriptionally regulated [27], another question is what kind of stimuli upregulate occludin expression leading to the tight junction phenotype of brain endothelial cells. The occludin promoter should be interesting in this context.

Junctions and extravasation

Another interesting situation where endothelial junctions may be regulated is during extravasation. As described elsewhere in this volume, immune cells (e.g. neutrophils) bind to endothelial cells and transmigrate. Much is understood about the binding of immune cells and endothelial activation, which involves selectins, integrins and immunoglobulin superfamily members [96]. More recently, the actual process of transmigration is being considered. There are two possible ways for cells to transmigrate: through the endothelial cells or around them. We favour the latter mechanism, but this is still a controversial issue. Interestingly, attachment of neutrophils to endothelial cells triggers endothelial signalling processes. This signalling appears to be similar to that initiated by some of the classic inflammatory agents, histamine and thrombin, known to alter endothelial permeability, suggesting that neutrophil transmigration may involve regulation of endothelial cell-cell adhesion, and indeed may be a necessary part of transmigration [70, 97]. An initial study suggested that destruction of the cadherin/catenin complex occurred when neutrophils encountered endothelial cells [98] but this suggestion appears to be flawed for technical reasons [99]. Other paradigms of extravasation have suggested that tumour cell transmigration may involve tyrosine phosphorylation of junctional proteins [100], and that monocyte transmigration across endothelial cells may involve cadherin-mediated interactions between the two cell types [101]. Gotsch et al. [102] have shown that a neutralizing VE-cadherin antibody facilitates neutrophil transmigration *in vivo*, again suggesting that regulation of endothelial junctions are important in extravasation. Extravasation mechanisms are clearly an interesting topic for future research.

Conclusions

There has been much progress in the understanding of endothelial cell-cell junctions. There has been an exciting interplay of information gleaned from studies of development, directed cell biology studies and antibody approaches. With the identification of major components of endothelial junctions, progress is now being made in terms of signalling and regulation. There are bound to be more proteins identified but the information so far allows testing of new ideas and concepts. Importantly, the fact that signalling appears to be important in the regulation of cell-cell adhesion will allow novel therapeutic strategies to be developed.

Acknowledgements
We would like to thank Susan Staddon for editorial assistance.

117

References

1   Risau W (1995) Differentiation of endothelium. *FASEB J* 9: 926–933
2   Rubin LL (1992) Endothelial cells: adhesion and tight junctions. *Curr Opin Cell Biol* 4: 830–833
3   Dejana E, Corada M, Lampugnani MG (1995) Endothelial cell-to-cell junctions. *FASEB J* 9: 910–918
4   Nelson WJ (1992) Regulation of cell surface polarity from bacteria to mammals. *Science* 258: 948–955
5   Staddon JM, Rubin LL (1996) Cell adhesion, cell junctions and the blood-brain barrier. *Curr Opin Neurobiol* 6: 622–627
6   Gumbiner BM, Simons K (1986) A functional assay for proteins involved in establishing an epithelial occluding barrier: identification of a uvomorulin-like polypeptide. *J Cell Biol* 102: 457–468
7   Garcia JGN, Schaphorst KL (1995) Regulation of endothelial cell gap formation and paracellular permeability. *J Invest Med* 43: 117–126
8   Haselton FR, Heimark RL (1997) Role of cadherins 5 and 13 in the aortic endothelial barrier. *J Cell Physiol* 171: 243–251
9   Farquhar MG, Palade GE (1963) Junctional complexes in various epithelia. *J Cell Biol* 17: 375–412
10   Gumbiner BM (1996) Cell adhesion: the molecular basis of tissue architecture and morphogenesis. *Cell* 84: 345–357
11   Schneeberger EE, Lynch RD (1992) Structure, function and regulation of cellular tight junctions. *Am J Physiol* 262: L647–L661
12   Staehelin LA (1973) Further observations on the fine structure of freeze-cleaved tight junctions. *J Cell Sci* 13: 763–786
13   Citi S (1993) The molecular organisation of tight junctions. *J Cell Biol* 121: 485–489
14   Anderson JM, Van Itallie, CM (1995) Tight junctions and the molecular basis for regulation of paracellular permeability. *Am J Physiol* 269: G467–G475
15   Balda MS, Matter K (1998) Tight junctions. *J Cell Sci* 111: 541–547
16   Denker BM, Nigam SK (1998) Molecular structure and assembly of the tight junction. *Am J Physiol* 274: F1–F9
17   Tsukita Sh, Tsukita Sa (1989) Isolation of cell-to-cell adherens junctions from rat liver. *J Cell Biol* 108: 31–41
18   Stevenson BR, Siciliano JD, Mooseker MS, Goodenough DA (1986) Identification of ZO-1: a high molecular weight polypeptide associated with the tight junction (zonula occludens) in a variety of epithelia. *J Cell Biol* 103: 755–766
19   Rubin LL, Hall DE, Porter S, Barbu K, Cannon C, Horner HC, Janatpour M, Liaw CW, Manning K, Morales J et al (1991) A cell culture model of the blood-brain barrier. *J Cell Biol* 115: 1725–1735
20   Itoh M, Nagafuchi A, Yonemura S, Kitani-Yasuda T, Tsukita S, Tsukita S (1993) The 220-kD protein colocalizing with cadherins in non-epithelial cells is identical to ZO-1,

a tight junction-associated protein in epithelial cells: cDNA cloning and immunoelectron microscopy. *J Cell Biol* 121: 491–502

21   Gumbiner BM, Lowenkopf T, Apatira D (1991) Identification of a 160 kDa polypeptide that binds to the tight junction protein ZO-1. *Proc Natl Acad Sci USA* 88: 3460–3464

22   Willott E, Balda MS, Fanning AS, Jameson B, Van Itallie C, Anderson JM (1993) The tight junction protein ZO-1 is homologous to the Drosophila discs-large tumor suppressor protein of septate junctions. *Proc Natl Acad Sci USA* 15: 7834–7838

23   Jesaitis LA, Goodenough DA (1994) Molecular characterization and tissue distribution of ZO-2, a tight junction protein homologous to ZO-1 and the Drosophila discs-large tumor suppressor protein. *J Cell Biol* 124: 949–961

24   Beatch M, Jesaitis LA, Gallin WJ, Goodenough DA, Stevenson BR (1996) The tight junction protein ZO-2 contains three PDZ (PSD-95/Discs-Large/ZO-1) domains and an alternatively spliced region. *J Biol Chem* 271: 25723–25726

25   Balda MS, Anderson, JM (1993) Two classes of tight junctions are revealed by ZO-1 isoforms. *Am J Physiol* 264: C918–924

26   Kurihara H, Anderson JM, Farquhar MG (1992) Diversity among tight junctions in rat kidney: glomerular slit diaphragms and endothelial junctions express only one isoform of the tight junction protein ZO-1. *Proc Natl Acad Sci USA* 89: 7075–7079

27   Hirase T, Staddon JM, Saitou M, Ando-Akatsuka Y, Itoh M, Furuse M, Fujimoto K, Tsukita Sh, Rubin LL (1997) Occludin as a possible determinant of tight junction permeability in endothelial cells. *J Cell Sci* 110: 1603–1613

28   Sheth B, Fesenko I, Collins J, Moran B, Wild, A, Anderson JM, Fleming T (1997) Tight junction assembly during mouse blastocyst formation is regulated by late expression of ZO-1 alpha plus isoform. *Development* 124: 2027–2037

29   Gumbiner B (1993) Breaking through the tight junction barrier. *J Cell Biol* 123: 1631–1633

30   Furuse M, Hirase T, Itoh M, Nagafuchi A, Yonemura S, Tsukita S, Tsukita S (1993) Occludin: a novel integral membrane protein localizing at tight junctions. *J Cell Biol* 123: 1777–1788

31   Ando-Akatsuka Y, Saitou M, Hirase T, Kishi M, Sakakibara A, Itoh M, Yonemura S, Furuse M, Tsukita S (1996) Interspecies diversity of the occludin sequence: cDNA cloning of human, mouse, dog and rat-kangaroo homologues. *J Cell Biol* 133: 43–47

32   Furuse M, Itoh M, Hirase T, Nagafuchi A, Yonemura S, Tsukita S, Tsukita S (1994) Direct association of occludin with ZO-1 and its possible involvement in the localization of occludin at tight junctions. *J Cell Biol* 127: 1617–1626

33   Balda, MS, González-Mariscal L, Matter K, Cereijido M, Anderson JM (1993) Assembly of tight junctions: the role of diacylglycerol. *J Cell Biol* 123: 293–302

34   Itoh M, Yonemura S, Nagafuchi A, Tsukita S, Tsukita S (1991) A 220-kD undercoat-constitutive protein: its specific localization at cadherin-based cell-cell adhesion sites. *J Cell Biol* 115: 1449–1462

35   Balda MS, Whitney JA, Flores C, González S, Cereijido M, Matter K (1996) Functional dissociation of paracellular permeability and transepithelial resistance and disruption

of the apical-basolateral intramembrane diffusion barrier by expression of a mutant tight junction membrane protein. *J Cell Biol* 134: 1031–1049

36 McCarthy KM, Skare IB, Stankewich MC, Furuse M, Tsukita S, Rogers RA, Lynch RD, Schneeberger EE (1996) Occludin is a functional component of the tight junction. *J Cell Sci* 109: 2287–2298

37 Van Itallie CM, Anderson JM (1997) Occludin confers adhesiveness when expressed in fibroblasts. *J Cell Sci* 110: 1113–1121

38 Fanning AS, Anderson JM (1996) Protein-protein interactions: PDZ domain networks. *Curr Biol* 6: 1385–1388

39 Citi S, Sabanay H, Jakes R, Geiger B, Kendrick-Jones J (1988) Cingulin, a new peripheral component of tight junctions. *Nature* 333: 272–276

40 Zhong Y, Saitoh T, Minase T, Sawada N, Enomoto K, Mori M (1993) Monoclonal antibody 7H6 reacts with a novel tight junction associated protein distinct from ZO-1, cingulin and ZO-2. *J Cell Biol* 120: 477–483

41 Zahraoui A, Joberty G, Arpin M, Fontaine JJ, Hellio R, Tavitian A, Louvard D (1994) A small rab GTPase is distributed in cytoplasmic vesicles in non polarized cells but colocalizes with the tight junction marker ZO-1 in polarized epithelial cells. *J Cell Biol* 124: 101–115

42 Keon BH, Schäfer. S. Kuhn C, Grund C, Franke WW (1996) Symplekin, a novel type of tight junction plaque protein. *J Cell Biol* 134: 1003–1018

43 Citi S (1992) Protein kinase inhibitors prevent junction dissociation induced by low extracellular calcium in MDCK epithelial cells. *J Cell Biol* 117: 169–178

44 Schulze C, Smales C, Rubin LL, Staddon JM (1997) Lysophosphatidic acid increases tight junction permeability in cultured brain endothelial cells. *J Neurochem* 68: 991–1000

45 Takeichi M (1995) Morphogenetic roles of classic cadherins. *Curr Opin Cell Biol* 7: 619–627

46 Overduin M, Harvey TS, Bagby S, Tong KI, Yau P, Takeichi M, Ikura M (1995) Solution structure of the epithelial cadherin domain responsible for selective cell adhesion. *Science* 267: 386–389

47 Shapiro L, Fannon AM, Kwong PD, Thompson A, Lehmann MS, Grubel G, Legrand JF, Als-Nielsen J, Colman DR, Hendrickson WA (1995) Structural basis of cell-cell adhesion by cadherins. *Nature* 374: 327–337

48 Nagar B, Overduin M, Ikura M, Rini JM (1996) Structural basis of calcium-induced E-cadherin rigidification and dimerization. *Nature* 380: 360–364

49 Heimark RL, Degner M, Schwartz SM (1990) Identification of a Ca^{2+}-dependent cell-cell adhesion molecule in endothelial cells. *J Cell Biol* 110: 1745–1756

50 Lampugnani MG, Resnati M, Raiteri M, Pigott R, Piscane A, Houen G, Ruco LP, Dejana E (1992) A novel endothelial-specific membrane protein is a marker of cell-cell contacts *J Cell Biol* 118: 1511–1522

51 Suzuki S, Sano K, Tanihara H (1991) Diversity of the cadherin family: evidence for eight new cadherins in nervous tissue. *Cell Regul* 2: 261–270

52 Matsuyoshi N, Toda K, Horiguchi Y, Tanaka T, Nakagawa S, Takeichi M, Imamura S (1997) *In vivo* evidence of the critical role of cadherin-5 in murine vascular integrity. *Proc Assoc Am Physicians* 109: 362–371

53 Vittet D, Burchou T, Schweitzer A, Dejana E, Huber P (1997) Targeted null-mutation in the VE-cadherin gene impairs the organization of vascular-like structures in embryoid bodies. *Proc Natl Acad Sci USA* 94: 6273–6278

54 Liaw CW, Cannon C, Power MD, Kiboneka PK, Rubin LL (1990) Identification and cloning of two species of cadherins in bovine endothelial cells. *EMBO J* 9: 2701–2708

55 Salomon D, Ayalon O, Patel-king R, Hynes RO, Geiger B (1992) Extrajunctional distribution of N-cadherin in cultured human endothelial cells. *J Cell Sci* 102: 7–17

56 Aberle H, Schwartz H, Kemler R (1996) Cadherin-catenin complex: protein interactions and their implications for cadherin functions. *J Cell Biochem* 61: 514–523

57 Navarro P, Caveda L, Breviaro F, Mandoteanu I, Lampugnani MG, Dejana E (1995) Catenin-dependent and -independent functions of vascular endothelial cadherin. *J Biol Chem* 270: 30965–30972

58 Huber AH, Nelson WJ, Weis WI (1997) Three-dimensional structure of the armadillo repeat region of β-catenin. *Cell* 90: 871–882

59 Staddon JM, Smales C, Schulze C, Esch FS, Rubin LL (1995) p120, a p120-related protein (p100) and the cadherin/catenin complex. *J Cell Biol* 130: 369–381

60 Lampugnani MG, Corada M, Cavead L, Breviario F, Ayalon O, Geiger B, Dejana E (1995) The molecular organization of endothelial cell to cell junctions: differential association of plakoglobin, β-catenin, and α-catenin with vascular endothelial cadherin (VE-cadherin). *J Cell Biol* 129: 203–217

61 Lum H, Malik AB (1994) Regulation of vascular endothelial barrier function. *Am J Physiol* 267: 223–241

62 Daniel JM, Reynolds AB (1997) Tyrosine phosphorylation and cadherin/catenin function. *Bioessays* 19: 883–891

63 Reynolds AB, Herbert L, Cleveland JL, Berg ST, Gaut JR (1992) p120, a novel substrate of protein tyrosine kinase receptors and of p60[v-src], is related to cadherin-binding factors beta-catenin, plakoglobin and armadillo. *Oncogene* 7: 2439–2445

64 Peifer MS, Berg S, Reynolds AB (1994) A repeating amino acid motif shared by proteins with diverse cellular roles. *Cell* 76: 789–791

65 Mo YY, Reynolds AB (1996) Identification of murine p120 isoforms and heterogeneous expression of p120[cas] isoforms in human tumor cell lines. *Cancer Res* 56: 2633–2640

66 Reynolds AB, Daniel J, McCrea P, Wheelock MJ, Wu J, Zhang Z (1994) Identification of a new catenin: the tyrosine kinase substrate p120[cas] associates with E-cadherin complexes. *Mol Cell Biol* 14: 8333–8342

67 Shibamoto S, Hayakawa M, Takeuchi K, Hori T, Miyazawa K, Kitamura N, Johnson KR, Wheelock MJ, Matusyoshi N, Takeichi M, Ito F (1995) Association of p120, a tyrosine kinase substrate, with E-cadherin/catenin complexes. *J Cell Biol* 128: 949–957

68 Daniel JM, Reynolds AB (1995) The tyrosine kinase substrate p120[cas] binds directly to

E-cadherin but not to the adenomatous polyposis coli protein or α-catenin. *Mol Cell Biol* 9: 4819–4824

69 Lampugnani MG, Corada M, Andriopxoulou P, Esser S, Risau W, Dejana E (1997) Cell confluence regulates tyrosine phosphorylation of adherens junction components in endothelial cells. *J Cell Sci* 110: 2065–2077

70 Huang A, Manning TM, Bandak MC, Ratau KR, Hanser KR, Silverstein SC (1993) Endothelial cell cytosolic free calcium regulates neutrophil migration across monolayers of endothelial cells. *J Cell Biol* 120: 1371–1380

71 Parkos CA (1997) Molecular events in neutrophil transepithelial migration. *Bioessays* 19: 865–873

72 Wolburg H, Neuhasu J, Kniessel U, Krauss B, Schmid E-M, Öcalan M, Farrell C, Risau W (1994) Modulation of tight junction structures in blood-brain barrier endothelial cells. *J Cell Sci* 107: 1347–1357

73 Langeler EG, van Hinsbergh VW (1991) Norepinephrine and iloprost improve barrier function of human endothelial cell monolayers: role of cAMP. *Am J Physiol* 260: C1052–C1059

74 Goeckeler ZM, Wysolmerski RB (1995) Myosin light chain kinase-regulated endothelial contraction: the relationship between isometric tension, actin polymerization and myosin phosphorylation. *J Cell Biol* 130: 613–627

75 Warren JB, Wilson AJ, Lori RK, Coughlan ML (1993) Opposing roles of cyclic AMP in the vascular control of edema formation. *FASEB J* 7: 1394–1400

76 Suttorp N, Ehreiser P, Hippenstiel S, Fuhrmann M, Krull M, Tenor H, Schudt C (1996) Hyperpermeability of pulmonary endothelial monolayer: protective role of phosphodi-esterase isoenzymes 3 and 4. *Lung* 174: 181–194

77 Moolenaar WH (1995) Lysophosphatidic acid, a multifunctional phospholipid messen-ger. *J Biol Chem* 270: 12949–12952

78 Kimura K, Ito M, Amano M, Chihara K, Fukata Y, Nakafuku M, Yamamori B, Feng J, Nakano T, Okawa K, Iwamatsu A, Kaibuchi K (1996) Regulation of myosin phos-phatase by Rho and Rho-associated kinase (Rho-kinase). *Science* 273: 245–248

79 Narumiya S, Ishizaki T, Wtanabe N (1997) Rho effectors and reorganization of the actin cytoskeleton. *FEBS Lett* 410: 68–72

80 Hall A (1998) Rho GTPases and the actin cytoskeleton. *Science* 279: 509–514

81 Braga VMM, Machesky L, Hall A, Hotchin NA (1997) The small GTPases Rho and Rac are required for the establishment of cadherin-dependent cell-cell contacts. *J Cell Biol* 137: 1421–1431

82 Takata K, Singer SJ (1988) Phosphotyrosine-modified proteins are concentrated at the membranes of epithelial and endothelial cells during tissue development in chick embryos. *J Cell Biol* 106: 1757–1764

83 Tsukita S, Oishi K, Akiyama T, Tamanishi Y, Yamamoto T, Tsukita S (1991) Specific proto-oncogenic tyrosine kinases of the src family are enriched in cell-to-cell adherens junction where the level of tyrosine phosphorylation is elevated. *J Cell Biol* 113: 867–879

84 Matsuyoshi N, Hamaguchi M, Taniguchi S, Nagafuchi A, Tsukita S, Takeichi M (1992) Cadherin-mediated cell-cell adhesion is perturbed by v-src tyrosine phosphorylation in metastaic fibroblasts. *J Cell Biol* 118: 703–714

85 Takeda H, Nagafuchi A, Yonemura S, Tsukita S, Behrens J, Birchmeier W, Tsukita S (1995) V-src kinase shifts the cadherin-based cell adhesion from the strong to the weak state and β-catenin is not required for the shift. *J Cell Biol* 131: 1839–1847

86 Zondag GCM, Moolenaar WH, Gebbink MFBG (1996) Lack of association between receptor protein tyrosine phosphatase RPTPμ and cadherins. *J Cell Biol* 134: 1513–1517

87 Brady-Kalnay SM, Rimm DL, Tonks NK (1995) Receptor protein tyrosine phosphatase PTPμ associates with cadherins and catenins *in vivo*. *J Cell Biol* 130: 977–986

88 Balsamo J, Leung TC, Ernst H, Zanin MKB, Hoffman S, Lilien J (1996) Regulated binding of a PTP 1B-like phosphatase to N-cadherin: control of N-cadherin-mediated adhesion by dephosphorylation of β-catenin. *J Cell Biol* 134: 801–813

89 Fuchs M, Muller T, Lerch MM, Ullrich A (1996) Association of human protein tyrosine phosphatase k with members of the Armadillo family. *J Biol Chem* 271: 16712–16719

90 Kypta RM, Su H, Reichardt LF (1996) Association between a transmembrane protein tyrosine phosphatase and the cadherin-catenin complex. *J Cell Biol* 134: 1519–1529

91 Staddon JM, Herrenknecht K, Smales C, Rubin LL (1995) Evidence that tyrosine phosphorylation may increase tight junction permeability. *J Cell Sci* 108: 609–619

92 Ayalon O, Geiger B (1997) Cyclic changes in the organization of cell adhesions and the associated cytoskeleton, induced by stimulation of tyrosine phosphorylation in bovine aortic endothelial cells. *J Cell Sci* 110: 547–556

93 Ratcliffe MJ, Rubin LL, Staddon JM (1997) Dephosphorylation of the cadherin-associated p100/p120 proteins in response to activation of protein kinase C in epithelial cells. *J Biol Chem* 272: 31894–31901

94 Sakakibara A, Furuse M, Ando-Akatstuka Y, Tsukita Sh (1997) Possible involvement of phosphorylation of occludin in tight junction formation. *J Cell Biol* 137: 1393–1401

95 Satoh H, Zhong Y, Isomura H, Saitoh M, Enomoto K, Sawada N, Mori M (1996) Localization of 7H6 tight junction-associated antigen along the cell border of vascular endothelial cells correlates with paracellular barrier function against ions, large molecules, and cancer cells. *Exp Cell Res* 222: 269–274

96 Albelda SM, Smith CW, Ward PA (1994) Adhesion molecules and inflammatory injury. *FASEB J* 8: 504–512

97 Hixenbaugh EA, Goeckeler ZM, Papaiya NN, Wysolmerski RB, Silverstein SC, Huang AJ (1997) Stimulated neutrophils induce myosin light chain phosphorylation and isometric tension in endothelial cells. *Am J Physiol* 273: H981–H988

98 Del Maschio A, Zanetti A, Corada M, Rival Y, Ruco L, Lampugnani MG, Dejana E (1996) Polymorphonuclear leukocyte adhesion triggers the disorganization of endothelial cell-to-cell adherens junctions. *J Cell Biol* 135: 497–510

99 Moll T, Dejana E, Vestweber D (1998) *In vitro* degradation of endothelial catenins by a neutrophil protease. *J Cell Biol* 140: 403–407

100 Lewalle JM, Bajou K, Desreux J, Mareel M, Dejana E, Noel A, Foidart JM (1997) Alteration of interendothelial adherens junctions following tumor cell-endothelial cell interaction *in vitro. Exp Cell Res* 237: 347–356

101 Sandig M, Negrou E, Rogers KA (1997) Changes in the distribution of LFA-1, catenins and F-actin during transendothelial migration of monocytes in culture. *J Cell Sci* 110: 2807–2818

102 Gotsch, U, Borges E, Bosse R, Böggemeyer E, Simon M, Mossmann H, Vestweber D (1997) VE-cadherin antibody accelerates neutrophil recruitment *in vivo. J Cell Sci* 110: 583–588

The role of PECAM in leukocyte emigration

William A. Muller

Department of Pathology and the Center for Vascular Biology, Weill Medical College of Cornell University, 1300 York Avenue, New York, NY 10021, USA

Transendothelial migration is a molecularly dissectible step in leukocyte emigration

The process of leukocyte emigration into a site of inflammation involves a number of sequential and coordinated adhesive interactions between the leukocyte and underlying endothelium. As has been made clear in previous chapters, emigration can be dissected into the steps of tethering, rolling, activation, firm adhesion, and transendothelial migration. These interactions typically involve distinct families of cell adhesion molecules (CAMs). It is our ability to block the actions of these molecules by specific monoclonal antibodies (mAb), soluble recombinant CAMs or their ligands, or genetic disruption that has identified these as distinct steps [1, 2].

This chapter will focus on the passage of leukocytes between the tightly apposed endothelial cells (EC) comprising the vascular lining (diapedesis) and their subsequent migration across the subendothelial basal lamina. These two processes have been defined as distinct steps in leukocyte emigration by the ability of reagents that block function of platelet/endothelial cell adhesion molecule-1 (PECAM). Anti-PECAM reagents selectively block transendothelial migration without interfering with the preceding steps of emigration (e.g. rolling or adhesion). In fact, distinct domains of the PECAM molecule are responsible for diapedesis and migration across the basal lamina [1, 3]. As will be reviewed below, reagents selective for these domains can block diapedesis without blocking migration across basal lamina and vice-versa.

Molecular structure and cellular distribution of PECAM

PECAM-1 (PECAM, CD31) is a member of the immunoglobulin gene superfamily [4–6]. It is a Type I transmembrane protein, spanning the membrane once. Its extracellular region, comprised of six C-2 type domains, is heavily N-glycosylated, with carbohydrate residues accounting for approximately 40% of its apparent M_r of

Vascular Adhesion Molecules and Inflammation, edited by J. D. Pearson
© 1999 Birkhäuser Verlag Basel/Switzerland

130 kDa [4]. The 118-residue cytoplasmic tail contains several serine and tyrosine residues that may be phosphorylated. In particular, phosphorylation of tyrosines at positions 663 and 686 has been reported to form functional SH2 domains [7–9] that are postulated to play roles in PECAM-related signal transduction [7–10] (see below). The murine [11] and bovine [12] counterparts are structurally homologous to the human form.

PECAM is constitutively expressed on all continuous endothelia *in situ* [13] as well as by megakaryocytes and platelets, neutrophils, monocytes [4], natural killer cells [14], and subsets of T cells [15]. It is diffusely distributed on the surfaces of subconfluent cultured human EC, but becomes concentrated at the borders between EC as they become confluent and make functional junctions with each other [13]. This behavior is recapitulated by cells transfected with PECAM [16]. These data suggested that PECAM was involved in the recognition and/or adhesion of endothelial cells to each other and that such interactions might be important for maintenance of the endothelial cell monolayer. Since circulating leukocytes bear PECAM diffusely on their surfaces, it was postulated that homophilic interactions between leukocyte PECAM and endothelial cell PECAM might play a role in transendothelial migration [1]. This chapter will focus on aspects of PECAM biology relevant to transendothelial migration. For details on other aspects of the biology of PECAM the reader is referred to recent reviews [17, 18].

Adhesive functions of PECAM are related to distinct molecular domains

PECAM has been demonstrated to be involved in three general types of adhesive interaction. PECAM can bind to itself in a homophilic manner [16, 19, 20]. PECAM on one cell binds to some other molecule on an apposing cell or in the extracellular matrix (heterophilic) [3, 21, 22]. On leukocytes, PECAM has been shown to be involved in an adhesion cascade: ligation of leukocyte PECAM results in the upregulation of leukocyte integrin function [14, 15, 23, 24]. The ability of a cell to participate in these interactions is not mutually exclusive. Indeed, leukocyte emigration involves at least two, and possibly all three of these PECAM-dependent interactions.

Early work with cultured endothelial cells [13, 25] and PECAM transfectants [16, 26] suggested that PECAM on apposing cells interacted in a homophilic manner. However, direct proof awaited the development of soluble recombinant PECAM/Fc fusion proteins. These were demonstrated to bind specifically to PECAM on transfected cells as well as on human umbilical vein EC [19, 20]. Anti-PECAM mAb whose epitopes mapped to domains 1 and/or 2, but not other domains [3, 27], completely blocked this adhesion, demonstrating that it is these amino-terminal domains of cellular PECAM that interact in homophilic adhesion [19, 20]. Subsequent work in a different model system demonstrated that domains 1 and 2 were both necessary for adhesion, and were sufficient, if they were presented on an inert scaffold of murine PECAM domains 3–6 (murine PECAM does not bind to human PECAM in this system) [28]. The amino acid residues of domain 1 critical for adhesion have been mapped [29].

PECAM-transfected L cell fibroblasts, when mixed in suspension, spontaneously aggregate in a divalent cation-dependent, temperature-sensitive, manner [21]. This adhesion requires the expression of PECAM by the transfectants [16, 21], and in particular requires expression of amino acids in the cytoplasmic tail encoded by exon 14 [28]. However, in this adhesion, PECAM-bearing cells bind equally well to nontransfected parental cells or controls expressing an anti-sense PECAM construct [21]. Hence PECAM on these transfectants must be binding to another molecule on the apposing cells. In contrast to homophilic adhesion described above, mAb against domains 1 and/or 2 have no effect on this heterophilic aggregation, but mAb against domain 6, the membrane-proximal domain, block [30]. Thus, two distinct portions of the extracellular region of PECAM participate in homophilic and heterophilic adhesion (see Fig. 1).

What is the heterophilic ligand for PECAM? It was postulated that heparan sulfate-containing glycosaminoglycans (GAGs) were the ligand, since the heterophilic aggregation assay could be blocked by heparin or heparan sulfate, but not by structurally unrelated sulfated GAGs, and by heparinase treatment of the nontransfected cells in the assay mixture [22]. However, recent studies have demonstrated that PECAM does not bind directly to heparin in several *in vitro* assays [31]. Therefore, a unifying hypothesis is that GAGs may be necessary, but not sufficient, to mediate binding of PECAM to some other yet-unidentified heterophilic ligand(s).

Two independent laboratories have reported that PECAM binds to the vitronectin receptor, the integrin $\alpha_v\beta_3$ [32, 33]. However, two other groups found no evidence of this interaction [19, 20]. It is clear that cellular PECAM interacts in a defined manner with non-PECAM ligands. The identity of these ligands remains unclear.

Participation of leukocyte PECAM in an adhesion cascade, culminating in the activation of leukocyte integrins, will be discussed in the section on signal transduction later in this chapter.

Role of PECAM in transmigration: Studies *in vitro*

One must be careful, when studying this phenomenon, to distinguish between reagents that block transendothelial migration *per se* and those that block migration of leukocytes in a "transmigration assay" [34]. This is not a semantic argument. In a typical *in vitro* transmigration assay, leukocytes are placed on top of an endothelial cell monolayer (often grown on a permeable filter support over a reservoir of chemoattractant-containing medium) at the start of the assay. What ends up below the monolayer (or in the reservoir) is called transmigration, and anything that

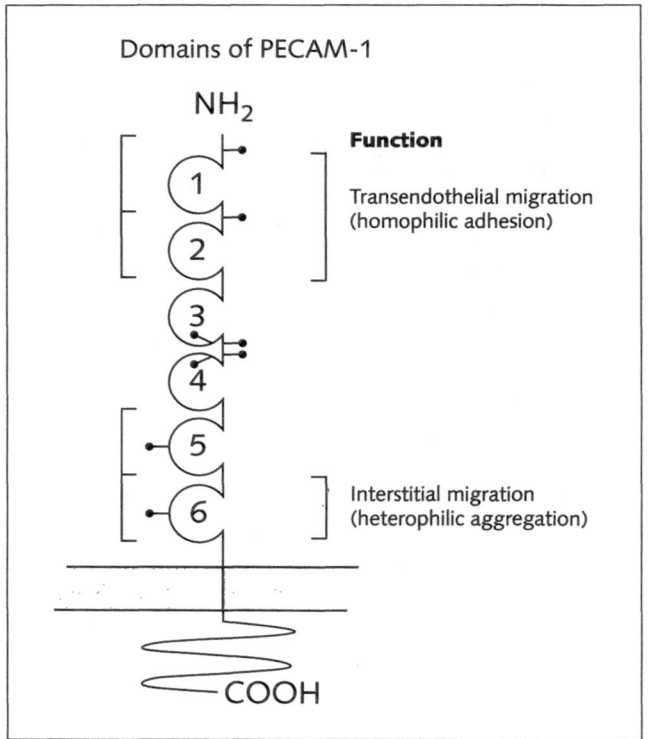

Figure 1
Schematic diagram of the immunoglobulin domain structure of PECAM identifying the domains responsible for transendothelial migration and migration across basal lamina (interstitial migration). Reproduced from [3] by copyright permission of The Rockefeller University Press.

decreases the number of leukocytes emerging would be an inhibitor of transmigration. However, it should be obvious that anything which interferes with the ability of leukocytes to bind to the apical surface of the endothelium, move to the junctions, migrate between the endothelial cells, migrate across the endothelial basal lamina, move through the support (often many times thicker than the cells), or detach from the support would produce a readout of decreased transmigration. It is therefore very difficult to distinguish any role for the β_2 integrins or VLA-4 on leukocytes, or their counterparts ICAM-1 and VCAM-1 on endothelial cells, in transendothelial migration independent of their well-documented role in the adhesion of leukocytes to the apical surface of endothelium. In this regard, PECAM is unique. It has no apparent role in adhesion of leukocytes to endothelium. Neither do anti-PECAM reagents inhibit the ability of leukocytes to migrate in response to a chemotactic gradient [1]. Rather, PECAM functions specifically in the diapedesis of leukocytes and their subsequent migration across the subendothelial basal lamina [1, 3].

Our group has developed a transmigration assay in which the adhesion and transmigration components can be physically separated [35]. In addition, direct visualization of the monolayers allows for fine distinctions between whether an adherent leukocyte is just above or just below the endothelial monolayer [1, 3]. Anti-PECAM reagents have no effect on the adhesion of leukocytes to the apical surface of cultured endothelial cells. The same number of leukocytes remain with the cultures in anti-PECAM-treated and control samples. The only difference is in the position of the leukocytes with regard to the endothelial monolayer. Seventy to 90% of those treated with mAb against PECAM domains 1 and/or 2 are arrested on the apical surface of the monolayer directly over the inter-endothelial junctions [1, 3]. This block is maintained as long as there is sufficient anti-PECAM reagent in the environment, and is reversible upon removal of the anti-PECAM reagent. The leukocytes rapidly resume transmigration and have all migrated below the endothelial monolayer within 1.5 h of mAb washout. In contrast, treatment of leukocytes with mAb that recognize PECAM domain 6 has no effect on their ability to migrate across the endothelial monolayer. However, over 80% of them remain directly below the endothelial cells, with many trapped between the undersurface of the endothelium and the endothelial basal lamina [3].

The specificity of antibody blockade described above is reminiscent of the specificity for blocking homophilic and heterophilic interactions, respectively (see Fig. 1). Indeed, several pieces of evidence demonstrate that diapedesis involves homophilic interaction between the amino terminal domains of PECAM on the leukocyte and the same domains on endothelial PECAM. (1) Transmigration can be blocked equally well by adding anti-PECAM mAb to either the leukocytes or to the endothelial cells, and adding to both cell types does not block any better than blocking either one alone [1]. (2) Transmigration is blocked only by mAb whose epitopes are in domains 1 and/or 2 – the same mAb that block homophilic adhesion [3]. 3. Transmigration is blocked by presenting monocytes with soluble PECAM molecules (mimicking interaction with endothelial PECAM) containing domain 1, but not by those lacking domains 1 and 2 [20].

When mAb that bind the membrane-proximal domain(s) of PECAM are added to suspensions of monocytes, the migrating cells are arrested between the undersurface of the endothelial cell and the endothelial basal lamina [3, 36]. These mAb are blocking an interaction of leukocyte PECAM, since addition of the same mAb to the endothelial cells has no effect [3, 37]. The relevant interaction of leukocyte PECAM seems to be with some molecule in the extracellular matrix, since the same results are obtained when monocytes are allowed to migrate into the collagen gels across basal lamina from which the endothelial cells have been non-enzymatically removed (unpublished observations). Similar to other heterophilic interactions that have been described above, the migration of monocytes across basal lamina was inhibited by treatment of the co-cultures with heparin but not dextran sulfate [3]. These observations provided the first evidence that migration of leukocytes across the subendothelial basal lamina was a distinct and separable step in the emigration process [3].

While the migration of leukocytes across basal lamina has not been extensively studied, several observations *in vivo* demonstrate that the role of PECAM in this process is not an *in vitro* curiosity. Investigators using a polyclonal antibody against human PECAM that cross-reacts with rat PECAM demonstrated that while a substantial number of leukocytes were indeed arrested intravascularly, at the ultrastructural level, a significant proportion of them were arrested between the endothelial cells and the underlying basal lamina [38]. Presumably this antiserum contained significant reactivity against membrane-proximal domains of rat PECAM. Mice with a gene-targeted deletion of PECAM have a very mild phenotype [55]. This is not unexpected, as will be discussed shortly. However, the most striking abnormality in these mice is the arrest of neutrophils between the vascular endothelium and the basement membrane of inflamed mesenteric microvessels. This arrest is transient, as normal numbers of leukocytes eventually enter the peritoneal cavity, but it is reproducible and statistically significant.

The importance of PECAM in transendothelial migration has been demonstrated for monocytes [1], neutrophils [1, 39], natural killer cells [14], and T cells [40]. Monocytes spontaneously migrate across resting HUVEC monolayers grown on hydrated collagen gels, while lymphocytes and neutrophils do not [35]. These non-activated HUVEC do not express E-selectin or VCAM-1, and express low levels of ICAM-1 [35]; however, they do make basal levels of chemoattractants [35] including MCP-1 [41]. When such monolayers are treated with IL-1 or TNFα, they are induced to express these markers of endothelial cell activation [35] and are now capable of supporting neutrophil adhesion and transendothelial migration. Under cytokine-activated conditions, monocyte adhesion and transmigration is more rapid than under resting conditions. Lymphocytes adhere, but still transmigrate poorly over the first few hours [35]. Under all of these conditions, transendothelial migration was selectively inhibited by preincubation of leukocytes or endothelial cells with mAb against domain 1 and/or 2 of PECAM, or by soluble recombinant PECAM-IgG containing at least domain 1 [1, 3, 20]. Two independent groups have described that transmigration of vitamin D_3-differentiated HL60 cells (a monocytoid cell line) across HUVEC grown on filters was inhibited by anti-PECAM antibodies [39, 42]. Rival et al. [39] also described that incubation of HUVEC with a combination of IFNγ and TNFα produced a down-regulation of PECAM expression. Coincident with this roughly 50% decrease in PECAM expression by HUVEC, transendothelial migration of neutrophils across these monolayers was reduced by roughly 50% compared to cultures treated with TNFα alone. This decrease in transmigration was in the face of a four-fold increased neutrophil adhesion to these same monolayers, presumably due to an increase in their expression of ICAM-1 and other apical adhesion molecules [39]. Thus, expression of ICAM-1 or other cytokine-inducible adhesion molecules on HUVEC was insufficient to support transendothelial migration in the absence of functioning PECAM under these conditions.

Natural killer (NK) cell transmigration across resting HUVEC monolayers was blocked by 50% by anti-PECAM mAb [14]. Similar to the findings with monocytes and neutrophils, mAb that bound to domain 1 of PECAM blocked well. However, some mAb that bind to an epitope comprised of domains 1 and 2 did not block transmigration of NK cells nearly as well, despite their ability to maximally block transmigration of monocytes. This finding with NK cells was similar to our experience with neutrophils (PMN) [1]. Whether these subtle differences in mAb susceptibility reflect real differences in the subdomains of PECAM involved leukocyte-endothelial cell interactions of these various cell types during transmigration or just reflect trivial variations in posttranslational modification of PECAM is not known. Reagents targeting PECAM domain 1 block PMN migration maximally *in vivo* [20, 37, 43]; mAb to murine PECAM selectively recognising epitopes in domains 1 and 2 are not yet available.

The role of PECAM in transendothelial migration of lymphocytes may be controversial; it is certainly difficult to study. One reason may be that peripheral blood lymphocytes do not migrate well in most *in vitro* systems. However, circulating lymphocytes are really a mixture of diverse cell populations that may each have different migratory properties that vary in physiologically relevant ways. Migration of only 3% of the total T cells added to the endothelial monolayer may therefore be relevant if those 3% of cells make up $\geq 90\%$ of the circulating pool of the proper subset. Using a filter migration system, one study found that PECAM was not enriched on T cells that migrated compared to the starting population, and concluded that PECAM had no obligatory role in T cell transmigration [44]. There is one report of T cells spontaneously (albeit slowly – peak migration occurred at 4 h) migrating across monolayers of PECAM-transfected murine fibroblasts in a manner that was inhibitable by anti-PECAM mAb [40].

Role of PECAM in transmigration: Studies *in vivo*

The importance of PECAM for transendothelial migration of neutrophils and monocytes has been confirmed by a number of different investigators using a variety of models of acute inflammation in several different species. Bogen et al. blocked recruitment of neutrophils and monocytes into the peritoneal cavity of mice for 24–48 h with a single 50 µg injection of anti-murine PECAM mAb [43] that binds domain 1 of murine PECAM [20]. Perhaps most interesting was the finding that the leukocytes blocked from entering the peritoneal cavity were seen in association with the lumenal surface of mesenteric venules, apparently bound but unable to transmigrate [43]. A similar block, both quantitatively and qualitatively, was seen when Liao et al. inhibited inflammation in the same model using soluble recombinant murine PECAM domain 1 as an Fc chimera [20], confirming the requirement for domain 1 in transendothelial migration *in vivo*. This was highly reminiscent of the appearance of leukocytes arrested on the apical surface of HUVEC monolayers by anti-PECAM reagents *in vitro* [1, 3]. In both cases neutrophil transmigration was blocked by at least 80% and monocyte transmigration was reduced to background levels. The block *in vivo* was at least as complete, if not better, than the block obtained using *in vitro* models [1, 3, 20, 43].

Vaporciyan et al. [45] used a rabbit anti-human PECAM polyclonal antibody that cross-reacts with rat PECAM to block neutrophil influx in several acute inflammation models in the rat. Intravenous administration of 200 μg of the IgG or F(ab')$_2$ form blocked neutrophil emigration into the peritoneum in response to glycogen, or into the alveoli of the lung in response to intratracheally instilled immune complexes, for 4 h. The same antibody also blocked the ability of murine leukocytes to emigrate into human skin grafts placed on SCID mice and stimulated with TNFα [45]. In a separate publication it was reported to block migration of feline leukocytes into the peritoneal cavity in response to glycogen [46].

An unambiguous role for neutrophil PECAM was subsequently demonstrated in the human skin graft to SCID mouse model using mAb against murine PECAM [37]. In fact, in this model, the role of the amino terminal domains of PECAM in transmigration was again confirmed *in vivo*, since mAb hec7 (against domains 1+2) but not 4G6 (against domain 6) was effective at blocking transendothelial migration (albeit of murine neutrophils) across human endothelium [37]. On the other hand, the results with mAb against murine leukocyte PECAM were apparently contradictory: mAb MEC13.3 blocked murine PMN emigration while mAb 390 did not; both recognize domain 1 of murine PECAM. However, mAb 390 may be the exception that proves the rule. This mAb does not block homophilic PECAM-PECAM adhesion in the same *in vitro* assays in which MEC13.3 does [47].

Infusion of anti-PECAM antibodies has been shown to protect animals against neutrophil-dependent damage in cardiac ischemia-reperfusion models [46, 48]. In a feline model a rabbit anti-PECAM antibody given after 90 min of ischemia reduced necrosis 4.5 h after reperfusion by 58% compared to control IgG, without a decrease in tissue leukocyte accumulation (inferred from tissue myeloperoxidase activity) [46]. The authors postulated that, as in other *in vivo* models, the decreased damage was due to the inability of the leukocytes to transmigrate once they arrived at the site of damage. The rat model [48] employed 30 min of ischemia followed by 2 h of reperfusion. In this shorter-term model, 5 mg/kg of an F(ab')$_2$ fragment of a different rabbit anti-human platelet antibody was perfused. The authors observed nearly the same degree of protection (54% reduction in infarct size compared to controls) [48]. However, in this model total myeloperoxidase activity in tissues was reduced by 83% in the anti-PECAM treated rats compared to controls. This was assumed to reflect decreased leukocyte retention in the tissues. The basis of this discrepancy between the results in the rat [48] and cat [46] models is not certain. It may reflect differences in the species, duration of the protocol, or type of antibody given (intact IgG vs. F(ab')$_2$). Both studies relied on the ability of an antibody against human PECAM to cross react with an unrelated species. Whatever the mechanism, it is clear that in many animal models, blockade of PECAM function is a promising target for anti-inflammatory therapy.

Signal transduction via PECAM: Implications for adhesion cascades

During transmigration there is an obligatory increase in intracellular calcium within the endothelial cell. Buffering the intracellular calcium rise blocked PMN transmigration without affecting the ability of the PMN to adhere to the apical surface of the endothelial cells [49]. This apparently selective action on transmigration is reminiscent of the effects of anti-PECAM reagents. The rise in intracellular calcium has been linked to a phosphorylation of myosin light chain kinase, presumed to be necessary for the traction of the endothelial cytoskeleton, facilitating the separation of the endothelial cells from each other during passage of the leukocyte [50].

Does PECAM play a role in any of these processes? There is one recent report that ligation of endothelial PECAM by certain mAb (or Fab fragments) led to a rise in intracellular free calcium [51]. This calcium rise was somewhat atypical in that it occurred after a several minute delay, was slow, and was sustained relative to the response to thrombin. In addition, it was blocked by the tyrosine kinase inhibitor genistein [51]. These data suggest that the calcium rise might not be a direct effect, but secondary to other PECAM-mediated signal transduction events. However, when evaluating these data, one must consider that the HUVEC in these studies were subconfluent, and the mAb, 4G6, which was the best stimulator of calcium flux in these experiments, binds to PECAM domain 6 and has no effect on transendothelial migration *in vitro* [3] or *in vivo* [37].

What exactly is the function of PECAM in diapedesis, and how does PECAM carry out this action? The answers are not known, but several *in vitro* models suggest how PECAM might play a role. As mentioned above, ligation of leukocyte PECAM by antibodies stimulates an adhesion cascade in which leukocyte integrin function is upregulated. This has been shown for the β_1 integrins (especially CD49d/CD29) on T cells [15] and CD34$^+$ progenitor cells [52] and the β_2 family of integrins (especially CD11b/CD18) on neutrophils, monocytes, NK cells and T cells [14, 15, 23, 24, 53]. This occurs through intracellular signaling in an "inside-out" fashion, since the number of cell surface integrin molecules does not increase enough to account for the increase in adhesion. We postulated that during passage of the

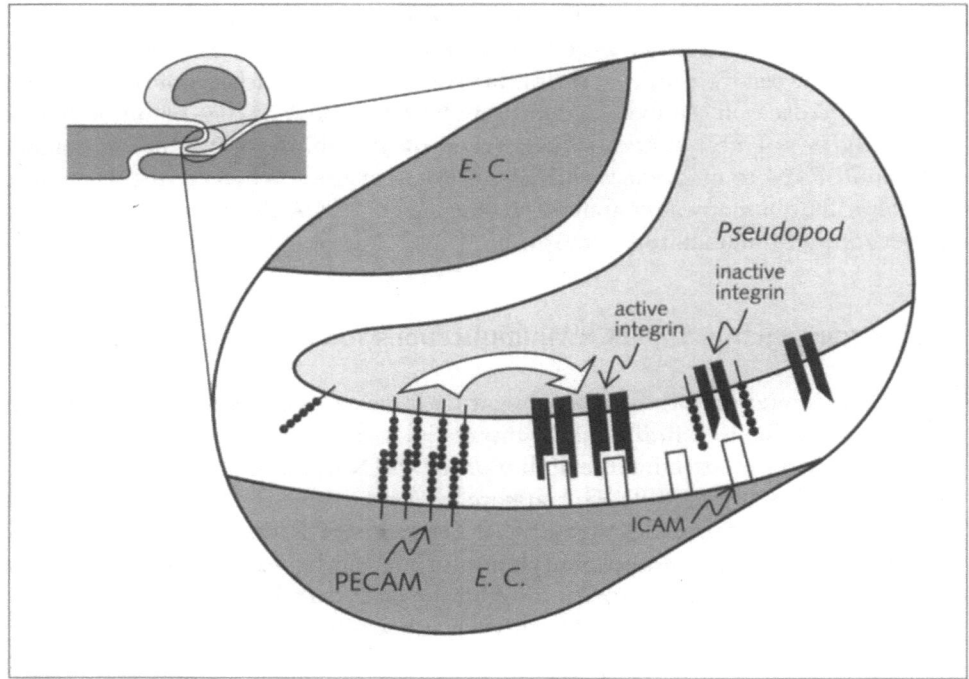

Figure 2

Hypothesized function of PECAM in an adhesion cascade. This figure illustrates a schema-tized leukocyte pseudopod entering an endothelial cell junction where PECAM is highly con-centrated. Adhesive interactions between leukocyte PECAM at the front of the pseudopod and endothelial cell PECAM stimulate a signal transduction pathway (perhaps involving phosphorylation of PECAM and interaction with SHP-2, see text) that causes the leukocyte integrin to assume its active conformation and bind to endothelial counter-receptors, pic-tured here as ICAM, providing traction. After transient activation, the integrin would resume its inactive conformation, allowing detachment and further extension of the pseudopod for more rounds of PECAM-stimulated adhesion as the leukocyte moves through the junction.

leukocyte through the junction, the densely-packed endothelial PECAM may act in a manner similar to the antibodies in the studies described above, engaging leuko-cyte PECAM and stimulating adhesion of leukocyte integrins to their counter-recep-tors in the junctions between the endothelial cells [1] (see Fig. 2).

How might ligation of leukocyte PECAM transduce this signal or generate a cal-cium flux? Reports from several laboratories have identified tyrosine 686 on the cytoplasmic tail of PECAM as crucial for PECAM signaling in various models. In a model of cell aggregation by PECAM-transfected L cells, phosphorylation or muta-tion of this residue converted heterophilic adhesion to homophilic adhesion [54]. Expression of PECAM in transfected cells is associated with a decrease in migration rate in those cells. Transfectants in which Y^{686} is mutated to F show a strongly reduced block in migration, implicating phosphorylation of this residue as crucial to the reduction in migration [10].

More recently, PECAM phosphorylated on tyrosines 686 and 663 has been shown to bind to SH2 domains of the protein tyrosine phosphatase SHP-2 and the tyrosine kinase c-src in platelet [7] and endothelial cell [8] lysates, respectively. Moreover, phosphorylation of both residues was required for SHP-2 binding [9]. SHP-2 is believed to be a positive regulator of β_3 integrin activation in platelets and other cells. These authors [8, 9] noted homologies between the cytoplasmic tail of PECAM in the region bearing tyrosines 663 and 686 and immunoregulatory tyro-sine-based activation motifs (ITAMs)[1] in other molecules, including the T cell recep-tor, B cell receptor and Fc receptor. These molecules, like PECAM, have no inherent kinase activity. However, when phosphorylated, they bind the SH2 domains of cyto-plasmic tyrosine kinases that propagate the signals. Considering the number of adhesive functions that PECAM has been demonstrated to mediate in the variety of cell types that express it, it is likely that PECAM participates in a variety of signal transduction pathways that are cell-type and function-specific.

Elegant as the above studies are, the signal transduction pathways relevant to transendothelial migration are not known. Endothelial cells concentrate about one million molecules of PECAM in the narrow junction between them. Alterations in PECAM phosphorylation pertinent to transmigration may be limited to the small fraction of those molecules directly interacting with the leukocyte. Therefore, it may be very difficult to discern appropriate PECAM-derived signals or changes in phos-phorylation status in the large ocean of cellular PECAM. Similarly, it may be very difficult to block these signals in wild-type endothelial cells using anti-sense con-structs or dominant negative mutations due to the large reservoir of functional PECAM. This remains a challenge for future studies.

PECAM-independent transmigration

Even in the best defined *in vitro* and *in vivo* models, anti-PECAM reagents never block transmigration completely at any concentration or dosage schedule tested. Blockade of neutrophil transmigration is often no better than 80%. Blockade of monocyte emigration into the peritoneal cavity has been reduced to background lev-els [20, 43], but this may reflect the difference between new monocyte influx and

---

[1] Note added in proof: Recently one of these authors has published a commentary stating that these domains of CD31 are more appropriately classified as immunoreceptor tyrosine-based inhibitory (ITIM) domains. Newman PJ (1999) Switched at birth: A new family for PECAM-1. *J Clin Invest* 103: 5–9

resident peritoneal macrophage turnover. *In vitro* blockade of monocyte transmigration ranges from 70–90%, and is usually closer to 70% than 90% [1, 3, 20]. Thus, even in these systems, it is apparent that PECAM-independent mechanisms of transendothelial migration exist.

Moreover, there are some models in which anti-PECAM reagents do not block well at all. Wakelin et al. [38] used rabbit anti-PECAM antibody to block emigration of rat leukocytes from mesenteric vessels stimulated with IL-1β. However, in the same model, the same anti-PECAM antibody failed to block neutrophils recruited by direct peritoneal instillation of the chemoattractant N-formyl-methionyl-leucyl-phenylalanine (fMLP). Similarly, employing *in vitro* models, A. Issekutz (personal communication) found that whereas anti-PECAM antibodies partially inhibited migration of PMN across IL-1 activated HUVEC grown on porous filters, neutrophil transmigration across such monolayers in response to the chemoattractants C5a or IL-8 placed in the lower chamber was PECAM-independent. It may be a general phenomenon that PECAM's role in transmigration can be bypassed by providing a strong chemoattractant. The role of the chemoattractant may be to directly activate the leukocyte integrins (bypassing the usual requirement for PECAM in this role, as proposed above) or to coerce it to follow a PECAM-independent pathway that would normally be a secondary route.

It may come as no surprise, therefore, that PECAM "knockout" mice do not have an overt phenotype. They respond to inflammatory challenges to the same degree as wild-type littermates [55]. These mice, deprived of PECAM since conception, have presumably learned to use their natural PECAM-independent pathways and expanded them so that the "road less traveled by" constitutes their main mode of transendothelial migration. Since 80% or more of transendothelial migration in wild-type mice is PECAM-dependent, it would be difficult to uncover the PECAM-independent modes of transendothelial migration in normal mice. On the other hand, the PECAM deficient mice will provide good subjects for these studies.

Acknowledgments
Supported by NIH grant HL46849. WAM is an Established Investigator of the American Heart Association. The author thanks Dr. Miriam E. Berman for permission to reproduce Figure 2 from her PhD thesis.

References

1   Muller WA, Weigl SA, Deng X, Phillips DM (1993) PECAM-1 is required for transendothelial migration of leukocytes. *J Exp Med* 178: 449–460
2   Muller WA (1995) Migration of leukocytes across the vascular intima Molecules and mechanisms. *Trends Cardiovasc Med* 5: 15–20

3   Liao F, Huynh HK, Eiroa A, Greene T, Polizzi E, Muller WA (1995) Migration of mono-
     cytes across endothelium and passage through extracellular matrix involve separate
     molecular domains of PECAM. *J Exp Med* 182: 1337–1343

4   Newman PJ, Berndt MC, Gorski J, White II GC, Lyman S, Paddock C, Muller WA
     (1990) PECAM-1 (CD31) cloning and relation to adhesion molecules of the
     immunoglobulin gene superfamily. *Science* 247: 1219–1222

5   Simmons DL, Walker C, Power C, Pigott R (1990) Molecular cloning of CD31, a puta-
     tive intercellular adhesion molecule closely related to carcinoembryonic antigen. *J Exp
     Med* 171: 2147–2152

6   Stockinger H, Gadd SJ, Eher R, Majdic O, Schreiber W, Kasinrerk W, Strass B, Schnabl
     E, Knapp W (1990) Molecular characterization and functional analysis of the leukocyte
     surface protein CD31. *J Immunol* 145: 3889–3897

7   Jackson DE, Ward CM, Wang R, Newman PJ (1997) The protein-tyrosine phos-
     phatase SHP-2 binds platelet/endothelial cell adhesion molecule-1 (PECAM-1) and
     forms a distinct signaling complex during platelet aggregation. *J Biol Chem* 272:
     6986–6993

8   Lu TT, Barreuther M, Davis S, Madri JA (1997) Platelet/endothelial cell adhesion mol-
     ecule-1 (PECAM-1/CD31) is phosphorylatable by c-src, binds src-SH2 domain and
     exhibits ITAM-like properties. *J Biol Chem* 272: 14442–14446

9   Jackson DE, Kupcho KR, Newman PJ (1997) Characterization of phosphotyrosine
     binding motifs in the cytoplasmic domain of platelet/endothelial cell adhesion mole-
     cule-1 (PECAM-1) that are required for the cellular association and activation of the
     protein-tyrosine phosphatase, SHP-2. *J Biol Chem* 272: 24868–24875

10   Lu TT, Yan LG, Madri JA (1996) Integrin engagement mediates tyrosine dephosphory-
     lation on platelet-endothelial cell adhesion molecule 1. *Proc Natl Acad Sci USA* 93:
     11808–11813

11   Xie Y, Muller WA (1993) Molecular cloning and adhesive properties of murine platelet/
     endothelial cell adhesion molecule-1. *Proc Natl Acad Sci USA* 90: 5569–5573

12   Stewart RJ, Kashour TS, Marsden PA (1996) Vascular endothelial platelet endothelial
     cell adhesion molecule-1 (PECAM-1) expression is decreased by TNFα and IFNγ. *J
     Immunol* 156: 1221–1228

13   Muller WA, Ratti CM, McDonnell SL, Cohn ZA 1989 A human endothelial
     cell-restricted, externally disposed plasmalemmal protein enriched in intercellular junc-
     tions. *J Exp Med* 170: 399–414

14   Berman ME, Xie Y, Muller WA (1996) Roles of platelet/endothelial cell adhesion mole-
     cule-1 (PECAM-1, CD31) in natural killer cell transendothelial migration and beta 2
     integrin activation. *J Immunol* 156: 1515–1524

15   Tanaka Y, Albelda SM, Horgan KJ, Van Seventer GA, Shimizu Y, Newman W, Hallam
     J, Newman PJ, Buck CA, Shaw S (1992) CD31 expressed on distinctive T cell subsets
     is a preferential amplifier of beta1 integrin-mediated adhesion. *J Exp Med* 176:
     245–253

16   Albelda SM, Muller WA, Buck CA, Newman PJ (1991) Molecular and cellular proper-

ties of PECAM-1 (endoCAM/CD31): A novel vascular cell-cell adhesion molecule. *J Cell Biol* 114: 1059–1068

17 Newman PJ (1997) The biology of PECAM-1. *J Clin Invest* 99: 3–8

18 Delisser HM, Baldwin HS, Albelda SM (1997) Platelet endothelial cell adhesion molecule 1 (PECAM-1/CD31): A multifunctional vascular cell adhesion molecule. *Trends Cardiovasc Med* 7: 203–210

19 Sun Q-H, Delisser HM, Zukowski MM, Paddock C, Albelda SM, Newman PJ (1996) Individually distinct Ig homology domains in PECAM-1 regulate homophilic binding and modulate receptor affinity. *J Biol Chem* 271: 11090–11098

20 Liao F, Ali J, Greene T, Muller WA (1997) Soluble domain 1 of platelet-endothelial cell adhesion molecule (PECAM) is sufficient to block transendothelial migration *in vitro* and *in vivo*. *J Exp Med* 185: 1349–1357

21 Muller WA, Berman ME, Newman PJ, Delisser HM, Albelda SM (1992) A heterophilic adhesion mechanism for platelet/endothelial cell adhesion molecule-1 [CD31]. *J Exp Med* 175: 1401–1404

22 Delisser HM, Yan HC, Newman PJ, Muller WA, Buck CA, Albelda SM (1993) Platelet/endothelial cell adhesion molecule-1 (CD31)-mediated cellular aggregation involves cell surface glycosaminoglycans. *J Biol Chem* 268: 16037–16046

23 Piali L, Albelda SM, Baldwin HS, Hammel P, Gisler RH, Imhof BA (1993) Murine platelet endothelial cell adhesion molecule (PECAM-1/CD31) modulates beta2 integrins on lymphokine-activated killer cells Eur. *J Immunol* 23: 2464–2471

24 Berman ME Muller, WA (1995) Ligation of platelet/endothelial cell adhesion molecule 1 (PECAM-1/CD31) on monocytes and neutrophils increases binding capacity of leukocyte CR3 (CD11b/CD18). *J Immunol* 154: 299–307

25 Albelda S, Oliver PD, Romer LH, Buck CA (1990) EndoCAM: a novel endothelial cell-cell adhesion molecule. *J Cell Biol* 110: 1227–1237

26 Muller W A (1992) PECAM-1: an adhesion molecule at the junctions of endothelial cells. In: R van Furth, ZA Cohn, S Gordon (eds): *Mononuclear phagocytes*. The proceedings of the Fifth Leiden Meeting on mononuclear phagocytes. Blackwell Publishers, London, 138–148

27 Yan H-C, Pilewski JM, Zhang Q, Delisser HM, Romer L, Albelda SM (1995) Localization of multiple functional domains on human PECAM-1 (CD31) by monoclonal antibody epitope mapping. *Cell Adhesion and Communication* 3: 45–66

28 Sun J, Williams J, Yan H, Amin KM, Albelda SM, Delisser HM (1996) Platelet/endothelial cell adhesion molecule-1 (PECAM-1) homophilic adhesion is mediated by immunoglobulin-like domains 1 and 2 and depends on the cytoplasmic domain and the level of surface expression. *J Biol Chem* 271: 18561–18570

29 Newton JP, Buckley CD, Jones EY, Simmons DL (1997) Residues on both faces of the first immunoglobulin fold contribute to homophilic binding sites of PECAM-1/CD31. *J Biol Chem* 272: 20555–20563

30 Delisser HM, Chilkotowsky J, Yan H-C, Daise ML, Buck CA, Albelda SM (1994) Deletions in the cytoplasmic domain of platelet-endothelial cell adhesion molecule-1

[PECAM-1, CD31] result in changes in ligand binding properties. *J Cell Biol* 124: 195–203

31   Sun Q-H, Paddock C, Visentin GP, Zukowski MM, Muller WA, Newman PJ (1998) Cell surface glycosaminoglycans do not serve as ligands for PECAM-1 PECAM-1 is not a heparin-binding protein. *J Biol Chem* 273: 11483–11490

32   Piali L, Hammel P, Uherek C, Bachmann F, Gisler RH, Dunon D, Imhof BA (1995) CD31/PECAM-1 is a ligand for $\alpha_v\beta_3$ integrin involved in adhesion of leukocytes to endothelium. *J Cell Biol* 130: 451–460

33   Buckley CD, Doyonnas R, Newton JP, Blystone SD, Brown EJ, Watt SM, Simmons DL (1996) Identification of alpha v beta 3 as a heterotypic ligand for CD31/PECAM-1. *J Cell Science* 109: 437–445

34   Muller WA (1996) Transendothelial migration of leukocytes. In: G Peltz (ed): *Leukocyte recruitment in inflammatory disease*. RG Landis Company, Austin, TX 3–18

35   Muller WA, Weigl S (1992) Monocyte-selective transendothelial migration: Dissection of the binding and transmigration phases by an *in vitro* assay. *J Exp Med* 176: 819–828

36   Muller WA, Greene T, Liao F (1998) Transendothelial migration and interstitial migration of monocytes are mediated by separate domains of monocyte CD31. In: T Springer (ed): *Leukocyte typing VI*. Proceedings of the VIth International Leukocyte Differentiation Antigen Workshop, Kobe, Japan, 1997. Garland Publishers, London, 370–372

37   Christofidou-Solomidou M, Nakada MT, Williams J, Muller WA, Delisser HM (1997) Neutrophil platelet endothelial cell adhesion molecule-1 participates in neutrophil recruitment at inflammatory sites and is down-regulated after leukocyte extravasation. *J Immunol* 158: 4872–4878

38   Wakelin M W, M-J Sanz A Dewar, S M Albelda S W Larkin, N Boughton-Smith T J Williams, S Nourshargh (1996) An anti-platelet/endothelial cell adhesion molecule-1 antibody inhibits leukocyte extravasation from mesenteric microvessels *in vivo* by blocking the passage through basement membrane. *J Exp Med* 184: 229–239

39   Rival Y, Del Maschio A, Rabiet M-J, Dejana E, Duperray A (1996) Inhibition of platelet endothelial cell adhesion molecule-1 synthesis and leukocyte transmigration in endothelial cells by the combined action of TNFα and IFNγ. *J Immunol* 157: 1233–1241

40   Zocchi MR, Ferrero E, Biagio EL, Rovere P, Bianchi E, Toninelli E, Pardi R (1996) CD31/PECAM-1-driven chemokine-independent transmigration of human T lymphocytes. *Eur J Immunol* 26: 759–767

41   Randolph GJ, Furie MB (1995) A soluble gradient of endogenous monocyte chemoattractant protein-1 promotes the transendothelial migration of monocytes *in vitro*. *J Immunol* 155: 3610–3618

42   Rattan V, Shen Y, Sultana C, Kumar D, Kalra VK (1996) Glucose-induced transmigration of monocytes is linked to phosphorylation of PECAM-1 in cultured endothelial cells. *Am J Physiol* 271: E711–E717

43   Bogen S, Pak J, Garifallou M, Deng X, Muller WA (1994) Monoclonal antibody to murine PECAM-1 [CD31] blocks acute inflammation *in vivo*. *J Exp Med* 179: 1059–1064

44   Bird IN, Spragg JH, Ager AH, Matthews N (1993) Studies of lymphocyte transendothelial migration: Analysis of migrated cell phenotypes with regard to CD31 (PECAM-1),
CD45RA and CD45RO. *Immunology* 80: 553–560

45   Vaporciyan AA, Delisser HM, Yan H-C, Mendiguren II, Thom SR, Jones ML, Ward PA,
Albelda SM (1993) Involvement of platelet-endothelial cell adhesion molecule-1 in neutrophil recruitment *in vivo*. *Science* 262: 1580–1582

46   Murohara T, J A Delyani, S M Albelda, A M Lefer (1996) Blockade of platelet endothelial cell adhesion molecule-1 protects against myocardial ischemia and reperfusion
injury in cats. *J Immunol* 156: 3550–3557

47   Yan H-C, Baldwin HS, Sun J, Buck CA, Albelda SM, Delisser HM (1995) Alternative
splicing of a specific cytoplasmic exon alters the binding characteristics of murine pla-
telet/endothelial cell adhesion molecule-1 (PECAM-1). *J Biol Chem* 270: 23672– 23680

48   Gumina RJ, Schultz JE, Yao Z, Kenny D, Warltier DC, Newman PJ, Gross GJ (1996)
Antibody to platelet/endothelial cell adhesion molecule-1 reduces myocardial infarct size
in a rat model of ischemia-reperfusion injury. *Circulation* 94: 3327–3333

49   Huang AJ, Manning JE, Bandak TM, Ratau MC, Hanser KR, Silverstein SC (1993)
Endothelial cell cytosolic free calcium regulates neutrophil migration across monolayers
of endothelial cells. *J Cell Biol* 120: 1371–1380

50   Hixenbaugh EA, Goeckeler ZM, Papaiya NN, Wysolmerski RB, Silverstein SC, Huang
AJ (1997) Chemoattractant-stimulated neutrophils induce regulatory myosin light chain
phosphorylation and isometric tension development in endothelial cells. *Am J Physiol*
273: H981–H988

51   Gurubhagavatula I, Amrani Y, Pratico D, Ruberg FL, Albelda SM, Panettieri RA, Jr
(1998) Engagement of human PECAM-1 (CD31) on human endothelial cells increases
intracellular calcium ion concentration and stimulates prostacyclin release. *J Clin Invest*
101: 212–222

52   Leavesley DI, Oliver JM, Swart BW, Berndt MC, Haylock DN, Simmons PJ (1994) Signals from platelet/endothelial cell adhesion molecule enhance the adhesive activity of the
very late antigen-4 integrin of human CD34+ hemopoietic progenitor cells. *J Immunol*
153: 4673–4683

53   Kuwabara H, Tanaka S, Sakamoto H, Oryu M, Uda H (1996) Antibody-mediated ligation of platelet/endothelial cell adhesion molecule-1 (PECAM-1) on neutrophils
enhances adhesion to cultured human dermal microvascular endothelial cells. *Kobe J
Med Sci* 42: 233–241

54   Famiglietti J, Sun J, Delisser HM, Albelda SM (1997) Tyrosine residue in exon 14 of the
cytoplasmic domain of platelet endothelial cell adhesion molecule-1 (PECAM-1/CD31)
regulates ligand binding specificity. *J Cell Biol* 138: 1425–1435

55   Duncan GS, Andrew DP, Takimoto H, Kaufman SA, Yoshida H, Spellberg J, de la
Pompa JL, Elia A, Wakeham A, Karan-Tamir B et al (1999) Genetic evidence for functional redundancy of platelet/endothelial cell adhesion molecule-1 (PECAM-1): CD31-
deficient mice reveal PECAM-1-dependent and PECAM-1-independent functions. *J
Immunol* 162: 3022–3030

Selective lymphocyte migration into secondary lymphoid organs and inflamed tissues

Mark A. Jutila

Veterinary Molecular Biology, Montana State University, Bozeman, MT 59717, USA

Introduction

An important aspect of the immune system is the delivery of lymphocytes from the blood to organs of the lymphoid system (secondary lymphoid organs) and extra-lymphoid sites of inflammation. It is in the former that most naive lymphocytes initially respond to foreign antigen. On a continual basis, most mature, naive B and T cells recirculate from the blood into secondary lymphoid organs, such as lymph nodes and Peyer's patches, and back into the blood via the lymphatics. This recirculation process provides the naive lymphocyte a mechanism to continuously access the organs of the body that collect antigen from epithelial surfaces, somatic tissues, and blood. Once lymphocytes respond to antigen, become activated, proliferate, and eventually develop into memory cells, they are thought to exhibit different trafficking behaviors, such as acquiring the increased capacity to migrate into extra-lymphoid tissues. In some instances, memory cells preferentially target and/or accumulate in certain organs. For example, it has been shown that certain lymphocyte subsets preferentially target the gut lymphoid tissues, such as Peyer's patches and lamina propria, peripheral sites, such as peripheral lymph nodes, and the inflamed skin [1–7]. In order for lymphocytes to enter a tissue, they must bind and migrate through the vascular endothelium, which involves a multi-step process regulated by specific receptor/ligand interactions. The intent of this chapter is to (1) define the interactions of lymphocytes with the vascular endothelium, (2) outline the cell types involved and briefly discuss tissue-selective lymphocyte recirculation, and (3) provide an overview of some of the molecules that are involved in tissue-selective lymphocyte trafficking.

Lymphocyte/endothelial cell interactions involved in T cell trafficking

The precise mechanisms accounting for tissue-selective accumulation of T cells are not completely understood, but likely involve interactions between the circulating

Vascular Adhesion Molecules and Inflammation, edited by J. D. Pearson lymphocyte and vascular endothelial cells lining vessels within the tissue, which will be the focus of the discussion below. Pabst and colleagues have suggested that trafficking mechanisms are a minor contributor to organ-specific migration and that tissue-selective survival is an important mechanism [8,9]. These studies suggest that lymphocyte trafficking may not account for the tissue-specific accumulation of lymphocyte subsets in all situations: however, a role for tissue selective trafficking cannot be excluded, because, for one of many reasons, tissue-restrictive adhesion molecules, which were predicted by *in vivo* and *in vitro* functional assays, have been defined at the molecular level (see discussion below).

To discuss lymphocyte trafficking, one must have an appreciation of the biological process of a cell getting out of the vascular system and into a tissue, which involves a complex series of events that leads to the recruitment of cells from the rapid flow of blood into specific tissues. Lymphocytes enter tissues via specialized postcapillary venules. In secondary lymphoid organs of humans and mice, these postcapillary venules exhibit a distinctive plump, or high, morphology and are called high endothelial venules (HEV). Lymphocytes follow at least three distinct steps in their migration through HEV, which involves (1) initial recognition of the vessel wall during blood flow (represented by capture and rolling of the lymphocyte along the vessel wall), (2) subsequent tight adhesion to endothelial cells, and, finally, (3) transendothelial migration and accumulation in the underlying tissue (Fig. 1). Endothelial cells serve as the primary substrate for capture and rolling, but *in vitro* assays have shown that immobilized platelets and neutrophils may also contribute to this event and are depicted in Figure 1 as well [10]. Importantly, initiation of rolling does not always lead to extravasation: some cells release and re-enter the circulation after initial attachment. Also, rolling interactions are not obligatory for all cells. Some "pre-activated" lymphocytes, which have increased adhesive potential, can bind and stop on the endothelium in the absence of significant rolling.

Molecularly distinct receptor/ligand interactions control each step of the extravasation process. In secondary lymphoid tissues, rolling interactions are controlled by lymphocyte adhesion molecules, which are constitutively expressed and recognize constitutively expressed ligands on endothelial cells. In inflamed tissues, rolling interactions are controlled by induced ligands on endothelial cells or immobilized cells, such as leukocytes or platelets. The transition of a rolling cell to one that tightly adheres to the endothelial cell surface is thought to be regulated by specific signaling events in the leukocyte induced by soluble activating factors (chemokines) or by the molecules involved in the rolling interaction itself. The signaling events lead to the functional upregulation of other adhesion receptors, which mediate tight binding. Different combinations of receptor/ligand pairs and different chemokines are thought to regulate constitutive, inflammation-induced, as well as tissue-selective trafficking of different lymphocyte subsets. The reader is directed to other chapters in this volume as well as reviews that outline various presentations of this model [10–15]. Direct support for this process has come from *in vitro* adhesion assays

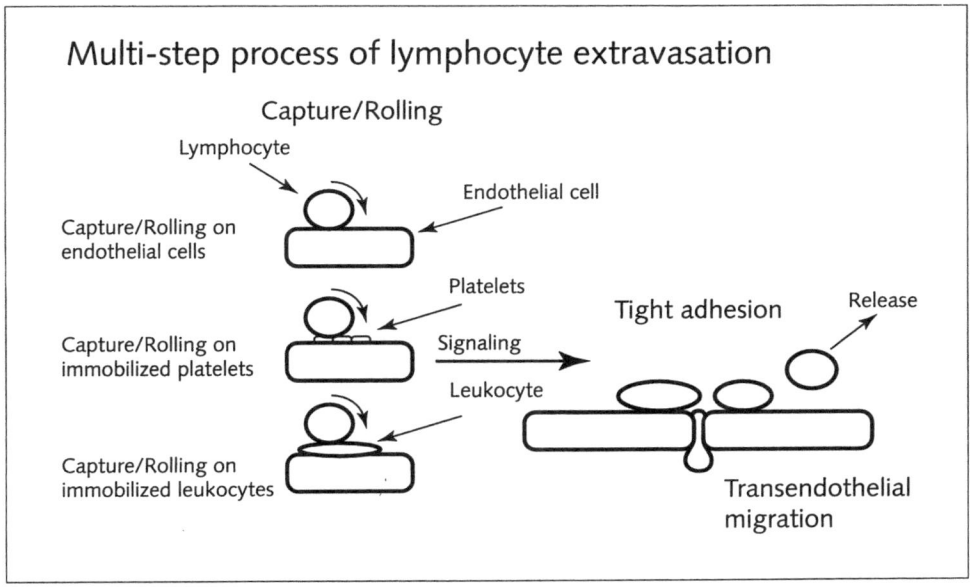

Figure 1
Multi-step process of lymphocyte extravasation. To leave the blood and enter a tissue, lymphocytes normally follow three distinct steps: 1) initial recognition of the vessel wall, which captures the leukocyte from the flow of blood and leads to a rolling interaction, 2) tight adhesion, and 3) transendothelial cell migration. Some cells do not continue with extravasation after rolling, and release back into the flow of blood. Endothelial cells are the predominant substrate for rolling, but in vitro *assays have shown that immobilized platelets and leukocytes can also participate in the capture and rolling event.*

done under physiological flow and also from intravital microscopy experiments where the interactions of lymphocytes with the vascular wall are directly examined *in vivo* [16–25].

Recirculation of naive and memory T cells

For simplicity, the discussion of lymphocyte trafficking will focus on T cells. The majority of T cells in circulation in most animals are α/β T cells, which are defined by their T cell receptor for antigen (Tcr). After export from the thymus and prior to exposure to antigen, α/β T cells exhibit a "naive" phenotype, which is defined by a number of parameters discussed below. Once naive α/β T cells encounter antigen they undergo expansion and eventually mediate some type of effector response. As this effector response subsides, the α/β T cell enters the memory T lymphocyte stage [1, 2, 3, 5]. Memory α/β T cells have the capacity for a more rapid and vigorous response to recall antigen, which then leads to the development of a second effector stage. These secondary effector cells produce large quantities of cytokines and are extremely potent immune cells [5].

Detection of different CD45 isoforms by immunofluorescence staining can be used to help distinguish naive and memory T cells in a mixed population, but the separation is not absolute. In general, naive α/β T cells express high molecular mass forms of CD45 called CD45RB in mice and CD45RA in humans. Memory α/β T cells preferentially express lower molecular mass isoforms called CD45RO [1, 5, 6]. Revertants and cells in transition complicate the identification of memory cells based solely on CD45 expression.

Of particular relevance to this chapter, naive and memory α/β T cells can also be distinguished by their expression of various adhesion molecules. Memory T cells express high levels of leukocyte integrins, such as CD11a/CD18 (LFA-1), α_4/β_1 and, on some cells, α_4/β_7. They also express high levels of CD44, a receptor for hyaluronate. In contrast, naive T cells express low levels of these adhesion molecules, but homogeneously express high levels of L-selectin [1, 3–5, 7]. After conversion to an effector/memory T lymphocyte, L-selectin is selectively downregulated on some cells [1, 4, 5]. Some memory α/β T cells, which are found in cutaneous sites of inflammation, express an adhesion molecule called cutaneous lymphocyte antigen (CLA) [4, 26–29]. Memory T cells from the gut express high levels of α_4/β_7 integrin [4, 30–32]. The altered expression of adhesion proteins is important in regulating the unique trafficking behavior of memory T cells, which will be addressed below.

Once naive T cells leave the thymus, they enter the blood where they exhibit the functional capacity to enter all secondary lymphoid tissues [1-5,33-35]. Naïve T cells are normally not found in extralymphoid sites of inflammation, however, under certain circumstances extralymphoid tissue trafficking can occur [8]. Once a naive T cell enters a secondary lymphoid organ, it responds to specific antigen, if it is present, and undergoes conversion to an effector and, eventually, a memory cell. If antigen is not encountered, the lymphocyte enters the lymphatic system and re-enters the circulation via the thoracic duct to begin the process again. Importantly, naive T cells exhibit minimal tissue preference during recirculation.

Memory and/or activated lymphocytes, as defined above, exhibit a different pattern of recirculation [1, 4, 5]. Unlike naive lymphocytes, memory T cells exhibit a unique capacity to migrate into extralymphoid tissues as well as secondary lymphoid organs [1, 4, 5, 33, 36, 37]. Indeed, memory α/β T cells are the predominant lymphocyte isolated from the lymphatics draining extralymphoid sites of inflammation, such as in the skin [1, 37]. The issue of whether memory T cells migrate into secondary lymphoid organs, such as lymph nodes, via the vascular system or simply collect there through the lymphatics has been somewhat controversial in recent

Table 1 - Lymphocyte trafficking pathways

Pathway[a]				Receptor/ligand
Blood	→ gut	→ lymphatics	→ blood	$\alpha_4\beta_7$/MAdCAM-1
				L-selectin
Blood	→ lymph node	→ lymphatics	→ blood	L-selectin/PNAd
Blood	→ skin	→ lymphatics	→ blood	E-selectin/CLA
Blood	→ inflammation	→ lymphatics	→ blood	Multiple

aThese examples represent only some of the pathways lymphocytes follow during recirculation. Lymphocytes can migrate into other sites, such as lung and spleen, whose discussion is beyond the scope of this chapter. The receptor/ligands are those defined in the context of these tissue pathways, which are predominantly involved in rolling. Other adhesion molecules also participate in the extravasation process (see text).

years [5, 9, 36–39]. Though the issue is still not completely clear, recent studies have shown that memory or activated lymphocytes have the capacity to enter secondary lymphoid organs via the vascular system [9, 36, 39]. The question remains whether memory T cells can migrate via the vascular system into secondary lymphoid organs as efficiently as naive T cells; some memory T cells likely do not, primarily due to a lack of expression of certain adhesion molecules.

Of particular relevance to this chapter, the migration of some memory or activated T cells through secondary lymphoid organs, either via the vascular bed in the specific tissue or via the draining lymphatics, exhibits tissue selectivity. Functional studies have suggested that tissue-selective lymphocyte recruitment can occur in at least three, and likely more, different sites (Tab. 1). These pathways are not mutually exclusive and many cells, particularly naive cells, have the capacity to enter into each of the sites; however, certain cell populations have been shown to be preferentially recruited to each of these tissues. For example, memory or activated T cells from mucosal tissues preferentially migrate back to mucosal sites when reinfused into the animal [1, 4, 30, 40–44]. Likewise, memory cells isolated from peripheral sites preferentially migrate back to those tissues [37, 43]. Phenotypic studies further support the existence of lymphocyte subsets which are unique to specific tissues, such as the skin [see discussion below].

It was hypothesized that the tissue-specific migration of memory T cells contributes to the efficiency of the immune response, by ensuring that cells that have previously contacted antigen in a tissue preferentially migrate back to the same tissue when they re-enter the circulation [1, 4]. In this model, after the naive T cell encounters specific antigen in a given tissue, proliferates, mediates its specific function, and becomes a memory cell, it preferentially expresses a homing phenotype for the tissue it encountered antigen in. This hypothesis has recently been tested in two different settings using human cells. In the first, it has been shown that antigen recall responses by circulating lymphocytes to rotavirus infection, a gut-specific pathogen, reside in the cells with a mucosal homing phenotype [45]. In the second study, Kantele et al. [46] showed that mucosal immunization leads to the appearance of antigen-specific cells exhibiting a mucosal homing phenotype, whereas peripheral immunization leads to the generation of antigen-specific cells with a preference for peripheral sites.

To summarize the trafficking profiles of naive and memory T cells, naive T cells constitutively recirculate through all secondary lymphoid organs via specialized post-capillary venules (see discussion below). If they encounter antigen, they proliferate, mediate their specific function, and eventually become memory T cells. These cells then acquire an increased capacity to migrate through extralymphoid tissue as well as, in many situations, retain the ability to migrate into secondary lymphoid sites via the vascular system. Some memory T cells exhibit tissue-specificity in their migration pathways. This phenomenon is thought to increase the efficiency of secondary immune responses. In the sections below, I outline three different settings where tissue-selective lymphocyte trafficking has been shown and tissue-selective adhesion molecules have been defined. A brief discussion of inflammation-associated lymphocyte trafficking is also provided. As a caveat, it is important to point out that tissue-selective trafficking is not universally accepted [8], nor are the pathways which have been defined completely separate – there is considerable overlap between them.

Adhesion molecules involved in tissue-selective lymphocyte trafficking

Though, as stated above, tissue-specific lymphocyte trafficking is not absolute, the pathways depicted in Table 1 have been described functionally and receptor/ligand adhesion interactions involved in these pathways have been characterized at the molecular level. Analysis of the expression of these various adhesion molecules is useful in gaining insight into tissue-specific immune responses (see [45, 46] for examples). Below, I describe adhesion molecules in the context of the pathways depicted in Table 1. Since inflammation is important in regulating lymphocyte trafficking into a variety of sites, adhesion molecules which may not be involved in tissue-specificity, but are important in inflammation-specific recruitment, will also be outlined.

Trafficking to peripheral lymph nodes (L-selectin/PNAd)

Both naive and memory T cells migrate from the blood through HEV and into peripheral lymph nodes. L-selectin on the circulating lymphocyte is required for this

146

pathway. L-selectin was the first lymphocyte adhesion molecule implicated in tissue-selective recirculation [33, 47–49]. Anti-L-selectin mAb almost completely block lymphocyte adhesion to high endothelial venules (HEV) in peripheral and mesenteric lymph nodes, whereas it only partially blocks adhesion to HEV in Peyer's patches [47]. *In vivo* studies using mAbs as well as experiments using L-selectin-deficient mice have clearly shown the importance of this molecule in lymphocyte traffic to peripheral lymph nodes [4, 48, 49, 50]. The *in vivo* studies also showed that L-selectin participates to a lesser extent in the accumulation of naive T cells into Peyer's patches, which will be discussed below.

L-selectin belongs to the selectin family of adhesion molecules, which also includes E- and P-selectin expressed by endothelial cells. All selectins have an N-terminal mammalian C-type lectin domain which recognizes defined carbohydrate moieties on target cells (reviewed in the chapter by Ley in this volume; see also [48, 49, 51]). L-selectin carbohydrate ligands are expressed on multiple large molecular mass glycoproteins produced by HEV in peripheral lymph nodes. Gut lymphoid tissue HEV can also express these ligands, though to a lesser extent, which accounts for L-selectin-dependent trafficking to the Peyer's patches (some of the cross-over between the gut- and peripheral-specific migration pathways mentioned above) [52, 53]. The MECA79 mAb recognizes these glycoproteins, which have been collectively called the peripheral lymph node addressin (PNAd). Two of the predominant PNAd species have been molecularly characterized: GlyCAM-1 [54] and CD34 [55, 56]. Though L-selectin binds each of these molecules, they apparently are not essential to trafficking, since GlyCAM-1 is secreted and lymphocyte homing in mice deficient in CD34 is not reduced [57]. Other large molecular mass glycoproteins of 90 kDa and 200 kDa have also been shown to bind L-selectin, which could be the essential ligands, but these molecules have not been molecularly characterized [57, 58].

As discussed above, naive α/β T cells express high levels of L-selectin which they use to enter secondary lymphoid organs. However, cutaneous lymphocyte antigen (CLA)-positive, as well as other memory α/β T cells, are also L-selectin bright [28, 48, 59, 60]. These cells likely use L-selectin in migration through lymph nodes, but they may also use it in migration to extralymphoid sites of inflammation as well. PNAd can be induced on vessels in chronically inflamed human and bovine skin, where it can potentially mediate extralymphoid, L-selectin-dependent lymphocyte recruitment ([61]; M.A. Jutila, unpublished observations). We have done limited mAb blocking experiments in calves and found that anti-L-selectin mAb block a significant portion of the migration of leukocytes into a skin lesion induced by endotoxin (M.A. Jutila, unpublished observations). Additional evidence that L-selectin is involved in the migration of T cells into inflamed skin has come from studies of L-selectin-deficient mice, where lymphocyte migration to skin during allograft rejection was shown to be reduced [50].

Though it is generally assumed that the primary role of L-selectin in mediating leukocyte extravasation is adhesion to endothelial cells, it does mediate another type of adhesive interaction which likely contributes to the magnitude of the inflammatory response. We showed in 1994 that once neutrophils become immobilized on the vascular endothelium, they can serve as the adhesive substrate for continual recruitment of newly arriving neutrophils (Fig. 1) [25]. This neutrophil/neutrophil interaction is completely blocked by anti-L-selectin mAbs [25]. One leukocyte ligand for L-selectin is P-selectin glycoprotein ligand-1 (PSGL-1) [51, 62], but antibodies that completely block PSGL-1 function only partially inhibit leukocyte-on-leukocyte rolling, suggesting that other ligands likely exist [62].

Though leukocyte-on-leukocyte rolling is accepted for neutrophils, less work as been done on lymphocytes and the importance of the interaction is unclear. Human lymphocytes can roll on monolayers of neutrophils (M.A. Jutila, unpublished observations), but results have been inconsistent in showing whether monolayers of lymphocytes can support rolling. We have shown that adherent bovine γ/δ T cells avidly support rolling interactions of other γ/δ T cells, which is completely blocked by anti-L-selectin mAb [63]. In contrast, studies by other groups have been unable to demonstrate L-selectin ligands on human peripheral blood lymphocytes [64]. However, subsets of human memory T cells express functional PSGL-1 [65]; therefore, under certain circumstances, human lymphocytes have the potential to interact with each other via L-selectin.

A series of *in vitro* and *in vivo* assays has conclusively shown that the L-selectin/PNAd interaction initiates the tethering or rolling of naive α/β T lymphocytes along HEV [24, 53, 66]. A rather striking feature of the L-selectin interaction is that it is dependent upon a threshold shear to mediate an adhesive interaction. Specifically, *in vitro* flow assays and *in vivo* intravital microscopy experiments show that L-selectin interactions occur in a defined range of shear values. If shear is too low or absent, L-selectin does not function [67]. Following L-selectin-dependent rolling, the adhesive activity of the lymphocyte is upregulated by G-protein-dependent signaling events triggered by L-selectin binding itself or by factors such as chemokines immobilized along the vessel wall [4, 22, 23]. This upregulation of adhesion involves adhesion proteins belonging to the integrin family on the lymphocyte, such as LFA-1 [68], and the Ig superfamily on the endothelium, such as intercellular adhesion molecule-1 (ICAM-1) [22, 23]. Integrins are heterodimeric proteins consisting of an α and β chain, and the family members are grouped together by the use of common β chains. In the context of lymphocytes, β_1, β_2 and β_7 integrins are important in trafficking (see [4] and also below).

Lymphocyte trafficking to Peyer's patches (α_4/β_7/MAdCAM-1)

T cells recirculate through HEV of the gut Peyer's patches and lamina propria, much like they do in peripheral lymph nodes. In contrast to peripheral lymph nodes, mucosal lymphoid tissue HEV selectively express a molecule called mucosal addressin cell adhesion molecule-1 (MAdCAM-1), which serves as a ligand for lymphocyte rolling as well as tight adhesion [69, 70]. MAdCAM-1 is a member of the immunoglobulin (Ig) superfamily and has domains similar to domains found in intercellular adhesion molecule-1 (ICAM-1) and vascular cell adhesion molecule-1 (VCAM-1). Another interesting feature of MAdCAM-1 is that it also has a region that can be decorated by PNAd carbohydrate structures [69, 70]. PNAd expression appears restricted to MAdCAM-1 in the Peyer's patch, where naive T cells are recruited, whereas MAdCAM-1 in the lamina propria lacks PNAd, where large numbers of memory cells are found. Thus, MAdCAM-1 has the potential of interacting with multiple receptors on the surface of different lymphocyte subsets.

· α_4/β_7 on naive and memory lymphocytes is one of the major counterreceptors for MAdCAM-1 expressed either in the Peyer's patches or lamina propria. This integrin was originally defined as a mucosal homing receptor and given the name lymphocyte Peyer's patch adhesion molecule (LPAM) [71]. α_4/β_7 is expressed at moderate levels on naive T cells, sufficient to mediate interactions with MAdCAM-1 [4, 22]. On the other hand, α_4/β_7 is expressed at high levels on memory cells, particularly those stimulated in the gut [45]. The higher levels lead to a more avid interaction with MAdCAM-1, which is characterized by both rolling and tight adhesion [4, 22, 72, 73]. α_4/β_7 can also bind vascular cell adhesion molecule-1 (VCAM-1), but this interaction is not important in mucosal homing [74].

L-selectin can also serve as a receptor for MAdCAM-1, but only for MAdCAM-1 in the Peyer's patch, which is decorated by PNAd [22, 70]. In this setting, L-selectin and α_4/β_7 act cooperatively in mediating homing of naive T cells to the Peyer's patches, which was shown in intravital microscopy experiments [22]. This is another direct illustration that tissue-selective adhesion systems that have been defined do show overlap.

Lymphocyte trafficking to inflamed skin (E-selectin/CLA)

Most discussions of tissue-selective lymphocyte trafficking focus on peripheral lymph nodes and gut lymphoid tissues. However, studies have shown that skin is also an important lymphoid tissue and may constitute another site of tissue-selective trafficking of memory T cells. Though many inducible endothelial cell adhesion proteins have been shown on skin vessels and likely contribute to the recruitment of cells to this site, E-selectin has been suggested to be uniquely involved in the recruitment of skin-specific memory T cells. E-selectin, another member of the selectin family, is upregulated on endothelial cells by inflammatory mediators, such as TNFα or IL-1 [48, 49, 51]. E-selectin was originally defined as a myeloid cell adhesion molecule, but in 1990 two different groups showed that subsets of human memory T cells avidly bind E-selectin [27, 75]. Later it was shown that E-selectin supports rolling interactions of human memory T cells and bovine γ/δ T cells [16–19].

Functional and immunohistological studies suggest that E-selectin is uniquely involved in the traffic of T cell subsets into the skin. Though E-selectin can be found in multiple tissues and sites of T cell accumulation [26, 27, 76, 77], immunohistological studies suggest that skin is a predominant site for expression [26, 27]. We have done extensive immunohistological analysis of E-selectin in calves and have found similar results: E-selectin is commonly found in inflamed skin and lymph nodes draining inflamed skin, but is rare in gut associated tissues (M.A. Jutila, unpublished observations). *In vivo* studies also support a role for E-selectin in skin. For example, anti-E-selectin mAbs block the migration of α/β and γ/δ T cells into delayed-type hypersensitivity (DTH) reactions induced by phytohaemaglutinin (PHA) in pigs [34, 78, 79]. E-selectin has been shown to be important in directing cells to DTH reactions in primates [80]. Lymphocyte (Th1 cytokine producing T helper cells) migration into inflamed mouse skin can also be blocked by anti-E-selectin mAbs [81]. A mAb directed against both L-selectin and E-selectin blocks the migration of bovine γ/δ T cells into acute dermal lesions induced by lipopolysaccharide (LPS) (M.A. Jutila, unpublished observations). Gene knockout mice have also supported an important role for E-selectin in directing T cell migration to chronic inflammation associated with DTH reactions [82].

E-selectin recognizes specific carbohydrate structures expressed on either glycoproteins or glycolipids on the surface of the T cell. Picker and colleagues showed that cutaneous lymphocyte associated (CLA) antigen, which is preferentially expressed by T cells that accumulate in diverse inflammatory reactions in the skin [26], comprises a group of glycoproteins that support E-selectin binding [83]. CLA is recognized by the HECA 452 monoclonal antibody. The HECA 452 epitope has been shown to be a specific carbohydrate moeity, suggested to be the site or close to the site bound by E-selectin. In peripheral blood and appendix, CLA is found on only a small subset of memory cells. It is not found on memory T cells from the gut, but can be found on > 50% of the memory cells from peripheral lymph nodes, particularly those draining cutaneous sites. Interestingly, all CLA positive T cells are also L-selectin positive [28, 29].

Recently, two different groups have suggested that PSGL-1 is CLA on human and mouse T cells [84, 85]. PSGL-1 is a 230 kDa glycoprotein under non-reducing conditions, comprised of two identical monomers covalently bound by disulfide bonds. PSGL-1 is expressed by all blood leukocytes and when appropriately modified by specific carbohydrates can mediate selectin-dependent binding. Though PSGL-1 can likely interact with E-selectin, it is unclear whether it represents the only glycoprotein ligand on human T cells and whether it comprises all of the CLA molecular species. For example, function blocking anti-PSGL-1 mAbs have little or no effect on E-selectin-dependent adhesion [49]. In western blot analyses, HECA 452 recognizes multiple bands in lysates of peripheral blood lymphocytes, with two prominent bands at 200 kDa and 125 kDa [26]. Using a recombinant E-selectin/Ig chimera we have shown that E-selectin can precipitate ligands of 200 kDa and

130 kDa from human lymphocytes [86]. In co-precipitation experiments, we show that PSGL-1 can account for a portion of the 200 kDa smear, but not the 130 kDa band (M.A. Jutila, unpublished observations). Thus, PSGL-1 is likely one CLA glycoprotein, but others also exist.

Inflammation-associated lymphocyte trafficking

Though lymphocytes constitutively migrate into certain tissues on a continual basis, inflammatory signals dramatically increase the magnitude of migration. Inflammation can occur in all tissues, including secondary lymphoid organs. A number of different adhesion receptor/ligand pairs have been shown to be important in inflammation-associated lymphocyte recruitment. In many situations, these molecules function cooperatively with the tissue-selective molecules outlined above, but can also mediate interactions directly. Here I discuss additional adhesion molecules which regulate lymphocyte trafficking, but unlike L-selectin/PNAd, α_4/β_7/MAd-CAM-1, and E-selectin/CLA, they have not been directly implicated in tissue-selective recruitment.

The third member of the selectin family, P-selectin, is also involved in the recruitment of T cells into extralymphoid sites of inflammation. Like E-selectin, P-selectin is expressed by inflamed endothelial cells, but it can also be expressed by platelets [49, 51]. It is stored in granules of both cell types and can be rapidly translocated to the cell surface, where it mediates adhesion by binding specific carbohydrates on target cells. Subsets of memory T cells and other T cells, such as γ/δ T cells, bind P-selectin [16–18, 65]. A major difference between E- and P-selectin is that the binding to P-selectin does not correlate with CLA expression on lymphocytes [16, 17]. Furthermore, P-selectin is found on vessels in a greater number of tissues than E-selectin; thus, it has the potential of regulating a greater array of inflammatory reactions. Antibody blocking studies in mice have shown that the migration of Th1 T cells into inflamed skin is blocked by anti-P-selectin mAbs [81]. Similar findings in the skin have also been shown in other studies [87]. Studies using gene knockout mice have also supported a role for P-selectin in regulating T cell migration into DTH reactions in mouse skin [82].

As described above, PSGL-1 is the P-selectin ligand expressed on T cells [51, 65]. Unlike the E-selectin interaction, it is clear that PSGL-1 is the major if not only P-selectin glycoprotein ligand on T cells. PSGL-1 contains a mucin domain, which is a region of densely clustered O-linked sialylated carbohydrates that is sensitive to O-sialoglycoprotease treatments [51]. O-sialoglycoprotease treatment of T cells blocks their binding to P-selectin [16,17]. Furthermore, using P-selectin/Ig chimeras we can precipitate PSGL-1 from T cell detergent lysates and show that an anti-PSGL-1 mAb blocks T cell binding to P-selectin (M.A. Jutila, unpublished observations).

Another very important inflammation-associated adhesion system of relevance to T cells is the α_4/β_1/VCAM-1 interaction [4, 88–95]. Indeed, a search of literature databases on VCAM-1 reveals publications numbering in the thousands; however, here I only briefly outline characteristics of this adhesive interaction. VCAM-1/α_4/β_1 interactions are generally restricted to mononuclear cells, though recent studies suggest that neutrophils in some animals may also use this pathway [96]. VCAM-1 is expressed on endothelial cells in a variety of different inflammatory lesions where it avidly supports T cell binding via α_4/β_1 [4, 92]. A requisite for this interaction is high expression of α_4/β_1 on the T cell, which is a common feature of memory cells [4, 92]. The α_4/β_1/VCAM-1 interaction can result in selectin-independent lymphocyte rolling as well as supporting tight adhesion [4, 93]. Since α_4/β_1 is expressed at high levels on most, if not all, memory T cells, selective inhibition of memory T cell subset migration most likely cannot be accomplished by targeting this interaction. It would be predicted that far more general effects on T cell migration would be achieved. Indeed, this has been shown *in vivo*. α_4/β_1/VCAM-1 interactions are important in psoriasis [97] and other cutaneous inflammatory lesions [95]. One of the more impressive *in vivo* effects of blocking this interaction has been shown in the brain, where antibodies against α_4/β_1 prevent experimental autoimmune encephalomyelitis [94].

There are many other receptor/ligand interactions involved in lymphocyte trafficking. The interactions of CD11a/CD18 (LFA-1) with ICAM-1, ICAM-2, and/or ICAM-3 are critical in both constitutive and inflammation-induced trafficking of T cells [98]. Vascular adhesion protein-1 (VAP-1) is another adhesion molecule thought to be important in regulating T cell traffic into some inflammatory lesions [99]. Functional analyses and other studies of adhesion molecule expression on memory T cells suggests that other undefined adhesion molecules exist. For example, memory T cells from inflamed lung lack L-selectin and CLA, suggesting they use other adhesion systems to enter this tissue [28]. Jones et al. have shown that T cell rolling on 24 h *in vitro* stimulated endothelial cells is independent of the known adhesion proteins [100]. We have recently shown that γ/δ T cell rolling on 24 h cytokine activated endothelial cells is not blocked by anti-E-selectin or -L-selectin mAbs and may involve a previously undescribed molecule [101]. Finally, interactions between lymphocyte and the extracellular matrix as well as transendothelial cell migration involve adhesion molecules which have not been discussed here.

Conclusion

Lymphocyte migration into tissues is essential for effective immune responses against various infectious pathogens. Though naive T cells can recirculate through most tissues, some lymphocytes (memory cells) follow tissue-selective and/or inflammation-associated pathways. The selective accumulation of certain T cell subsets into given non-inflamed and inflamed tissues is a fascinating aspect of the mammalian immune system which is conserved in animals as diverse as mice, sheep, cows, and humans. Adhesion proteins expressed by endothelial cells lining venules in tissues and the circulating lymphocyte contribute to the specificity of the lymphocyte trafficking response, though other mechanisms, such as tissue-selective survival, most likely are involved as well. Understanding the molecular mechanism contributing to tissue-specific lymphocyte recruitment may give insight to better methods of stimulating tissue-specific immune responses.

Ackowledgements

Helpful and critical comments of Kemal Aydintug and Jeff Leid are greatly appreciated. Some of the work summarized here was supported by grants from USDA NRI 96-35204-3580, NIH 1RO1 AI41671-01, and the Montana Agricultural Experiment Station.

References

1   Mackay CR (1993) Homing of naive, memory and effector lymphocytes. *Curr Opin Immunol* 5: 423–427

2   Mackay CR (1991) T-cell memory: the connection between function, phenotype and migration pathways. *Immunol Today* 12: 189–192

3   Bradley LM, Watson SR (1996) Lymphocyte migration into tissue: the paradigm derived from CD4 subsets. *Curr Opin Immunol* 8: 312–320

4   Butcher EC, Picker LJ (1996) Lymphocyte homing and homeostasis. *Science* 272, 60–66

5   Swain SL, Croft M, Dubey C, Haynes L, Rogers P, Zhang X, Bradley LM (1996) From naive to memory T cells. *Immunol Rev* 150: 143–167

6   LaSalle JM, Hafler DA (1991) The coexpression of CD45RA and CD45RO isoforms on T cells during the S/G2/M stages of cell cycle. *Cell Immunol* 138: 197–206

7   Mackay CR, Imhof BA (1993) Cell adhesion molecules in the immune system. *Immunol Today* 14: 99–102

8   Westermann J, Pabst R (1996) How organ-specific is the migration of "naive" and "memory" T cells? *Immunol Today* 17: 278–282

9   Bode U, Wonigeit K, Pabst R, Westermann J (1997) The fate of activated T cells migrating through the body: rescue from apoptosis in the tissue of origin. *Eur J Immunol* 27: 2087–2093

10   Jutila MA (1997) Recruitment of γ/δ T cells and other T cell subsets to sites of inflammation. In: C Serhan, P Ward (ed): *Molecular and Cellular Basis of Inflammation*. Humana Press, Totawa, 193–214

11   Butcher EC (1991) Leukocyte-endothelial cell recognition: Three (or more) steps to specificity and diversity. *Cell* 67: 1033–1036

12   Zimmerman G A, Prescott SM, McIntyre TM (1992) Endothelial cell interactions with granulocytes: Tethering and signaling molecules. *Immunol Today* 13: 93–100

13   Springer TA (1994) Traffic signals for lymphocyte recirculation and leukocyte emigration: The multistep paradigm. *Cell* 76: 301–314

14   Kishimoto TK (1991) A dynamic model for neutrophil localization to inflammatory sites. *J NIH Res* 3: 75–77

15   Jutila MA (1997) Leukocyte trafficking. In: DA Lawrence (ed): *Comprehensive toxicology*, vol 5. Elsevier, New York, 201–214

16   Jutila MA, Bargatze RF, Kurk S, Warnock RA, Ehsani N, Watson S, Walcheck B (1994) Cell surface P- and E-selectin support shear-dependent rolling of bovine γ/δ T cells. *J Immunol* 153: 3917–3928

17   Alon R, Rossiter H, Wang X, Springer TA, Kupper TS (1994) Distinct cell surface ligands mediate T lymphocyte attachment and rolling on P- and E-selectin under physiological flow. *J Cell Biol* 127: 1485–1495

18   Lichtman AH, Ding H, Henault L, Vachino G, Camphausen R, Cumming D, Luscinskas FW (1997) CD45RA-RO+ (memory) but not CD45RA+RO– (naive) T cells roll efficiently on E- and P-selectin and vascular cell adhesion molecule-1 under flow. *J Immunol* 158: 3640–3650

19   Jones DA, McIntire LV, Smith CW, Picker LJ (1994) A two-step adhesion cascade for T cell/endothelial cell interactions under flow conditions. *J Clin Invest* 94: 2443–2450

20   Luscinskas FW, Ding H, Lichtman AH (1995) P-selectin and vascular cell adhesion molecule-1 mediate rolling and arrest, respectively, of CD4$^+$ T lymphocytes on tumor necrosis factor alpha-activated vascular endothelium under flow. *J Exp Med* 181: 1179–1186

21   Diavcoc-TG, Roth SJ, Morita CT, Rosat JP, Brenner MB, Springer TA (1996) Interactions of human alpha/beta and gamma/delta T lymphocyte subsets in shear flow with E-selectin and P-selectin. *J Exp Med* 183: 1193–1203

22   Bargatze RF, Jutila MA, Butcher EC (1995) Distinct roles for L-selectin, α4 integrin, and LFA-1 in lymphocyte interactions with HEV *in situ*: the multi-step model confirmed and refined. *Immunity* 3: 99–108

23   Bargatze RF, Butcher EC (1993) Rapid G protein-regulated activation event involved in lymphocyte binding to high endothelial venules. *J Exp Med* 178: 367–372

24   Warnock RA, Skari S, Butcher EC, von Andrian UH (1998) Molecular mechanisms of lymphocyte homing to peripheral lymph nodes. *J Exp Med* 187: 205–216

25   Bargatze RF, Kurk S, Butcher EC, Jutila MA (1994) Neutrophils roll on adherent neutrophils bound to cytokine-stimulated endothelium via L-selectin on the rolling cells. *J Exp Med* 180: 1785–1792

26   Picker LJ, Michie SA, Rott LS, Butcher EC (1990) A unique phenotype of skin-associated lymphocytes in humans: Preferential expression of the HECA-452 epitope by benign and malignant T cells at cutaneous sites. *Am J Pathol* 136: 1053–1068

27   Picker LJ, Kishimoto TK, Smith CW, Warnock RA, Butcher EC (1991) ELAM-1 is an adhesion molecule for skin-homing T cells. *Nature* 349: 796–799

28   Picker LJ, Martin RJ, Trumble A, Newman LS, Collins PA, Bergstresser PR, Leung DYM (1994) Differential expression of lymphocyte homing receptors by human memory/effector T cells in pulmonary versus cutaneous immune effector sites. *Eur J Immunol* 24: 1269–1277

29   Picker LJ, Treer JR, Ferguson-Darnell B, Collins PA, Bergstresser PR, Terstappen LWMM (1993) Control of lymphocyte recirculation in man II Differential regulation of the cutaneous lymphocyte-associated antigen, a tissue-selective homing receptor for skin homing T cells. *J Immunol* 150: 1122–1136

30   Abitorabi MA, Mackay CR, Jerome EH, Osorio O, Butcher EC, Erle DJ (1996) Differential expression of homing molecules on recirculating lymphocytes from sheep gut, peripheral, and lung lymph. *J Immunol* 156: 3111–3117

31   Farsted IN, Halstensen TS, Kvale D, Fausa O, Brandtzaeg P (1997) Topographic distribution of homing receptors on B and T cells in human gut-associated lymphoid tissue: relation of L-selectin and integrin alpha 4 beta 7 to naive and memory phenotypes. *Am J Pathol* 150: 187–199

32   Rott LS, Briskin MJ, Andrew DP, Berg EL, Butcher EC (1996) A fundamental subdivision of circulating lymphocytes defined by adhesion to mucosal addressin cell adhesion molecule-1   Comparison with vascular cell adhesion molecule-1 and correlation with beta 7 integrins and memory differentiation. *J Immunol* 156: 3727–3736

33   Picker LJ, Butcher EC (1992) Physiological and molecular mechanisms of lymphocyte homing. *Ann Rev Immunol* 10: 561–591

34   Binns RM, Whyte A, License ST (1996) Constitutive and inflammatory lymphocyte trafficking. *Vet Immunol Immunopath* 54: 97–104

35   Girard JP, Springer TA (1995) High endothelial venules (HEVs): specialized endothelium for lymphocyte migration. *Immunol Today* 16: 449–457

36   Williams MB, Butcher EC (1997) Homing of naive and memory T lymphocyte subsets to Peyer's patches, lymph nodes and spleen. *J Immunol* 159: 1746–1752

37   Mackay CR, Marston W, Dudler L (1992) Altered patterns of T cell migration through lymph nodes and skin following antigen challenge. *Eur J Immunol* 22: 2205–2210

38   Bradley LM, Arkins GG, Swain SL (1992) Long-term CD4+ memory T cells from the spleen lack MEL-14, the lymph node homing receptor. *J Immunol* 148: 324–331

39   Westermann J, Geismar U, Sponholz A, Bode U, Sparshott SM, Bell EB (1997) CD4+ T cells of both the naive and memory phenotype enter rat lymph nodes and Peyer's patches via high endothelial venules: within the tissue their migratory behavior differs. *Eur J Immunol* 27: 3174–3181

40   Mackay CR, MarstonWL, Dudler L (1990) Naive and memory T cells show distinct pathways of lymphocyte recirculation. *J Exp Med* 171: 801–817

41   Cahill RN, Poskitt DC, Frost DC, Trnka Z (1977) Two distinct pools of recirculating T lymphocytes: migratory characteristics of nodal and intestinal T lymphocytes. *J Exp Med* 130: 1427–1451

42 Ottaway CA, Husband AJ (1994) The influence of neuroendocrine pathways on lymphocyte migration. *Immunol Today* 15: 511–517

43 Hall JG, Hopkins J, Orlans E (1977) Studies of the lymphocytes in sheep II Destination of lymph-borne immunoblasts in relation to their tissue of origin. *Eur. J Immunol* 7: 30–37

44 Chin W, Hay JB (1980) A comparison of lymphocyte migration through intestinal lymph nodes, subcutaneous lymph nodes, and chronic inflammatory sites of sheep. *Gastroenterology* 79: 1231–1242

45 Rott LS, Rose JR, Bass D, Williams MB, Greenberg HB, Butcher EC (1997) Expression of mucosal homing receptors α4/β7 by circulating CD4⁺ cells will memory for intestinal rotavirus. *J Clin Invest* 100: 1204–1208

46 Kantele A, Kantele JM, Savilaht E, Westerholm M, Arvilommi H, Lazarovits A, Butcher EC, Makela PH (1997) Homing potentials of circulating lymphocytes in humans depend on the site of activation. Oral, but not parenteral, typhoid vaccination induces circulating antibody-secreting cells that all bear homing receptors directing them to the gut. *J Immunol* 158: 574–579

47 Gallatin WM, Weissman IL, Butcher EC (1983) A cell surface molecule involved in organ-specific homing of lymphocytes. *Nature* 304: 30–34

48 Tedder TF, Steeber DA, Chen A, Engel P (1995) The selectins: vascular adhesion molecules. *FASEB J* 9: 866–873

49 Kansas GS (1996) Selectins and their ligands: Current concepts and controversies. *Blood* 88: 3259–3287

50 Tang ML, Hale LP, Steeber DA, Tedder TF (1997) L-selectin is involved in lymphocyte migration to sites of inflammation in the skin: delayed rejection of allografts in L-selectin-deficient mice. *J Immunol* 158: 5191–5199

51 McEver RP, Cummings RD (1997) Role of PSGL-1 binding to selectins in leukocyte recruitment. *J Clin Invest* 100: 485–492

52 Streeter PR, Rouse BTN, Butcher EC (1988) Immunologic and functional characterization of a vascular addressin involved in lymphocyte homing into peripheral lymph nodes. *J Cell Biol* 107: 1853–1862

53 Berg EL, Robinson MK, Warnock RA, Butcher EC (1991) The human peripheral lymph node vascular addressin is a ligand for LECAM-1, the peripheral lymph node homing receptor. *J Cell Biol* 114: 343–349

54 Lasky LA, Singer MS, Dowbenko D, Imai Y, Henzel WJ, Grimley C, Fennie C, Gillett N, Watson SR, Rosen SD (1992) An endothelial ligand for the lymphocyte homing receptor. *Cell* 69: 927–938

55 Baumheuter S Singer, MS Henzel, W Renz, M Rosen, SD, Lasky L (1993) Binding of L-selectin to the vascular sialomucin, CD34. *Science* 262: 436–438

56 Puri KD, Finger EB, Gaudernack G, Springer TA (1995) Sialomucin CD34 is the major L-selectin ligand in human tonsil high endothelial venules. *J Cell Biol* 131: 261–270

57 Suzuki A, Andrew DP, Gonzalo JA, Fukumoto M, Spellberg J, Hashiyama M, Takimoto H, Gerwin N, Webb I, Molinex G et al (1996) CD34-deficient mice have reduced

eosinophil accumulation after allergen exposure and show a novel crossreactive 90-kD protein. *Blood* 87: 3550–3562

58   Hoke D, Mebius RE, Dybdal N, Dowbenko D, Gribling P, Kyle C, Baumhueter S, Watson SR (1995) Selective modulation of the expression of L-selectin ligands by an immune response. *Curr Biol* 5: 670–678

59   Tedder TF, Matsuyama T, Rothstein D, Schlossman SF, Morimoto C (1990) Human antigen-specific memory T cells express the homing receptor (LAM-1) necessary for lymphocyte recirculation. *Eur J Immunol* 20: 1351–1355

60   Picker LJ, Treer JR, Ferguson-Darnell B, Collins PA, Buck D, Terstappen LWMM (1993) Control of lymphocyte recirculation in man I Differential regulation of the peripheral lymph node homing receptor L-selectin on T cells during virgin to memory cell transition. *J Immunol* 150: 1105–1121

61   Michie SA, StreeterPR, Bolt PA, Butcher EC, Picker LJ (1993) The human peripheral lymph node vascular addressin: An inducible endothelial antigen involved in lymphocyte homing. *Am J Pathol* 143: 1688–1698

62   Walcheck B, Moore KL, McEver RP, Kishimoto TK (1996) Neutrophil-neutrophil interactions under hydrodynamic shear stress involve L-selectin and PSGL-1. A mechanism that amplifies initial leukocyte accumulation on P-selectin *in vitro*. *J Clin Invest* 98: 1081–1087

63   Jutila MA, Kurk S (1996) Analysis of bovine γ/δ T cell interactions with E-, P-, and L-selectin: Characterization of lymphocyte on lymphocyte rolling and the effects of O-glycoprotease. *J Immunol* 156: 289–296

64   Alon R, Fuhlbrigge RC, Finger EB, Springer TA (1996) Interactions through L-selectin between leukocytes and adherent leukocytes nucleate rolling adhesions on selectins and VCAM-1 in shear flow. *J Cell Biol* 135: 849–865

65   Moore KL, Thompson LF (1992) P-selectin (CD62) binds to subpopulations of human memory T lymphocytes and natural killer cells. *Biochem Biophys Res Comm* 186: 173–181

66   von Andrian UH (1996) Intravital microscopy of the peripheral lymph node microcirculation in mice. *Microcirculation* 3: 287–300

67   Finger EB, Puri KD, Alon R, Lawrence MB, von Andrian UH, Springer TA (1996) Adhesion through L-selectin requires a threshold hydrodynamic shear. *Nature* 379: 266–269

68   Hamann A, Jablonski-Westrich D, Duijvestijn A, Butcher EC, Baisch H, Harder R, Thiele H-G (1988) Evidence for an accessory role of LFA-1 in lymphocyte-high endothelium interaction during homing. *J Immunol* 140: 693–699

69   Briskin MJ McEvoy LM, Butcher EC (1993) MAdCAM-1 has homology to immunoglobin and mucin-like adhesion receptors and to IgA1. *Nature* 363: 461–464

70   Berg EL, McEvoy LM, Berlin C, Bargatze RF, Butcher EC (1993) L-selectin-mediated lymphocyte rolling on MAdCAM-1. *Nature* 366: 695–698

71   Hu MC, Crowe DT, Weissman IL, Holzmann B (1992) Cloning and expression of mouse integrin βp (β7): a functional role in Peyer's patch-specific lymphocyte homing. *Proc Natl Acad Sci* 89: 8254–8258

72   Berlin C, Berg EL, Briskin MJ, Andrew D, Kilshaw PJ, Holzmann B, Weissman IL,
      Hamann A, Butcher EC (1993) α4/β7 integrin mediates lymphocye binding to the
      mucosal vascular addressin MAdCAM-1. *Cell* 74: 185–195

73   Hamann A, Andrew DP, Jablonski-Westrich D, Holzmann B, Butcher EC (1994) Role
      of alpha 4-integrins in lymphocyte homing to mucosal tissues *in vivo*. *J Immunol* 152:
      3282–3293

74   Hahne M, Lenter M, Jager U, Isenmann S, Vestweber D (1993) VCAM-1 is not
      involved in LPAM-1 (apha 4 beta p/alpha 4 beta 7) mediated binding of lymphoma cells
      to high endothelial venules of mucosa-associated lymph nodes. *Eur J Cell Biol* 61:
      290–298

75   Shimizu Y, Shaw S, Graber N, Gopal TV, Horgan KJ, van Seventer GA, Newman W
      (1991) Activation-independent binding of human memory T cells to adhesion molecule
      ELAM-1. *Nature* 349: 799–803

76   Walcheck B, Watts G, Jutila MA (1993) Bovine gamma/delta T cells bind E-selectin via
      a novel glycoprotein receptor: First characterization of a lymphocyte/E-selectin interac-
      tion in an animal model. *J Exp Med* 178: 853–863

77   Kohem CL, Brezinschek RI, Wisbey H, Tortorella C, Lipsky PE, Oppenheimer-Marks N
      (1996) Enrichment of differentiated CD45RBdim, CD27- memory T cells in the periph-
      eral blood, synovial fluid, and synovial tissue of patients with rheumatoid arthritis.
      Arthritis Rheum 39: 844–854

78   Whyte A, License ST, Robinson MK, vanderLienden K (1996) Lymphocyte subsets and
      adhesion molecules in cutaneous inflammation induced inflammatory agonists: corre-
      lation between E-selectin and gamma/delta TcR+ lymphocytes. *Lab Invest* 75:
      439–449

79   Binns RM, Whyte A, License ST, Harrison AA, Tsang YT, Haskard DO, Robinson MK
      (1996) The role of E-selectin in lymphocyte and polymorphonuclear cell recruitment
      into cutaneous delayed hypersensitivity reactions in sensitized pigs. *J Immunol* 157:
      4094–4099

80   Silber A, Newman W, Sasseville VG, Pauley D, Beall D, Walsh DG, Ringler D J (1994)
      Recruitment of lymphocytes during cutaneous delayed hypersensitivity in nonhuman
      primates is dependent on E-selectin and vascular cell adhesion molecule 1. *J Clin Invest*
      93: 1554–1563

81   Austrup F, Vestweber D, Borges E, Lohning M, Brauer R, Herz U, Renz H, Hallmann
      R, Scheffold A, Radbruch A, Hamann A (1997) P- and E-selectin mediate recruitment
      of T-helper-1 but not T-helper-2 cells into inflamed tissues. *Nature* 385: 81–83

82   Staite ND, Justen JM, Sly LM, Beaudet AL, Bullard DC (1996) Inhibition of delayed-
      type contact hypersensitivity in mice deficient in both E-selectin and P-selectin. *Blood*
      88: 2973–2979

83   Berg EL, Yoshino T, Rott LS, Robinson MK, Warnock RA, Kishimoto TK, Picker LJ,
      Butcher EC (1991) The cutaneous lymphocyte antigen is a skin lymphocyte homing
      receptor for the vascular lectin endothelial cell-leukocyte adhesion molecule 1. *J Exp
      Med* 174: 1461–1466

84 Borges E, Tietz W, Steegmaier M, Moll T, Hallmann R, Hamann A, Vestweber D (1997) P-selectin glycoprotein-1 (PSGL-1) on T helper 1 but not on T helper 2 cells binds to P-selectin and supports migration into inflamed skin. *J Exp Med* 185: 573–578

85 Fuhlbrigge RC, Kieffer JD, Armerding D, Kupper TS (1997) Cutaneous lymphocyte antigen is a specialized form of PSGL-1 expressed on skin-homing T cells. *Nature* 389: 978–981

86 Jones W, Watts G, Robinson M, Vestweber D, Jutila MA (1997) Comparison of E-selectin binding glycoprotein ligands on human lymphocytes and neutrophils, and bovine gamma/delta T cells. *J Immunol* 159: 3574–3583

87 Tipping PG, Huang XR, Berndt MC, Holdsworth SR (1996) P-selectin directs T lymphocyte-mediated injury in delayed-type hypersensitivity responses: studies in glomerulonephritis and cutaneous delayed-type hypersensitivity. *Eur J Immunol* 26: 454–460

88 Newham P, Craig SE, Seddon GN, Schofield NR, Rees A, Edwards RM, Jones EY, Humphries MJ (1997) Alpha4 integrin binding interfaces on VCAM-1 and MAdCAM-1 Integrin binding sites that play a role in integrin specificity. *J Biol Chem* 272: 19429–19440

89 Groves RW, Ross EL, Barker JNWN, MacDonald DM (1993) Vascular cell adhesion molecule-1: Expression in normal and diseased skin and regulation *in vivo* by interferon gamma. *J Am Acad Dermatol* 29: 67–72

90 Abe Y, Sugisaki K, Dannenberg AM Jr (1996) Rabbit vascular endothelial adhesion molecules: ELAM-1 is most elevated in acute inflammation, whereas VCAM-1 and ICAM-1 predominate in chronic inflammation. *J Leuk Biol* 60: 692–703

91 Greenwood J, Wang Y, Calder VL (1995) Lymphocyte adhesion and transendothelial migration in the central nervous system: the role of LFA-1, ICAM-1, VLA-4, and VCAM-1. *Immunol* 86: 408–415

92 Picker LJ (1994) Control of lymphocyte homing. *Current Opin Immunol* 6: 394–406

93 Berlin C R, Bargatze RF, Campbell JJ, von Andrian UH, Szabo MC, Hasslen SR, Nelson RD, Berg EL, Erlandsen SL, Butcher EC (1995) α4 integrins mediate lymphocyte attachment and rolling under physiologic flow. *Cell* 80: 413–422

94 Yednock TA, Cannon C, Fritz LC, Sanchez-Madrid F, Steinman L, Karin N (1992) Prevention of experimental autoimmune encephalomyelitis by antibodies against alpha 4 beta 1 integrin. *Nature* 356: 63–66

95 Hakugawa J, Bae SJ, Tanaka Y, Katayama I (1997) The inhibitory effect of anti-adhesion molecule antibodies on eosinophil infiltration in cutaneous late phase response in Balb/c mice sensitized with ovalbumin. *J Dermatol* 24: 73–79

96 Reinhardt PH, Elliot JF, Kubes P (1997) Neutrophils can adhere via alpha4beta1-integrin under flow conditions. *Blood* 89: 3837–3846

97 Wakita H, Takigawa M (1994) E-selectin and vascular cell adhesion molecule-1 are critical for initial trafficking of helper-inducer/memory T cells in psoriatic plaques. *Arch Dermatol* 130: 457–463

98   Hogg N, Berlin C (1995) Structure and function of adhesion receptors in leukocyte trafficking. *Immunol Today* 16: 327–330
99   Arvilommi AM, Salmi M, Kalimo K, Jalkanen S (1996) Lymphocyte binding to vascular endothelium in inflamed skin revisited: a central role for vascular adhesion protein-1 (VAP-1). *Eur J Immunol* 26: 825–833
100   Jones DA, Smith CW, Picker LJ, McIntire LV (1996) Neutrophil adhesion to 24-hour IL-1 stimulated endothelial cells under flow conditions. *J Immunol* 157: 858–863
101   Jutila MA, Wilson E, Kurk S (1997) Identification and characterization of an adhesion molecule that mediates leukocyte rolling on 24-hour cytokine stimulated bovine endothelial cells under flow conditions. *J Exp Med* 186: 1701–1711

Oxidation-reduction sensitive regulation of vascular inflammatory gene expression

Xi-Lin Chen[1] and Russell M. Medford[1,2]

[1]Division of Cardiology, Department of Medicine, Emory University School of Medicine, Atlanta, GA 30322, USA;
[2]AtheroGenics, Inc., 8995 Westside Parkway, Alpharetta, GA 30004, USA

Introduction

Reactive oxygen species (ROS) have been implicated in the pathogenesis of a variety of diseases. Increased production of ROS is responsible for tissue damage during inflammation. Inflammatory cells such as neutrophils and macrophages play an important role in host defense, but may also contribute to tissue injury through the release of tissue damaging oxidants upon activation. Recently, however, it has been evident that production of ROS also occurs, although on a smaller scale, in non-phagocytic cells, such as fibroblasts, endothelial cells and smooth muscle cells. Under these condition, ROS play a role in signal transduction processes such as cell growth and posttranslational modification of proteins. It is now apparent that oxidants, antioxidants and other determinants of the intracellular reduction-oxidation (redox) state play an important role in the regulation of gene expression [1, 2].

Atherosclerosis is a chronic inflammatory disease characterized by early infiltration of monocytes into the arterial blood vessel wall. Recent studies suggest that intracellular ROS may serve as regulatory signals that modulate expression of inflammatory genes involved in early atherosclerosis [1, 3]. Consistent with this notion, activation of vascular cell adhesion molecule-1 (VCAM-1) and monocyte chemoattractant protein-1 (MCP-1) gene expression by diverse inflammatory signals occurs through a redox-sensitive mechanism that involves activation of redox-sensitive transcription factors such as nuclear factor κB (NF-κB) [4, 5]. The purpose of this review is to summarize recent advances in our understanding of the regulation of vascular inflammatory gene expression by oxidants, antioxidants and other redox-sensitive factors during the pathogenesis of vascular inflammatory diseases such as atherosclerosis.

Reactive oxygen species in vasculature: an overview

Oxidation-reduction refers to the transfer of electrons from an electron donor (the reducing agent or antioxidant) to an electron acceptor (the oxidizing agent). Reducing agents (antioxidants) differ from one another in their tendency to lose electrons, and oxidizing agents differ from one another in their tendency to gain electrons. The standard oxidation-reduction potential allows us to predict the direction in which electrons will tend to flow from one pair to another. Molecular oxygen has a very high affinity for electrons and is thus a good oxidizing agent. A wide variety of soluble cell components, capable of undergoing oxidation-reduction reactions in a neutral aqueous milieu, are quantitatively important contributors to intracellular free radical production. These include thiols, hydroquinones, catecholamines and flavins. In all cases superoxide anion (O_2^{-}) is the primary radical formed by one-electron reduction of molecular O_2. Hydrogen peroxide (H_2O_2) is a secondary product of one-electron autoxidations, via spontaneous or enzymatically catalyzed dismutation of O_2^{-} [6].

Oxygen free radicals and their by-products that are capable of causing oxidative damage are collectively referred to as reactive oxygen species (ROS). Eukaryotic cells continuously produce ROS such as O_2^{-}, H_2O_2 and hydroxyl radicals (OH·) as side products of electron transfer reactions. ROS can be produced by a variety of enzymatic reactions (e.g. NAD(P)H oxidase, xanthine oxidase, etc.) in mammalian organisms. However, cells are protected from ROS by antioxidant defense mechanisms. The major intracellular antioxidant defenses are superoxide dismutase (SOD), catalase and glutathione peroxidase. SOD removes O_2^{-} by converting it into H_2O_2 and O_2. Glutathione peroxidase and catalase catalyze the breakdown of H_2O_2 into H_2O and O_2. HO· can be generated by the reaction of H_2O_2 with O_2^{-} in the presence of metal ions such as iron. HO· is very reactive and very short lived. A common feature associated with inflammatory stimuli is their ability to generate ROS. When the rate of formation of ROS exceeds the capacity of antioxidant enzymes, a condition of oxidative stress occurs. However, even in the absence of global oxidant stress, locally or compartmentally generated ROS may serve as second messages to stimulate inflammatory gene expression.

There is a variety of potential cellular sources of ROS including mitochondria, membrane bound NAD(P)H oxidase, cyclooxygenase, lipoxygenase, xanthine oxidase, cytochrome p450 oxidase and nitric oxide synthase. However, strong evidence has shown that NAD(P)H oxidase accounts for greater than 90% of O_2^{-} production in the vasculature [7, 8]. NADPH oxidase has been extensively studied in neutrophils. The active membrane component of NADPH oxidase is cytochrome b558, which consists of two subunits, gp91^{phox} and p22^{phox}. In addition, three cytosolic proteins p47^{phox}, p67^{phox} and Rac, are required for the activation of NADPH oxidase in cell-free assays. mRNA encoding p22^{phox}, p47^{phox} and p67^{phox} has been detected in human fibroblasts. In addition, there are two Rac proteins, Rac1 and Rac2, which are 95% identical to each other at the amino acid level. Both Rac1 and Rac2 can activate NADPH oxidase. Rac1 is ubiquitously expressed, whereas Rac2 is expressed predominantly in cells of myeloid lineage, and is the predominant iso-form in human neutrophils [9]. p22^{phox} is a critical component of NAD(P)H oxidase for generating $O_2{}^-$ in vascular smooth muscle cells [10]. Rac1 is involved in the $O_2{}^-$ generation in response to a variety of stimuli, such as tumor necrosis factor-α (TNFα), IL-1β, lipopolysaccharide (LPS) and platelet derived growth factor (PDGF) in human fibroblasts [11].

Inflammation and pathogenesis of atherosclerosis

A central and one of the earliest features of the atherosclerotic plaque is the infil-tration of monocytes to discrete segments of the arterial wall, followed by their transformation into lipid-laden macrophages, or "foam cells" [12]. The recruitment of these monocytes into the lesion is mediated initially by an increased gradient of chemotactic activity, followed by monocyte adherence to the endothelium and migration into the neointima. Monocyte adherence is mediated, in part, by VCAM-1 and MCP-1 (see chapters by Smith et al. and Furie, this volume). VCAM-1 is an endothelial adhesion molecule that specifically binds cells expressing the integrin counter-receptor very late antigen-4 (VLA-4). Since VLA-4 is only expressed on the surface of monocytes and lymphocytes, but not neutrophils, VCAM-1 is important in mediating the selective adhesion of monocytes and lymphocytes [13]. MCP-1, a peptide chemokine synthesized and secreted by vascular smooth muscle and endothelial cells, is a chemoattractant for monocytes and lymphocytes *in vitro* and *in vivo* [14]. Both VCAM-1 and MCP-1 have been detected in human atheroscle-rotic lesions [15, 16], suggesting that they play a significant role in the pathogene-sis of atherosclerosis.

Redox-sensitive gene expression hypothesis: Oxidative signaling mechanisms in vascular inflammatory gene expression

Hyperlipidemia, smoking, diabetes mellitus and hypertension are well established risk factors for the development of atherosclerosis. However, the molecular and cel-lular mechanisms linking these risk factors into a common pathological pathway are still unclear. Modulation of the expression of a selective set of vascular inflammatory genes by intracellular oxidative signals may provide a molecular mechanism linking these seemingly diverse processes with the early pathogenesis of atherosclerosis [1]. This theory of redox-sensitive gene expression proposes that diverse pro-inflammatory or pro-oxidant stimuli directly stimulate or sensitize vascular cells to generate ROS, which in turn serve as regulatory signals and result in abnormally elevated expression of adhesion molecules such as VCAM-1 and other gene products involved in inflammation. These elevated gene products thus promote infiltration of monocytes into the vessel walls. Conversely, antioxidants may desensitize vascular cells to inflammatory stimuli by quenching or scavenging ROS and inhibit inflammatory gene expression in vasculature. In this context, ROS are coupled to specific regulatory factors and transduce metabolic signals (i.e. oxidation) into nuclear regulatory signals (i.e. expression of inflammatory gene products).

Consistent with this, activation of the endothelial VCAM-1 gene by diverse inflammatory signals occurs through a redox-sensitive mechanism that involves activation of the transcription factor NF-κB. Thiol antioxidants, pyrrolidine dithiocarbamate (PDTC) or N-acetylcysteine (NAC), inhibit VCAM-1 expression stimulated by diverse inflammatory stimuli such as the cytokines IL-1β and TNFα as well as the non-cytokines LPS and poly I:C in cultured endothelial cells [4, 17]. In contrast, the induction of other cell surface adhesion molecules such as intercellular adhesion molecule-1 (ICAM-1) and E-selectin does not exhibit such redox sensitivity, suggesting that oxidative signals selectively regulate a distinct set of inflammatory genes such as VCAM-1 [4, 17].

MCP-1 is also regulated by redox-sensitive regulatory mechanism(s). MCP-1 is secreted by both vascular endothelial cells and smooth muscle cells. Vascular smooth muscle is the major source of MCP-1 secretion, since vascular smooth muscle cells comprise more than 90% of vasculature. Similar to VCAM-1 expression, TNFα-induced MCP-1 expression can be blocked by either PDTC or NAC in human aortic smooth muscle and endothelial cells [5]. In mesangial cells, the induction of MCP-1 gene expression by cytokines or aggregated IgG is mediated by oxidative signals generated by NAD(P)H oxidase [18].

A common feature in the promoter regions of the human VCAM-1 and MCP-1 genes is the presence of multiple binding sites for transcription factors NF-κB and AP-1 [19, 20]. Transcription factors are proteins that activate or repress gene expression within the cell nucleus by binding to specific DNA sequences called "enhancer elements" that are generally near the region of the mRNA transcriptional start site called the "promoter". NF-κB is a ubiquitous transcription factor that induces the expression of a variety of genes in response to inflammatory agents [21]. As such, it plays a key role in mediating inflammatory and other stress signals to the nuclear regulatory apparatus. The increase in ROS observed in many conditions activates NF-κB. Activation of NF-κB by a large and diverse group of agents such as TNFα, IL-1β, LPS, and H_2O_2 can be specifically inhibited by the thiol antioxidants NAC and PDTC, suggesting that oxidative signals play an important role in the activation of NF-κB [22, 23]. Similarly, AP-1 activity is strongly induced by conditions causing a pro-oxidative state in cells [24]. Both an increase in AP-1 DNA binding, with induction of *c-jun* and *c-fos* (two major components of AP-1) mRNA, and modulation of the *c-jun* transcription domain have been observed in response to H_2O_2 and u.v. light [25]. Treatment of mouse skeletal myoblasts with H_2O_2 results in a dose-dependent induction of AP-1 binding activity, which can be inhibited by NAC [26]. Angiotensin II-induced AP-1 binding activity is also inhibited by NAC, suggesting a role for ROS in signal transduction initiated by this agonist [26].

Increased gene expression by ROS is also mediated by post-transcriptional mechanisms such as modulation of mRNA stability. Stability of mRNA transcripts plays an important role in the regulation of some inflammatory genes. Changes in turnover rate can affect steady state levels of mRNA over a relatively short period of time. For example, the rapid, hyperoxia-induced elevation of lung catalase mRNA in neonatal rats is due to enhanced stability of its mRNA but not an increased rate of transcription [27]. Similarly, exposure of alveolar macrophages to H_2O_2 produces a six-fold increase in macrophage inflammatory protein-1α (MIP-1α) mRNA half life [28]. The 3'-untranslated regions of the rat MIP-1α gene contains six copies of a reiterated AU-rich motif [29], implicated in mRNA stability and translational control. A cytoplasmic protein termed adenosine-uridine binding factor has been shown to bind specifically to the AUUUA motif of *in vitro* transcribed RNAs and form exceptionally stable complexes [30]. Moreover, the binding of adenosine-uridine binding factor to RNA templates is also redox-sensitive [31].

Thus, the alteration in vascular cell redox state is accompanied by an increased expression of a set of inflammatory genes that are involved in the pathogenesis of the atherosclerotic lesion. These data suggest that by activating redox-sensitive transcription factors and inducing inflammatory gene expression, ROS may serve as a common signaling and molecular pathway used by many of the risk factors, such as hyperlipidemia, smoking, hypertension, diabetes mellitus and other "causative" signals to contribute to the pathogenesis of atherosclerosis.

NAD(P)H oxidase

NAD(P)H oxidase is thought to be the most important source of superoxide production in both endothelial cells and vascular smooth muscle cells [7, 8]. TNFα activates membrane bound NAD(P)H oxidase activity in vascular endothelial cells and smooth muscle cells [32]. TNFα-induced superoxide generation in human aortic endothelial cells is inhibited by the flavin binding protein inhibitor diphenylene iodonium (DPI), an inhibitor of NAD(P)H oxidase [33]. Overexpression of a dominant negative Rac1, a critical component of activated NAD(P)H oxidase, inhibits $O_2^{.-}$ generation induced in fibroblasts by stimuli including TNFα, IL-1β and PDGF [11]. Antisense DNA against p22^{phox} inhibits angiotensin II-induced generation of $O_2^{.-}$ in vascular smooth muscle cells, suggesting that p22^{phox} is a critical component of NAD(P)H oxidase for generating $O_2^{.-}$ [10].

Activation of NAD(P)H oxidase and generation of ROS may serve as an oxidative signaling pathway associated with expression of inflammatory gene expression. In HeLa cells, overexpression of dominant positive Rac1 activates NAD(P)H oxidase and stimulates generation of $O_2^{.-}$, which in turn is coupled to activation of NF-κB. Conversely, expression of a dominant negative Rac1 mutant inhibits basal and IL-1β stimulated NF-κB activity [34]. NAD(P)H oxidase inhibition blocks both VCAM-1 and ICAM-1 gene expression in response to TNFα, IL-1β and LPS, but not to poly I:C, in human aortic endothelial cells [33]. Similarly, treatment with NAD(P)H oxidase inhibitors, DPI or apocynin, inhibited angiotensin II-induced MCP-1 and VCAM-1 gene expression in rat vascular smooth muscle cells [35]. TNFα-induced MCP-1 expression in mesangial cells is also mediated by ROS generated by NADPH oxidase [36]. These data suggest that NAD(P)H oxidase modulates redox-sensitive gene expression through generation of ROS.

Hyperlipidemia and fatty acid hydroperoxides

In early atherosclerosis, oxidative stress is manifested by the elevated production of ROS by endothelial and smooth muscle cells that results in the oxidative modification of low density lipoprotein (LDL) [37]. Oxidatively modified LDL (oxLDL) has been implicated as an important oxidative signal in the pathogenesis of atherosclerosis [37]. oxLDL accumulates preferentially at sites of the vascular wall predisposed to atherosclerosis [38]. oxLDL may promote the formation of atherosclerotic lesions by modulation of expression of vascular inflammatory genes. Hyperlipidemia and oxLDL may induce oxidative signals by lowering vascular cell glutathione levels, thus stimulating endothelial cells to generate superoxide anion [39]. Alterations in endothelial cell oxidant buffering capacity might explain the increased risk of atherosclerotic lesion formation in individuals who smoke, since such activity has been associated with the generation of oxidized lipids. Enhanced adhesion of monocytes to arterial endothelial cells has been demonstrated in hypercholesterolemic animals [40]. Treatment of cultured endothelial cells with oxLDL enhances monocyte adhesion [41]. Although still controversial, oxLDL has been shown to selectively increase VCAM-1 and ICAM-1 gene expression in human umbilical vein endothelial cells through a redox-sensitive mechanism [42]. Long term incubation with oxLDL augments cytokine-induced VCAM-1 gene expression in endothelial cells [43]. These data suggest that oxLDL and fatty acid hydroperoxides may play an important role in modulating redox-sensitive inflammatory gene expression in vasculature.

oxLDL is a complex structure containing several chemically distinct oxidants, each of which, alone or in combination, might modulate cytokine-activated adhesion molecule gene expression. Recent studies suggest that polyunsaturated fatty acids (PUFA) and their oxidized metabolites serve as important mediators of redox sensitive gene expression in the vasculature. Fatty acid hydroperoxides, notably 13-hydroperoxyoctadecadienoic acids (13-HPODE; derived from the polyunsaturated fatty acid linoleic acid), are abundant components of oxLDL. 13-HPODE has been shown to stimulate *c-fos*, *c-jun* and *c-myc* mRNA expression [44]. Chronic exposure to oxidized oxLDL or 13-HPODE augments TNFα-induced VCAM-1 expression [43]. These and other studies suggest a potential role for PUFA and their oxidative metabolites in the regulation of redox sensitive gene expression in the vasculature [45, 46].

Lipoxygenases and their products, fatty acid hydroperoxides, contribute to oxidant signals associated with development of atherosclerosis [47, 48]. Immunohistochemical studies demonstrate 15-lipoxygenase expression in human atheroma and in lesions of cholesterol-fed rabbits [49, 50]. Increased levels of fatty acid hydroperoxides are found in human atherosclerotic lesions [51–53]. Fatty acid hydroperoxides derived from lipoxygenase activity may act as signaling molecules for regulating gene expression. In endothelial cells, transient overexpression of human 15-lipoxygenase enhances TNFα-induced VCAM-1 expression [46]. 5-Lipoxygenase inhibitors, nordihydroguaiaretic acid or AA8861, inhibit IL-1β-induced VCAM-1 expression in vascular endothelial cells [54].

Hypertension and the renin-angiotensin system

Hypertension is an established risk factor for the development of atherosclerosis, however, the underlying molecular and cellular mechanisms are unclear . Experimental and clinical evidence suggests a potential role of the renin-angiotensin system in contributing to the pathogenesis of atherosclerosis. Angiotensin II (Ang II), an important component of the renin-angiotensin system and a vasoactive peptide, exerts numerous effects on the cardiovascular system. As noted earlier, Ang II induces oxidant stress by stimulating generation of $O_2{}^{.-}$ through membrane-bound NAD(P)H oxidase in cultured rat aortic smooth muscle cells [8]. $O_2{}^{.-}$ is generated by membrane-bound NAD(P)H oxidase in aortas from rats made hypertensive with Ang II, but not norepinephrine [55]. These studies suggest that Ang II can induce intracellular oxidative stress, with potential inflammatory consequences in the vasculature, independent of hypertension.

167

We recently demonstrated that Ang II may contribute to the pathogenesis of atherosclerosis through induction of vascular inflammatory gene expression. When rats were made hypertensive by infusion with Ang II or norepinephrine, both Ang II and norepinephrine induced a similar degree of hypertension after six days of infusion. Ang II induced a remarkable increase in both MCP-1 and VCAM-1 mRNA expression in the aortas of rats. In contrast, norepinephrine-treated rats had no increase in MCP-1 mRNA level and only a moderate increase in VCAM-1 mRNA [35,56]. The induction of VCAM-1 and MCP-1 expression in cultured vascular smooth muscle cells can be inhibited by the NAD(P)H oxidase inhibitors DPI or apocynin as well as by catalase [35], suggesting that NAD(P)H oxidase contributes to oxidative signals by generating H_2O_2. Ang II also activates nuclear NF-κB DNA binding activity and activates a κB-dependent promoter in cultured vascular smooth muscle cells (R.M. Medford, unpublished observation). These results suggest that Ang II contributes to the pathogenesis of atherosclerosis by activation of NF-κB and inducing expression of VCAM-1 and MCP-1 genes, both of which promote migration of monocytes into the vascular wall. These proinflammatory effects of Ang II may provide a potential molecular link between hypertension and atherosclerosis.

Diabetes

Accelerated atherosclerosis and microvascular disease are the major vascular complications of diabetes. Clinical evidence indicates that sustained hyperglycemia is a prerequisite for the development of vascular complications and other sequelae of diabetes. Hyperglycemia present in diabetes produces oxidative stress which leads to vascular dysfunction. Mechanisms that contribute to increased oxidative stress in diabetes include nonenzymatic glycosylation (glycation), autoxidative glycation and metabolic stress resulting from changes in energy metabolism, alterations in the sorbitol pathway and the status of antioxidant defense systems [57].

Prolonged exposure to pathologically high glucose alone has pro-oxidant effects. High concentrations of glucose stimulate superoxide generation and enhance cell mediated LDL peroxidation in cultured endothelial cells [58]. Incubation of endothelial cells with increased glucose concentration also results in activation of NF-κB [59, 60]. Enhanced VCAM-1 expression has been demonstrated in the aortic endothelium of alloxan-treated diabetic rabbits [61].

In diabetes, the extended interaction of aldose with proteins can lead to the formation of highly reactive advanced glycosylation endproducts of proteins (AGE) [62]. The steady accumulation of AGE on proteins with relatively long half-lives, such as sub-endothelial cell basement membrane proteins, may play an important role in the development of vascular complications associated with diabetes. AGE elicit their cellular effects by binding to specific cellular receptors. One of the receptors for AGE (RAGE) has been identified on endothelial cells and smooth muscle cells. Interaction of AGE with endothelial surface RAGE generates intracellular oxidative free radicals [63], decreases reduced glutathione levels and activates NF-κB [64]. Incubation of cultured endothelial cells with AGE induces expression of VCAM-1 and increased adhesivity of the monolayer for monocytes. These effects can be blocked by anti-RAGE antibody, PDTC or NAC [65]. Chronic AGE accumulation in animals promotes VCAM-1 expression and formation of atherosclerotic lesions independent of diabetic hyperglycemia. Infusion of low doses of AGE-modified rabbit serum albumin for four months results in enhanced endothelial adhesion of monocytes and positive focal expression of VCAM-1 and ICAM-1 in aortic endothelium. When animals were co-fed for a brief period (two weeks) with a cholesterol-rich diet, these AGE-induced changes were markedly enhanced. The lesions consisted of multifocal atheromas, foam cells, massive lipid droplets and strong endothelial expression of VCAM-1 and ICAM-1 [66]. These results suggest that diabetes, like many other risk factors for atherosclerosis, has the ability to generate reactive oxygen species, resulting in activation of NF-κB and initiation of vascular inflammatory gene expression leading to lesion formation.

Nitric oxide

Nitric oxide (NO) is an endogenously synthesized free radical, which exerts potent actions in the regulation of cell function and tissue viability. NO is produced by a variety of cells including endothelium, macrophages, smooth muscle cells, platelets and fibroblasts. NO may exhibit a dual redox function based on its interaction with reactive oxygen species. Depending on the concentrations present, NO has been shown to augment or inhibit oxygen-radical mediated tissue damage and lipid peroxidation. NO reacts with superoxide to produce peroxynitrite anion (ONOO⁻), which is a potent oxidant. However, NO can also play a cytoprotective role due to its ability to redirect the reactivity of partially reduced oxygen species [67].

Intracellular NO levels play an important role in the regulation of expression of inflammatory genes in the vasculature. Exogenous NO selectively inhibited cytokine-induced VCAM-1 gene expression as well as monocyte adhesion to endothelial monolayers [68]. Inhibition of endogenous NO production has been shown to induce or augment cytokine-induced VCAM-1 expression [68, 69]. Similarly, exogenous NO has been reported to inhibit both MCP-1 expression as well as chemotactic activity for monocytes in response to LPS and oxLDL in vascular endothelial cells and smooth muscle cells [39]. Inhibition of NO synthesis upregulated MCP-1 gene expression both in cultured vascular smooth muscle cells and in aortas of rabbits [39, 70]. Dietary L-arginine, the precursor of NO, inhibited activation of MCP-1 expression in aortas of rabbits fed with a high-cholesterol diet [39]. Chronic inhibition of NO production increased monocyte-endothelium interaction and markedly enhanced the development of atherosclerosis in cholesterol-fed rabbits [71]. Chronic provision of L-arginine in the diets of hypercholesterolemic rabbits has been shown to improve endothelium-dependent vasorelaxation and reduce atherogenesis [72]. These observations are consistent with anti-atherogenic effects of NO.

Attenuation of inflammatory gene expression by NO is mediated, at least in part, by its ability to inhibit activation of the redox-sensitive transcription factor NF-κB. Exogenous NO selectively inhibited cytokine-induced activation of NF-κB in vascular endothelial cells [68, 73]. Conversely, inhibition of endogenous NO production activated NF-κB in endothelial cells [70, 73]. NO induces the expression of IκB, an inhibitory factor for NF-κB, and inhibits degradation of IκB in response to cytokines [73]. In addition, NO can directly inhibit the DNA binding activity of recombinant NF-κB p50 and p65 homodimers and p50-p65 heterodimers to their consensus κB sequence. This inhibitory effect involves modification of the Cys-62 in p50 by nitrosylation [74].

NO may also exert its effects by reducing intracellular oxidative stress. NO has been shown to reduce superoxide generation by endothelium in response to cytokines and oxLDL [39]. NO can redirect the reactivity of partially reduced oxygen species and can react with superoxide to produce $ONOO^-$ [67]. Although $ONOO^-$ itself is a highly reactive free radical, it is possible that $ONOO^-$ could subsequently nitrosylate sulfhydryl groups to form nitrosothiols [75]. NO can also ameliorate oxidative stress by terminating the autocatalytic chain of lipid peroxidation that is initiated by oxLDL or intracellular generation of oxygen-derived free radicals. Exogenous NO inhibited copper-induced oxidation of LDL and delayed formation of lipid peroxides [76]. The modulation of the activity of NF-κB-like transcription factors by NO suggests a molecular link between an oxidant-sensitive transcriptional regulatory mechanism and NO synthesis in vascular cells.

Hemodynamic forces

The distribution of atherosclerotic lesions throughout the vascular tree is non-uniform. This non-uniformity is due to, at least in part, local alterations in hemodynamic forces impinging on the vascular tree. At sites vulnerable to plaque formation such as bends, branches and bifurcations, unidirectional laminar flow is disturbed, with an area of recirculation characterized by low and fluctuating shear stress. Endothelial cells form the interface between the circulating blood and the vessel wall, and as such they reside in a dynamic physical force environment, experiencing both a normal pressure force and tangential shearing force resulting from the flow of blood over the lumen surface [77]. Recent studies indicate that the tractive force of fluid flow has profound effects on redox status and gene expression in vascular endothelial cells [78, 79].

When endothelial cells were subjected to oscillatory shear stress, they exhibited a progressively increased NAD(P)H oxidase activity, associated with sustained upregulation of the redox-sensitive gene heme oxygenase-1 [78] and VCAM-1 mRNA accumulation (Varner and Medford, unpublished observation). This induction of heme oxygenase-1 is completely blocked by the antioxidant NAC, suggesting that continuous oscillatory shear causes a sustained increase in intracellular ROS generation resulting in redox-sensitive gene expression in endothelial cells. In contrast, when cultured endothelial cells were exposed to steady laminar shear for 24 hours and then exposed to IL-1β, expression of VCAM-1, but not ICAM-1 or E-selectin, was selectively inhibited [79]. Interestingly, NF-κB activation was not inhibited by chronic laminar shear stress [79]. Laminar shear may modulate VCAM-1 gene expression by specifically targeting oxidative signals mediating inflammatory gene expression. Consistent with this, the ability of laminar shear-preconditioned endothelial cells to synthesize fatty acid hydroperoxides, specifically 13-HPODE, is markedly reduced compare to static control cells (Varner and Medford, unpublished observation). These observations suggest that different types of shear stress may contribute to the focal nature of atherosclerosis by modulating endothelial redox status and inflammatory gene expression.

Summary

In the inflammatory response characteristic of early atherosclerosis, the interaction of monocytes with vascular cells is mediated by a complex amalgam of interacting regulatory signals. As shown in Figure 1, a common feature underlying these interactions involves redox-sensitive nuclear regulatory factors that modulate the expression of a set of inflammatory gene products. Many of the risk factors associated with atherosclerotic vascular disease, such as hyperlipidemia, diabetes and hypertension, promote vascular cells to generate ROS. The alteration in endothelial cell redox state is accompanied by increased adhesive interactions between the endothelium and inflammatory cells. Mechanistically, this change may occur because ROS can function as signaling molecules that mediate increased activity of transcription factors such as NF-κB. Activation of these transcription factors induces a coordinated up-regulation in the expression of inflammatory genes such VCAM-1 and MCP-1. Thus, the alteration in oxidative signaling mechanisms in vascular endothelial and smooth muscle cells may provide a molecular link between hyperlipidemia, hypertension, diabetes and atherosclerosis lesion formation. On the basis of these observations, therapeutic strategies that modulate the endothelial cell redox state are postulated to help reverse endothelial dysfunction and thereby prevent the progression of vascular diseases such as atherosclerosis.

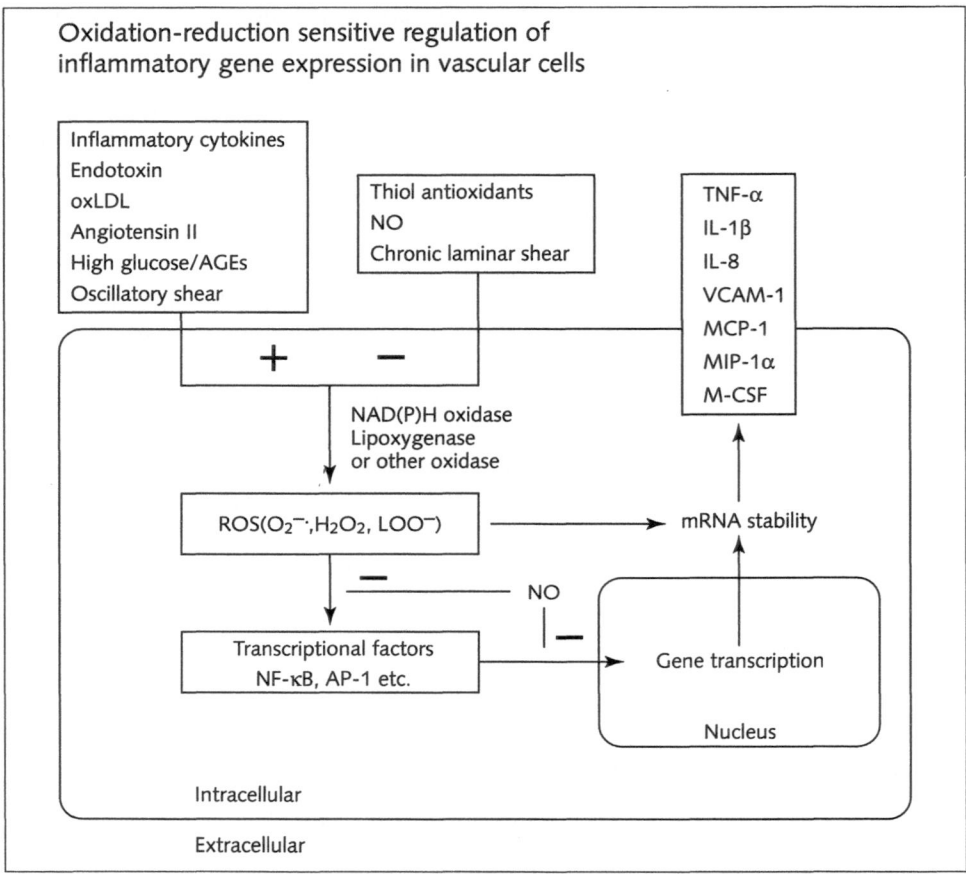

Figure 1

Schematic presentation of redox-sensitive gene expression theory. Extracellular stimuli such as cytokines, endotoxin, oxidized low density protein (oxLDL), angiotensin II, high glucose, advanced glycosylation endproducts of proteins (AGEs) or oscillatory shear stress stimulate or sensitize vascular cells to generate reactive oxygen species (ROS). ROS then activate transcription factors such as NF-κB and AP-1 and increase inflammatory gene transcription. ROS also increase mRNA stability in some inflammatory genes such as macrophage inflammatory protein-1 (MIP-1α). Thiol antioxidants, nitric oxide (NO) or laminar shear stress inhibit inflammatory gene expression by scavenging ROS or decreasing ROS generation in response to inflammatory stimuli. In addition, NO induces IκB expression and stabilizes IκB protein resulting in inhibition of NF-κB activation. NO also blocks DNA binding activity of activated NF-κB. O_2^{-}, superoxide anion; H_2O_2, hydrogen peroxide; LOO^{-}, fatty acid hydroperoxide; TNFα, tumor necrosis factor α; IL-1β, Interleukin-1β; IL-8, interleukin-8; M-CSF, monocyte-colony stimulating factor.

References

1   Offermann MK, Medford RM (1994) Antioxidants and atherosclerosis: a molecular perspective. *Heart Dis Stock* 3: 52–57

2   Sen CK, Packer L (1996) Antioxidant and redox regulation of gene transcription. *FASEB J* 10: 709–20

3   Collins T (1993) Endothelial nuclear factor-κB and the initiation of the athersclerotic lesion. *Lab Invest* 68: 499–508

4   Marui N, Offermann MK, Swerlick R, Kunsch C, Rosen CA, Ahmad M, Alexander RW, Medford RM (1993) VCAM-1 gene transcription and expression is regulated through an antioxidant sensitive mechanism in human vascular endothelial cells. *J Clin Invest* 92: 1866–1874

5   Chen XL, Tummala PE, Obrych MT, Medford RM (1996) Oxidation-reduction and proteasome dependent activation of monocyte chemotactic protein-1 gene expression in in human vascular cells. *Circ Res* 94: I276

6   Freeman BA, Capro JD (1982) Free radicals and tissue injury. *Lab Invest* 46: 412–426

7   Mohazzab KM, Kaminski PM, Wolin MS (1994) NADH oxidoreductase is a major source of superoxide anion in bovine coronary artery endothelium. *Am J Physiol* 266: H2568–H2572

8   Griendling K, Minieri C, Ollerenshw J, Alexander RW (1994) Angiotensin II stimulates NADH and NADPH oxidase activity in cultured vascular smooth muscle cells. *Circ Res* 74: 1141–1148

9   Ridley AJ, Paterson HF, Johnson CL, Diekmann D, Hall A (1992) The small GTP-binding protein rac regulates growth factor-induced membrane ruffling. *Cell* 70: 401–410

10   Ushio-Fukai M, Zafari AM, Fukui T, Ishizaka N, Griendling KK (1996) p22phox is a critical component of the superoxide-generating NADH/NADPH oxidase system and regulates angiotensin II induced hypertrophy in vascular smooth muscle cells. *J Biol Chem* 271: 23317–23321

11   Sunderasan M, Yu ZX, Ferrans VJ, Sulciner DJ, Gutkind JS, Irani K, Goldschmidt-Clermont P, Finkel T (1996) Regulation of reactive oxygen species generation in fibroblasts by Rac1. *Biochem J* 318: 379–382

12   Ross R (1993) The pathogenesis of atherosclerosis: a perspective for 1990s. *Nature* 362: 801–809

13   Bevilacqua MP (1993) Endothelial-leukocyte adhesion molecules. *Ann Rev Immunol* 11: 767–804

14   Leonard EJ, Yoshimura T (1991) Human monocyte chemoattractant protein-1 (MCP-1). *Immunol Today* 11: 97–101

15   Takeya M, Yoshimura T, Leonard EJ, Takahashi K (1993) Detection of monocyte chemoattractant protein-1 in human atherosclerotic lesions by an anti-monocyte chemoattractant protein-1 monoclonal antibody. *Hum Pathol* 24: 534–539

16   O'Brien KD, Allen MD, McDonald TO, Chait A, Harlan JM, Fishbein D, McCarty J, Ferguson M, Hudkins K, Benjamin CD et al (1993) Vascular cell adhesion molecule-1 is

expressed in human coronary atherosclerotic plaques. Implications for the mode of progression of advanced coronary atherosclerosis. *J Clin Invest* 92: 945–951

17 Weber C, Erl W, Pietsch A, Strobel M, Ziegler-Heitbrock H, Weber P (1994) Antioxidants inhibit monocyte adhesion by suppressing nuclear factor-κB mobilization and induction of vascular cell adhesion molecule-1 in endothelial cells stimulated to generate radicals. *Arterioscleros Thrombos* 14: 1665–1673

18 Satriano JA, Shuldiner M, Hora K, Xing Y, Shan Z, Schlondorff D (1993) Oxygen radicals as second messengers for expression of the monocyte chemoattractant protein, JE/MCP-1, and the monocyte colony-stimulating factor, CSF-1, in response to tumor necrosis factor-alpha and immunoglobulin G. Evidence for involvement of reduced nicotinamide adenine dinucleotide phosphate (NADPH)-dependent oxidase. *J Clin Invest* 92: 1564–1571

19 Iademarco MF, McQuillan JJ, Rosen GD, Dean DC (1992) Characterization of the promoter for vascular cell adhesion molecule-1 (VCAM-1). *J Biol Chem* 267: 16323–16329

20 Ueda A, Okuda K, Ohno S, Shirai A, Igarashi T, Matsunaga J, Kawamoto S, Ishigatsubo Y, Okubo T (1994) NF-κB and Sp1 regulate transcription of human monocyte chemoattractant protein-1 gene. *J Immunol* 153: 2052–2063

21 Baeuerle P, Henkel T (1994) Function and activation of NF-κB in the immune system. *Ann Rev Immunol* 12: 141–179

22 Schreck R, Albermann K, Baeuerle PA (1992) Nuclear factor kappa B: an oxidative stress-responsive transcription factor of eukaryotic cells. *Free Rad Res Commun* 17: 221–237

23 Schreck R, Baeuerle PA (1991) A role for oxygen radicals as second messengers. *Trends Cell Biol* 1: 39–42

24 Puri PL, Avantaggiati ML, Burgio VL, Chirillo P, Collepardo D, Natoli G, Balsano C, Levrero M (1995) Reactive oxygen intermediates (ROIs) are involved in the intracellular transduction of angiotensin II signal in C2C12 cells. *Ann NY Acad Sci* 752: 394–405

25 Devary Y, Gottlieb RA, Lau LF, Karin M (1991) Rapid and preferential activation of the c-jun gene during the mammalian UV response. *Mol Cell Biol* 11:2804–2811

26 Puri PL, Avantaggiati ML, Burgio VL, Chirillo P, Collepardo D, Natoli G, Balsano C, Levrero M (1995) Reactive oxygen intermediates mediate angiotensin II-induced c-Jun, c-Fos heterodimer DNA binding activity and proliferative hypertrophic responses in myogenic cells. *J Biol Chem* 270: 22129–22134

27 Clerch LB, Iqbal J, Massaro D (1991) Perinatal rat lung catalase gene expression: influence of corticosteroid and hyperoxia. *Am J Physiol* 260: L428–L433

28 Shi MM, Godleski JJ, Paulauskis JD (1996) Regulation of macrophage inflammatory protein-1alpha mRNA by oxidative stress. *J Biol Chem* 271: 5878–5883

29 Shi MM, Godleski JJ Paulauskis JD (1995) Molecular cloning and posttranscriptional regulation of macrophage inflammatory protein-1 alpha in alveolar macrophages. *Biochem Biophys Res Commun* 211: 289–295

30 Malter JS (1989) Identification of an AUUUA-specific messenger RNA binding protein. *Science* 246: 664–666

31   Malter JS, Hong Y (1991) A redox switch and phosphorylation are involved in the post-translational up-regulation of the adenosine-uridine binding factor by phorbol ester and ionophore. *J Biol Chem* 266: 3167–3171

32   Keulenaer GW, Ushio-Fukei M, Ishizaka N, Alexander RW, Griendling KK (1996) TNF-alpha activates a p22 phox-containing NADH oxidase in vascular smooth muscle cells. *Circulation* 94: I44

33   Tummala PE, Chen X, Medford RM (1996) Differential regulation of oxidation sensitive VCAM-1 gene expression and NF-κB activation by flavin binding proteins. *Circulation* 94: 1–45

34   Sulciner DJ, Irani K, Yu Z-X, Ferrans VJ, Goldschmidt-Claermont P, Finkel T (1996) Rac1 regulates a cytokine-stimulated redox-dependent pathway necessary for NF-κB activation. *Mol Cell Biol* 16: 7115–7121

35   Chen XL, Tummala PE, Laursen JB, Harrison DG, Alexander RW, Medford RM (1997) Direct activation of aortic monocyte chemoattractant protein-1 gene expression *in vivo* and ex vivo by angiotensin II in experimental hypertension. *Circ Res* 96: I285

36   Satriano JA, Hora K, Shan Z, Stanley ER, Mori T, Schlondorff D (1993) Regulation of monocyte chemoattractant protein-1 and macrophage colony-stimulating factor-1 by IFN-gamma, tumor necrosis factor-alpha, IgG aggregates, and cAMP in mouse mesangial cells. *J Immunol* 150: 1971–1978

37   Steinberg D, Parthasarathy S, Carew TE, Khoo JC, Witztum JL (1989) Beyond cholesterol: modifications of low-density lipoprotein that increase its atherogenicity. *N Engl J Med* 320: 915–924

38   Yla-Herttuala S, Pawlinski SW, Rosenfeld ME, Paratsarathy S, Carew TE, Butler S (1989) Evidence for the presence of oxidatively modified low densitiy lipoproteins in the pathogenesis of atherosclerosis lesion in rabbit and man. *J Clin Invest* 84: 1785–1792

39   Tsao PS, Wang B, Buitrago R, Shyy JY, Cooke JP (1997) Nitric oxide regulates monocyte chemotactic protein-1. *Circulation* 96: 934–940

40   Joris I, Zand T, Nunnari JJ, Krolikowski FJ, Majna G (1983). Adhesion and migration of mononuclear cells in the aorta of hypercholesterolemic rats. *Am J Pathol* 113: 341–358

41   Berliner JA, Territo MC, Sevanian A, Ramin S, Kim JA, Bahshad B, Esterson M, Fogelman AM (1990) Minimally modified low densitiy lipoprotein stimulates monocyte endothelial interactions. *J Clin Invest* 85: 1260–1266

42   Cominacini L, Ulisse G, Pasini AF, Davoli A, Campagnola M, Contessi GB, Pastorino A, Cascio VL (1997) Antioxidants inhibit the expression of intercellular cell adhesion molecule-1 and vascular cell adhesion molecule-1 induced by oxidized LDL on human umbilical endothelial cells. *Free Rad Biol Med* 22: 117–127

43   Khan BR, Parthasarathy SS, Alexander RW, Medford RM (1995) Modified low density lipoprotein and its constituents augment cytokine-activated vascular cell adhesion molecule-1 gene expression in human endothelial cells. *J Clin Invest* 95: 1262–1270

44   Rao GN, Alexander RW, Runge MS (1995) Linoleic acid and its metabolites, hydroperoxyoctadecadienoic acids, stimulate c-Fos, c-Jun, and c-Myc mRNA expression, mito-

gen-activated protein kinase activation, and growth in rat aortic smooth muscle cells. *J Clin Invest* 96: 842–847

45 Sultana C, Shen Y, Rattan V, Kalra VK (1996) Lipoxygenase metabolites induced expression of adhesion molecules and transendothelial migration of monocyte-like HL-60 cells is linked to protein kinase C activation. *J Cell Physiol* 167: 477–487

46 Wolle J, Welch KA, Devall LJ, Cornicelli JA, Saxena U (1996) Transient overexpression of human 15-lipoxygenase in aortic endothelial cells enhances tumor necrosis factor-induced vascular cell adhesion molecule-1 gene expression. *Biochem Biophy Res Commun* 220: 310–314

47 Hajjar DP, Pomerantz KB (1992) Signal transduction in atherosclerosis: integration of cytokines and the eicosanoid network. *FASEB J* 6: 2933–2941

48 Sigal E,. Laughton CW, Mulkins MA (1994) Oxidation, lipoxygenase, and atherogenesis. *Ann NY Acad Sci* 714: 211–224

49 Yla-Herttuala S, Rosenfield ME, Parthasarathy S, Glass K, Sigal E, Witztum JL, Steinberg D 1990. Colocalization of 15-lipoxygenase mRNA and protein with epitopes of oxidized low density lipoprotein in macrophage-rich areas of atherosclerotic lesions. *Proc Natl Acad Sci USA* 87: 6959–6963

50 Yla-Herttuala S, Rosenfield ME, Parthasarathy S, Sigal E, Sarkioja T, Witztum JL, Steinberg D (1991) Gene expression in macrophage-rich human atherosclerotic lesions: 15-lipoxygenase and acetyl LDL receptor mRNA colocalize with oxidation-specific lipid-protein adducts. *J Clin Invest* 87: 1146–1152

51 Pomerantz KB, Hajjar DP (1991) Role of eicosanoids and the cytokine network in transmembrane signaling in vascular cells. *Adv Exp Med Biol* 314: 159–83

52 Kuhn H, Heydeck D, Hugou I, Gniwotta C (1997) *In vivo* action of 15-lipoxygenase in early stages of human atherogenesis. *J Clin Invest* 99: 888–893

53 Folcik VA, Nivar-Aristy RA, Krajewski LP, Cathcart MK (1995) Lipoxygenase contributes to the oxidation of lipids in human atherosclerotic plaques. *J Clin Invest* 96: 504–510

54 Lee S, Felts KA, Parry GC, Armacost LM, Cobb RR (1997) Inhibition of 5-lipoxygenase blocks IL-1 beta-induced vascular adhesion molecule-1 gene expression in human endothelial cells. *J Immunol* 158: 3401–3407

55 Rajagopalan S, Kurz S, Munzel T, Tarpey M, Freeman BA, Griendling KK, Harrison DG (1996) Angiotensin II mediated hypertension in the rat increases vascular superoxide production via membrane NADH/NADPH oxidase activation: Contribution to alterations of vasomotor tone. *J Clin Invest* 97: 1916–1923

56 Chen XL, Tummala PE, Laursen JB, Harrison DG, Alexander RW, Medford RM (1998) Hypertension and regulation of vascular inflammatory genes: role of angiotensin II. *Circ Res* 94: I594

57 Baynes JW (1991) Role of oxidative stress in development of complications in diabetes. *Diabetes* 40: 405–412

58 Graier WF, Simecek S, Kukovetz WR, Kostner GM (1996) High D-glucose-induced

changes in endothelial Ca^{2+}/EDRF signaling are due to generation of superoxide anions. *Diabetes* 45: 1386–1395

59   Maziere C, Auclair M, Rose-Robert F, Leflon P, Maziere JC (1995) Glucose-enriched medium enhances cell-mediated low density lipoprotein peroxidation. *FEBS Lett* 363: 277–279

60   Pieper GM, Riaz-ul-Haq (1997) Activation of nuclear factor-kB in cultured endothelial cells by increased glucose concentration: prevention by calphostin C. *J Cardiovasc Pharm* 30: 528–532

61   Richardson M, Hadcock S, DeReske M, Cybulsky M (1994) Inreased expression *in vivo* of VCAM-1 and E-selectin by the aortic endothelium of normolipidemic and hyperlipi-demc diabetic rabbits. *Arterioscler Thrombos* 14: 760–769

62   Brownlee M, Cerami A, Vlassara H (1988) Advanced glycosylation end products in tis-sue and the biochemical basis of diabetic complications. *N Engl J Med* 318: 1315–1321

63   Yan SD, Schmidt AM, Anderson GM, Zhang J; Brett J, Zou YS, Pinsky D, Stern D (1994) Enhanced cellular oxidative stress by the interaction of advanced glycation end products with their receptors/binding proteins. *J Biol Chem* 269: 9889–9897

64   Bierhaus A, Chevion S, Chevion M, Hofmann M, Quehenberger P, Illmer T, Luther T, Berentstein E, Tritschler H, Muller M, Wajl P, Ziegler R, Nawroth PP (1997) Advanced glycation end product-induced activation of NF-κB is suppressed by α-lipoic acid in cul-tured endothelial cells. *Diabetes* 46: 1481–1490

65   Schmidt AM, Hori O, Chen JX, Li JF, Crandall J, Zhang J, Cao R, Yan SD, Brett J, Stern D (1995) Advanced endproducts interacting with their endothelial receptor induce expression of vascular cell adhesion molecule (VCAM-1) in cultured human endothelial cellls and in mice. *J Clin Invest* 96: 1395–1403

66   Vlassara H, Fuh H, Donnelly T, Cybulsky M (1995) Advanced glycation endproducts promote adhesion molecule (VCAM-1, ICAM-1) expression and atheroma formation in normal rabbits. *Mol Med* 1: 447–456

67   Rubbo H, Darley-Usmar V, Freeman BA (1996) Nitric oxide regulation of tissue free radical injury. *Chem Res Toxicol* 9: 809–820

68   Khan BV, Harrison DG, Olbrych MT, Alexander RW, Medford RM (1996) Nitric oxide regulates vascular cell adhesion molecule 1 gene expression and redox-sensitive tran-scriptional events in human vascular endothelial cells. *Proc Natl Acad Sci USA* 93: 9114–9119

69   Caterina RD, Libby P, Peng HB, Thannickal VJ, Rajavashisth TB, Gimbrone MA, Shin WS, Liao JK (1996) Nitric oxide decreases cytokine-induced endothelial activation: nitric oxide selectively reduces endothelial expression of adhesion molecules and proin-flammatory cytokines. *J Clin Invest* 96: 60–68

70   Zeiher AM, Fisslthaler B, Schray-Utz B, Busse R (1995) Nitric oxide modulates the expression of monocyte chemoattractant protein 1 in cultured human endothelial cells. *Circ Res* 76: 980–986

71   Cayette AJ, Palacino JJ, Horten K, Cohen RA (1994) Chronic inhibition of nitric oxide

prduction accelerates neointima formation and impairs endothelial function in hyperc-holeserolemic rabbits. *Arterioscleros Thrombos* 14: 746–752

72   Cooke JP, Singer AH, Tso P, Zera P, Rowan RA, Billingham ME (1992) Antiatherogenic effects of L-arginine in the hypercholesterolemic rabbit. *J Clin Invest* 90: 1168–1172

73   Peng HB, Libby P, Liao JK (1995) Induction and stabilization of I kappa B alpha by nitric oxide mediates inhibition of NF-kappa B. *J Biol Chem* 270: 14214–14219

74   Matthews JR, Botting CH, Panico M, Morris HR, Hay R (1996) Inhibition of Nf-kB binding by nitric oxide. *Nucleic Acid Res* 24: 2236–2242

75   Stamler JS, Simon DI, Osborne JA, Mullins ME, Jaraki O, Michel T, Singel DJ, Loscal-zo J (1992) S-nitrosylation of proteins with nitric oxide: synthesis and characterization of biologically active compounds. *Proc Natl Acad Sci USA* 89: 444–448

76   Hogg N, Kalyanaramer B, Joseph J, Struck A, Parthasarathy S (1993) Inhibition of low-density lipoprotein oxidation by nitric oxide – potential role in atherosclerosis. *FEBS Lett* 334: 170–174

77   Takahashi M, Ishida T, Traub O, Corson MA, Berk BC (1997) Mechanotransduction in endothelial cells: temporal signaling events in response to shear stress. *J Vasc Res* 34: 212–219

78   DeKeulenaer GW, Chappell DC, Ishizaka N, Nerem RM, Alexander RW, Griendling KK (1998) Oscillatory and steady laminar shear stress differentially affect human endothe-lial redox state – role of a superoxide producing NADH oxidase. *Circ Res* 82: 1094–1101

79   Varner SE, Chappell DC, Nerem RM, Offermann MK, Alexander RW, Medford RM. Chronic laminar shear stress differentially inhibits inflammatory activation of vascular endothelial cell VCAM-1 and NF-κB. *In preparation*

Quantification and imaging of vascular adhesion molecule expression in inflammatory diseases *in vivo*

Tanya Y. Huehns and Dorian O. Haskard

BHF Cardiovascular Medicine Unit, National Heart and Lung Institute (Hammersmith Hospital), Imperial College School of Medicine, Du Cane Road, London W12 0NN, UK

Introduction

Advances in our understanding of the molecular mechanisms involved in leukocyte-endothelial cell interactions have suggested novel methods for quantifying and imaging endothelial cell activation *in vivo* [1, 2]. Activated endothelial cells express several molecules related to leukocyte recruitment that provide possible targets [3]. Molecular probes to these might be clinically useful for imaging inflammation and provide more readily interpretable information than that supplied by existing techniques [4]. In this chapter we describe our experience evaluating E-selectin and vascular cell adhesion molecule-1 (VCAM-1) for this purpose.

E-selectin provides an attractive target for imaging, since expression is minimal on unstimulated cultured human or porcine endothelial cells but is transiently up-regulated by a protein synthesis-dependent mechanism following activation by factors such as interleukin-1α (IL-1α), tumour necrosis factor α (TNFα) or bacterial lipopolysaccharide (LPS) [5–7]. There are a number of studies in the literature (reviewed by Mason and Haskard [8]) which have used immunocytochemistry to show that endothelial cells express E-selectin during inflammatory responses *in vivo*. A feature of E-selectin expression that has turned out to be particularly relevant for our *in vivo* studies is that the molecule is predominantly removed from the cell surface by rapid internalisation into endosomes, at approximately 1.7% of membrane-bound antigen per minute [9]. Experiments using confocal laser scanning microscopy have shown that cytokine-activated endothelial cells internalise antibody to E-selectin along with antigen [10].

Like E-selectin, VCAM-1 is only minimally expressed by resting cultured human or porcine endothelial cells, and its expression by cultured human umbilical vein endothelial cells can be induced by stimulation with IL-1α, TNFα or LPS [6, 11, 12]. However, VCAM-1 expression differs from that of E-selectin *in vitro*, not only in terms of kinetics but also in terms of responsiveness to other mediators such as interleukin-4 [13]. VCAM-1 expression by microvascular dermal endothelial cells tends to be only weakly induced by IL-1α in comparison with TNFα, while E-selectin is readily induced by both mediators [14]. The poor response of dermal microvascular endothelial cells to IL-1α may be because of the presence of an IL-1α-mediated repressor of VCAM-1 transcription within these cells [15]. In contrast to E-selectin, VCAM-1 is expressed by other cells besides endothelial cells; it is also present on some epithelial, fibroblastic and dendritic cells [16]. Compared with E-selectin, there is little published information on the mechanisms by which VCAM-1 is cleared from the cell surface, but our own *in vivo* data (see below) suggest that it may occur along similar lines to that of intercellular cell adhesion molecule-1 (ICAM-1), which is predominantly shed rather than being internalised [17].

Studies in experimental models of inflammation

The *in vitro* studies referred to above suggest that E-selectin and VCAM-1 might be useful markers for studying the behaviour of endothelial cells during inflammatory responses *in vivo*, and for clinical imaging. Although the majority of *in vivo* studies on leukocyte-endothelial cell interactions have focused on small animal models, in the first instance we developed our targeting techniques in the pig. While in the beginning this decision was dictated largely by the availability of suitable monoclonal antibodies (mAb), the pig also offers a number of advantages over small animal models, amongst which are the cardiovascular and metabolic similarities between pigs and humans. Furthermore, resting leukocyte populations can be isolated relatively easily from pig peripheral blood in sufficient quantities for radiolabelling and intravenous infusion, and a background of work investigating the physiology of constitutive and cytokine-induced lymphocyte migration in the inbred pig already existed [18–20]. Lastly, insights from porcine models may have potential use in the field of xenotransplantation. Our studies used young Large White pigs, either outbred or from the Babraham swine leukocyte antigen b/b inbred herd. Pigs were fed standard chow and weighed 15–20 kg at the time of investigation. Experiments were carried out under anaesthesia, following Home Office and local guidelines.

The anti-E-selectin antibody used in these experiments, mAb 1.2B6 (mouse IgG1), was developed in our laboratory from a mouse immunised with TNF-activated human umbilical vein endothelial cells [6]. Studies using COS-7 cells transfected with porcine E-selectin cDNA demonstrate that mAb 1.2B6 also reacts with porcine E-selectin [7]. The antibody does not react with either human or pig L-selectin, as shown by the failure to stain leukocytes using flow cytometry. We have recently generated the cDNA and mAb for porcine P-selectin and have directly demonstrated that the mAb 1.2B6 does not bind pig P-selectin (unpublished observations). On the other hand, we have recently found that mAb 1.2B6 does weakly bind human P-selectin, albeit with an affinity that is significantly less than that for human E-selectin (manuscript in preparation).

The anti-porcine VCAM-1 antibody, mAb 10.2C7 (mouse IgG1), was generated from a mouse immunised with TNF-activated porcine aortic endothelial cells [21]. It specifically binds COS-7 cells transfected with porcine VCAM-1 cDNA and does not bind porcine peripheral blood leukocytes.

Of particular importance for the *in vivo* experiments described below has been the use of an isotype-matched control antibody to distinguish the specific tissue uptake of anti-E-selectin or anti-VCAM-1 from the non-specific accumulation of immunoglobulin through protein leakage into inflamed tissues. In porcine models this was usually achieved by simultaneously administering differentially-radiolabelled MOPC-21, a mouse IgG1 myeloma protein of undefined specificity.

Systemic vascular activation

In initial experiments we tested the capacity of anti-E-selectin and anti-VCAM-1 mAb to localise specifically to endothelium following systemic activation of the vasculature by intravenous injection of human IL-1α, given as a bolus (5 μg/kg), followed by an infusion of 6 μg/kg over 2 h. Clinically, pigs developed tachycardia and tachypnoea, together with a fall in the circulating leukocyte count. Immunocytochemistry demonstrated that both E-selectin and VCAM-1 were expressed on endothelial cells in all organs studied, albeit with variability in the degree of antigen expression between vessels of different size [21–23].

Clearance rates of the targeting antibodies were established by measuring antibody-associated radioactivity in blood samples taken at regular intervals following injection of radiolabelled antibodies [21–23]. About two-thirds of the injected control antibody, MOPC-21, remained in the circulation after 2 h, with the rate of antibody clearance being uninfluenced by injection of IL-1α. In unstimulated pigs, mAb 1.2B6 (anti-E-selectin) was cleared slightly faster than MOPC-21. Between 30 and 40 min after injection of IL-1α, circulating anti-E-selectin-associated radioactivity in plasma fell to less than 50% of the initial level and plateaued at a level of 16% after 90 min. These observations, together with the fact that uptake of radiolabelled mAb 1.2B6 into tissues could be inhibited by an excess of unlabelled antibody, indicated that the antibody was specifically binding E-selectin that had become newly expressed by endothelial cells in response to IL-1α.

Moreover, gamma camera imaging of animals receiving radiolabelled anti-E-selectin showed that IL-1α administration led to the disappearance of radioactivity from the blood pool, with a redistribution to tissues such as liver and the lungs [22]. There was a good relationship between organ distribution by gamma imaging, counts obtained post-mortem in tissue samples and immunocytochemical detection of antibody in tissue sections, using peroxidase- or alkaline phosphatase-conjugated rabbit anti-mouse immunoglobulin to locate the injected antibodies [22, 23]. In unpublished studies we have shown by immunoelectron microscopy that mAb

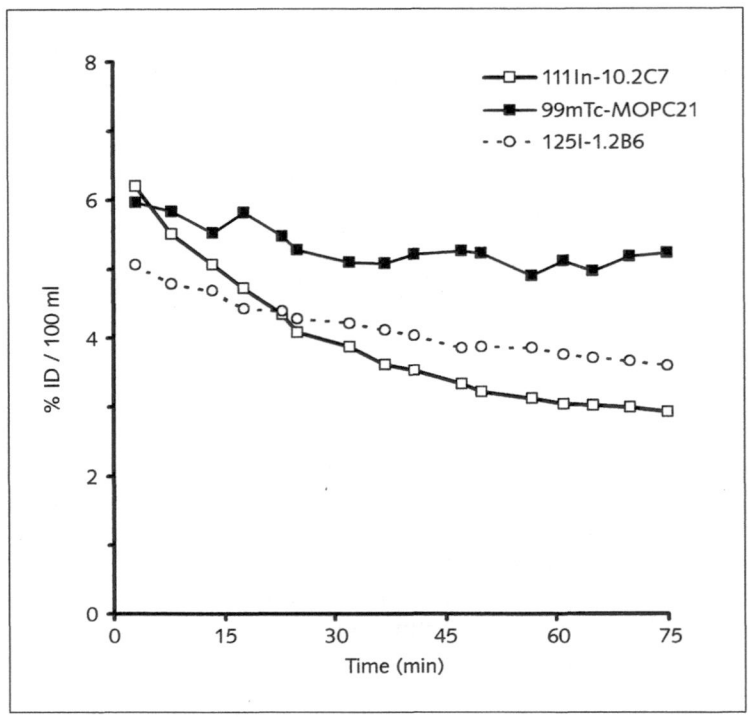

Figure 1
Kinetics of clearance of radiolabelled anti-E-selectin (1.2B6) and anti-VCAM-1 (10.2C7)
mAb from the circulation.
[111]Indium-labelled mAb 10.2C7, [125]Iodine-labelled mAb 1.2B6 and [99m]Technecium-
labelled mAb MOPC-21 were intravenously injected at time zero, and venous blood sam-
ples were taken at 5 min intervals. The data show the percent injected dose (ID) of the anti-
bodies per 100 ml of blood remaining in the circulation over time.
Reproduced with permission from [21].

1.2B6 is rapidly internalised into endothelial cells following binding to E-selectin *in vivo*.

When we directly compared the kinetics of clearance of mAb 1.2B6 (anti-E-selectin) with those of mAb 10.2C7 (anti-VCAM-1) we found that [111]Indium-labelled anti-VCAM-1 was cleared faster in unstimulated pigs than [125]Iodine-labelled anti-E-selectin (Fig. 1). Similar results were obtained when the radiolabels were reversed, indicating that the faster clearance of VCAM-1 was not related to the isotope used. The injected anti-VCAM-1 localised mainly to the liver, spleen, lung and bone marrow, as shown by gamma camera imaging and immunocytochemistry with alkaline phosphatase conjugated rabbit anti-mouse immunoglobulin [21]. Surprisingly, intravenous injection of IL-1α made no difference to the rate of clearance of anti-VCAM-1 mAb.

To investigate the fact that intravenous IL-1α did not alter the clearance kinetics of anti-VCAM-1 mAb 10.2C7, we performed studies to determine the immunoreactivities of the radiolabelled antibodies following injection. As a quantitative assay we used the antibody-associated radioactivity to study the capacity of antibody in timed blood samples still able to bind TNF-activated porcine aortic endothelial cells *in vitro*. In the case of mAb 1.2B6 (anti-E-selectin), the immunoreactivity of circulating antibody remained stable over the course of at least 2 h. In marked contrast, there was a dramatic reduction in the immunoreactivity of circulating anti-VCAM-1 over the same period, indicating that the antibody had become neutralised. The observation that there was a redistribution of radiolabelled antibody from lungs to spleen between 3 and 10 min following injection suggested that the loss of immunoreactivity of anti-VCAM-1 was at least partially attributable to shedding of antibody-antigen complexes from the cell surface following binding of anti-VCAM-1 to cell surfaces expressing VCAM-1. It is also possible that, in the pig, levels of soluble circulating VCAM-1 capable of neutralising antibody may be significantly higher than those of soluble circulating E-selectin, as is known to be true in humans [24].

The experiments investigating the clearance of radiolabelled anti-E-selectin and anti-VCAM-1 mAb in unstimulated and IL-1α-stimulated pigs therefore indicate (i) that mAb 1.2B6 specifically binds E-selectin expressed by activated endothelial cells *in vivo*, (ii) that E-selectin is expressed between 30–40 min following stimulation by IL-1α *in vivo*, consistent with the kinetics seen with cultured endothelial cells [5–7] and (iii) that anti-E-selectin and anti-VCAM-1 mAb show very different patterns of clearance *in vivo*, partly on account of differences in the distribution of antigen expression, but also because of differences in the fate of antibody-antigen complexes following antibody binding. The latter differences are very important when considering the relative potential of the two molecules as targets for imaging.

Cytokine-mediated inflammation in the skin

Pig skin has a number of similarities to human skin and provides a powerful model for dissecting mechanisms of leukocyte traffic [18, 19]. Since the surface area of skin is relatively large, a number of replicate inflammatory sites investigating several parameters, including time courses, can be simultaneously studied, with internal controls. By measuring the uptake of intravenously injected radiolabelled leukocytes and/or radiolabelled mAb into individual lesions, we determined the relationship between the kinetics of expression of E-selectin and VCAM-1 and the kinetics of recruitment of particular leukocyte populations. In the case of radiolabelled antibody uptake we tried to minimise any contribution from internalisation or shedding

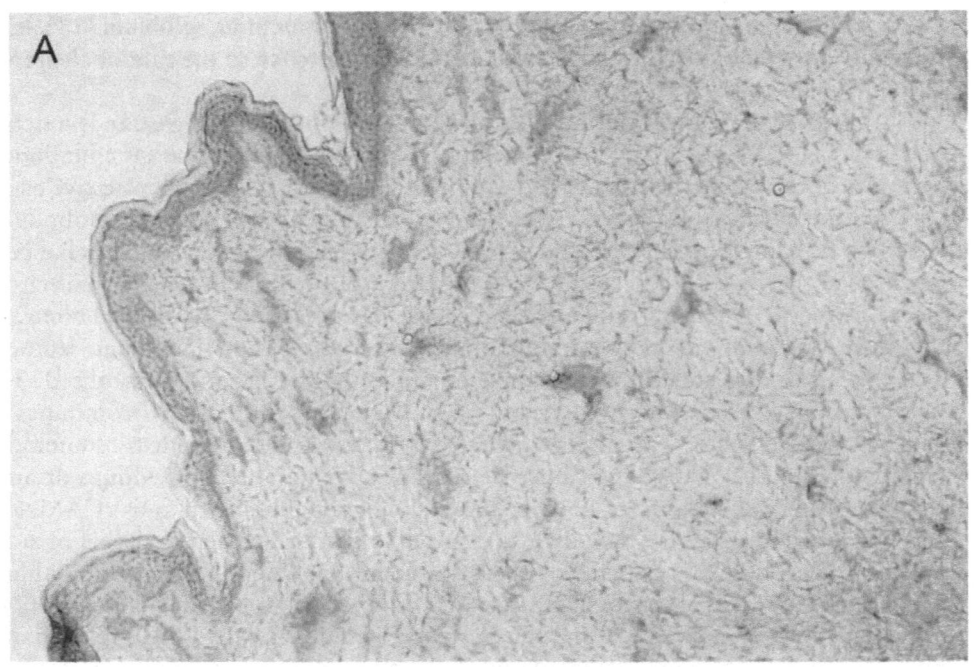

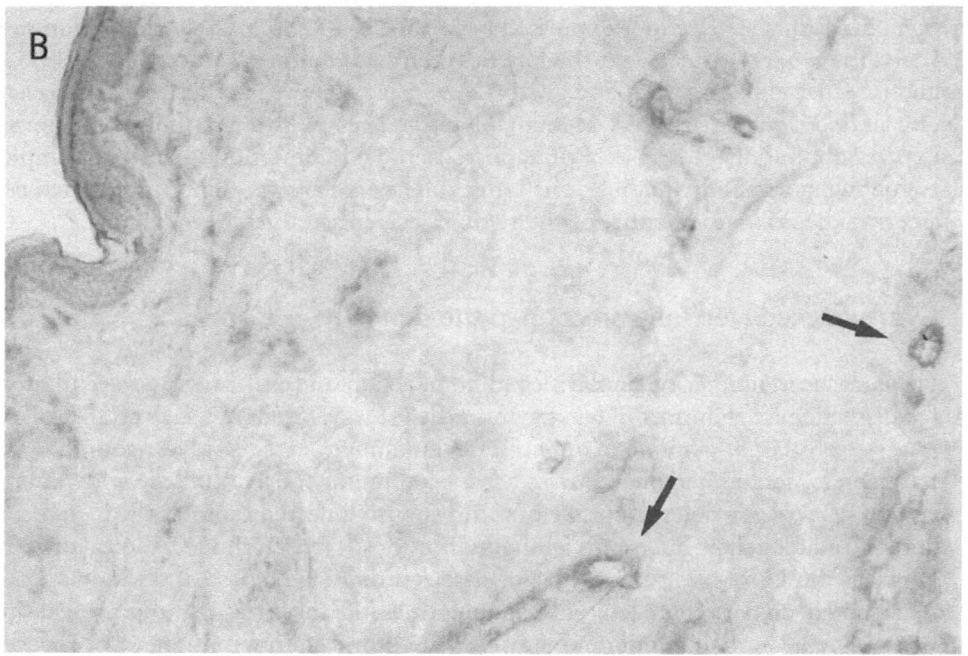

of antibodies following binding to endothelial cell-associated antigen by reducing the interval between antibody injection and the end of the experiment to as little as 3 min.

Uptake of labelled anti-E-selectin into unstimulated skin was greater than that of the simultaneously administered control antibody, consistent with the modest expression of E-selectin in the dermal venules of normal pig skin detected by immunocytochemistry [22]. Following injection of human recombinant IL-1α or human recombinant TNFα, increased uptake of anti-E-selectin could first be detected at 45 min, and was maximal at 2 h. E-selectin expression then decreased, falling more rapidly in IL-1α than in TNFα-stimulated lesions.

In contrast to the uptake of anti-E-selectin, radiolabelled anti-VCAM-1 was not taken up into unstimulated skin to any greater extent than control antibody [21]. However, anti-VCAM-1 localised to cytokine-stimulated skin in immunocytochemical studies on sections with alkaline phosphatase conjugated rabbit anti-mouse immunoglobulin (Fig. 2). In addition, the pattern of upregulation of VCAM-1 by different cytokines in skin measured by radiolabelled anti-VCAM-1 uptake was distinct from that of E-selectin. There was considerably greater uptake of anti-VCAM-1 into TNFα-induced lesions compared with that seen into lesions created by IL-1α injection. The difference between the effects of the two cytokines on VCAM-1 expression in the skin is consistent with observations on cultured human dermal microvascular endothelial cells (see above) [14]. In the case of the cutaneous endothelial cell response to TNFα, expression of E-selectin precedes that of VCAM-1, with the peak expression of VCAM-1 occurring after 8 h (Fig. 3). Again, this mirrors the pattern of expression of the two molecules by endothelial cells in culture [6].

By simultaneously injecting anti-E-selectin with differentially radiolabelled neutrophils and lymphocytes, we traced the relationship between the time-course of expression of this adhesion molecule and that of the recruitment of each leukocyte type. In the case of both IL-1α and TNFα, detailed analysis showed that there was a close relationship between the onset of E-selectin expression and neutrophil localisation, each starting 30–45 min after injection of the cytokine (Fig. 4). However, whilst neutrophil uptake peaked at 105 min and then rapidly declined, uptake of anti-E-selectin expression continued to increase for a period during which neu-

Figure 2
Localisation of intravenously injected anti-VCAM-1 in unstimulated and stimulated pig skin. Tissues were snap-frozen 3 min after intravenous injection of mAb 10.2C7 (anti-VCAM-1), and localisation of antibody was detected in sections using rabbit anti-mouse immunoglobulin. A: No antibody is detectable in unstimulated skin (x100); B: anti-VCAM-1 antibody is seen bound to endothelium in dermal vessels (arrows) in skin stimulated for 6 h with TNFα (2250 U) (x 200). Reproduced with permission from [21].

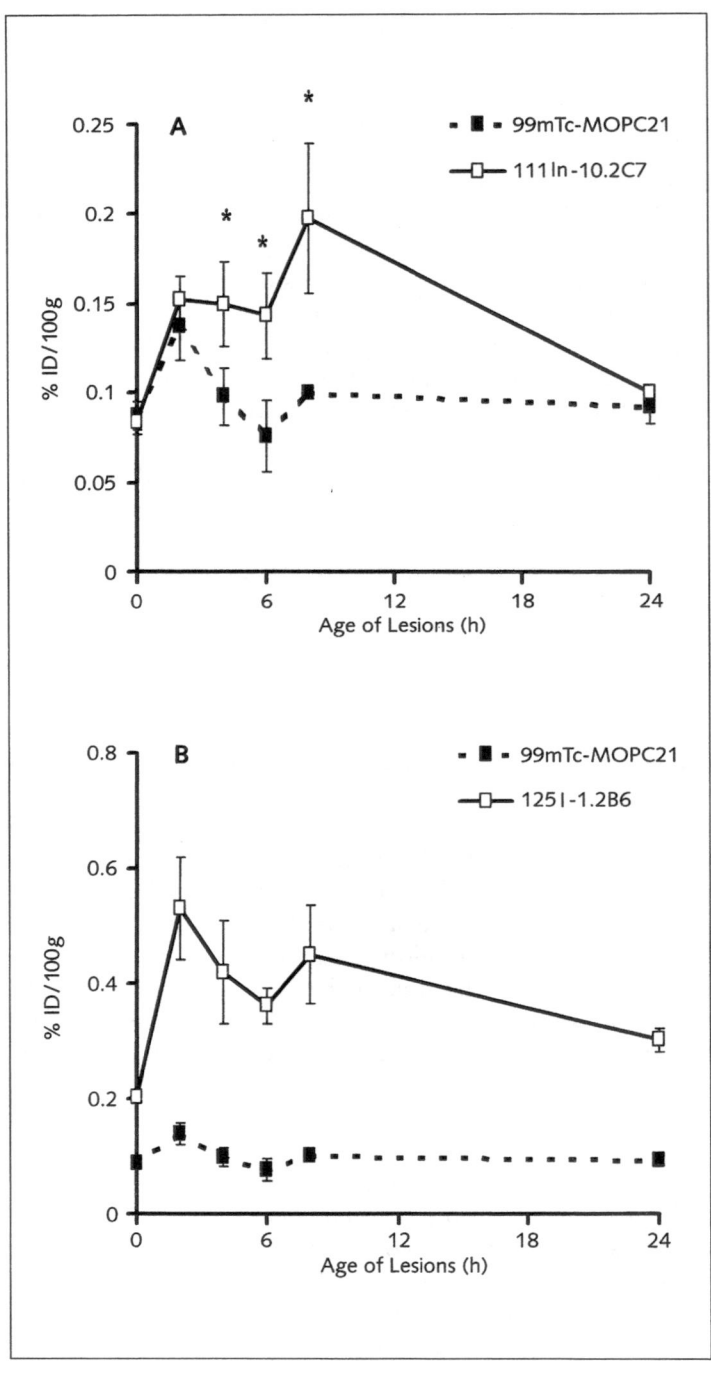

trophil localisation was falling. In contrast, the onset of lymphocyte uptake was found to be later than that of initial E-selectin expression and neutrophil recruitment, but was contemporaneous with the later stage of E-selectin expression.

Having determined the relationship between the kinetics of E-selectin expression and the kinetics of neutrophil and lymphocyte localisation in these skin lesions, we next investigated if either neutrophil and lymphocyte uptake required E-selectin, using saturating rather than tracer quantities of mAb 1.2B6 and using $F(ab')_2$ antibody fragments. The experiments demonstrated that the uptake of both neutrophils and lymphocytes was inhibited by anti-E-selectin to a degree comparable to inhibiting the β_2 integrin (CD18) subunit. Putting the inhibition data together with data on the kinetics of E-selectin expression and cell recruitment suggests that, in these simple cytokine-stimulated lesions, expression of E-selectin facilitates the recruitment of both neutrophils and lymphocytes while not fully determining the time-course of their uptake.

Cutaneous delayed-type hypersensitivity

We used two models of T cell-mediated immunity to study the endothelial cell expression of adhesion molecules in the skin in more complex inflammatory responses. In the first experimental model, pigs were sensitised by intradermal injection of bacillus Calmette-Guerin, and challenged 10–14 days later by intradermal injection of purified protein derivative (PPD). In the second model, pigs were both sensitised and challenged by topical application of 2,4-dinitro-1-fluorobenzene in acetone/dimethylsulphoxide. Both inflammatory responses were more prolonged than seen after injection of cytokines, and allowed comparisons to be made between the tissue irritant reaction in unsensitised naïve pigs and the immune response in pigs that had been previously sensitised to antigen.

Figure 3
Uptake of anti-VCAM-1 (10.2C7) (A) and anti-E-selectin (1.2B6) (B) mAb into cutaneous TNFα-induced inflammation.
Inflammatory lesions were elicited by intradermal injection of 2250 U TNFα at varying times before the end of the experiment. ^{111}Indium-labelled mAb 10.2C7, ^{125}Iodine-labelled mAb 1.2B6 and ^{99m}Technecium-labelled mAb MOPC-21 were intravenously injected 3 min before the end of the experiment, and uptake of isotopes was counted in excised skin post-mortem. Data points are mean ± SEM of the percent injected dose (ID) per 100 g of tissue from a total of 24 skin discs from three pigs.
*indicates p<0.05 for uptake of 10.2C7; uptake of 1.2B6 was significantly greater than that of MOPC-21 at all time points (p<0.05). Reproduced with permission from [21].

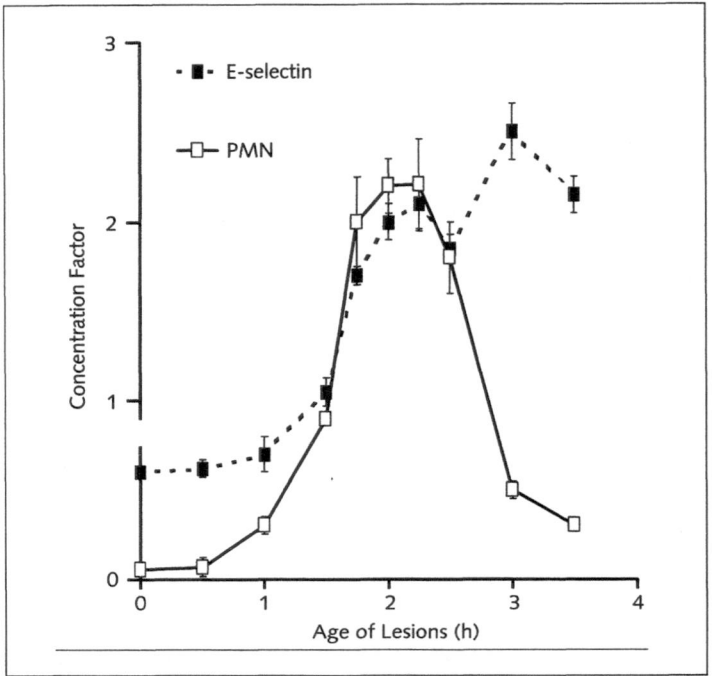

Figure 4
Comparison of time courses of localisation of polymorphonuclear leukocytes and expression of E-selectin after intradermal injection of TNFα.
Polymorphonuclear leukocyte accumulation starts after 30 min and correlates with increased expression of E-selectin; however, the leukocyte wave is short-lived, whereas E-selectin expression continues to increase in a biphasic response.
Reproduced with permission from [25].

In both models, three components to the inflammatory response could be distin-guished: (i) during the first 12 h there is a non-specific early phase demonstrated by the expression of E-selectin and by the uptake of neutrophils. This was similar in naïve and sensitised animals and is presumably a non-specific irritant response; (ii) uptake of lymphocytes during this early phase is greater in sensitised than in naïve pigs, indicating that even at this stage there is an immune-specific component to the response; and (iii) between 24 and 48 h after challenge there is a secondary phase of E-selectin expression and lymphocyte uptake in sensitised but not in naïve ani-mals, indicating a delayed effect of the immune response to antigen. As in the response to cytokine injection, optimal uptake of neutrophils and lymphocytes in both forms of immune-mediated response was dependent upon E-selectin expression, as shown by inhibition studies with saturating quantities of anti-E-selectin mAb.

So far we have only explored the expression of VCAM-1 in the response to PPD [21]. Unlike E-selectin, VCAM-1 expression is not detected during the early phase in animals not previously sensitised to PPD. In contrast, sensitised animals showed increased uptake of anti-VCAM-1 compared with uptake of non-specific antibody during both the early and late phases, correlating well with the increased uptake of lymphocytes. In view of the differential capacity of IL-1α and TNFα to induce VCAM-1 expression, we tested the hypothesis that expression of VCAM-1 during the response to PPD depended critically upon TNFα by using an inhibitory anti-TNFα mAb. Pigs pre-treated with anti-TNFα 2 h before antigen challenge had no significant uptake of anti-VCAM-1 mAb at 6 and 8 h compared with control antibody uptake. At 24 h there was some uptake of anti-VCAM-1 antibody, but this was significantly reduced compared with control pigs. In contrast, anti-TNFα had no significant effect on the uptake of anti-E-selectin in the same animals.

Thus, observations in cutaneous inflammatory studies indicate that E-selectin is expressed in response to both IL-1α and TNFα, and that this adhesion molecule plays a facilitating role in the uptake of neutrophils and lymphocytes, but does not independently determine the uptake of either. In comparison with E-selectin, VCAM-1 expression appears to be relatively more dependent upon TNFα, and its kinetics correlate well with the uptake of lymphocytes. Whether or not inhibiting VCAM-1 or TNFα in this model would influence lymphocyte recruitment remains to be tested.

Inflammatory arthritis

In pre-clinical experiments, we evaluated the imaging potential of anti-E-selectin antibody, either as the whole antibody molecule mAb 1.2B6 [26] or as a F(ab')$_2$ fragment [23, 27], using the monoarthritis induced by the injection of phyto-haemagglutinin or urate crystals as a model. Uptake and clearance of the F(ab')$_2$ fragment correlated well with those of whole antibody in experiments in which the two were differentially radiolabelled and injected into the same animals [24]. We found that the F(ab')$_2$ fragment mAb 1.2B6 was specifically taken up into inflamed synovium, with clear gamma camera images obtained within 3 h of antibody injection (Fig. 5). Images obtained with the F(ab')$_2$ fragment mAb 1.2B6 were significantly more localised than those with the radiolabelled F(ab')$_2$ fragment MOPC-21. Regional lymph nodes were also imaged in occasional animals as a result of endothelial expression of E-selectin, presumably in response to factors in afferent lymph draining inflamed synovial tissue.

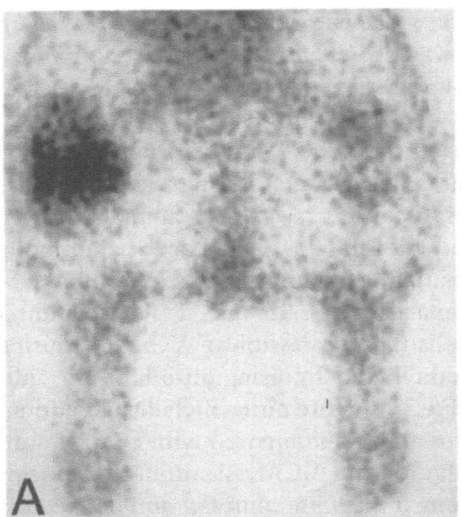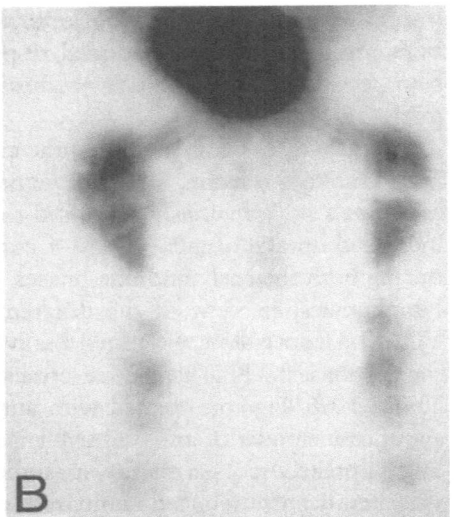

Figure 5
Scintigrams obtained 3 h after injection of ^{111}Indium-labelled 1.2B6 F(ab')$_2$ fragments (A)
and ^{99m}Technecium-labelled polymorphonuclear leukocytes (B) in a pig with phytohaemag-
glutinin-induced monoarthritis in the right knee.
Intense uptake of ^{111}Indium-labelled 1.2B6 F(ab')$_2$ fragments is visible in the right knee
compared with the left knee, into which buffer was injected. Faint filling of the joint space
of the right knee is observed with the ^{99m}Technecium-labelled polymorphonuclear leuko-
cytes, which accumulated in the subchondral bone marrow on either side. The body outline
is clearly delineated with the ^{111}Indium-labelled 1.2B6 F(ab')$_2$ fragments because of specif-
ic skin uptake of antibody. Reproduced with permission from [23].

In contrast to the successful imaging of porcine monoarthritis with anti-E-selectin, preliminary experiments have failed to show similar accumulation of radi-olabelled anti-VCAM-1 in inflamed synovium, probably because of shedding of antibody-antigen complexes into the circulation. For this reason we feel that imaging VCAM-1 will be more difficult than imaging E-selectin.

Clinical imaging

In clinical studies, we have employed the anti-E-selectin antibody mAb 1.2B6 to image E-selectin expression in patients. Again we used the F(ab')$_2$ fragment to reduce the possibility of induction of pro-inflammatory events, thrombosis or vasculitis through the binding of the Fc domain by leukocytes. When interpreting the images in patients, it should be noted that whilst mAb 1.2B6 specifically reacts with E-selectin in the pig, in humans it also reacts weakly with P-selectin (see above). Whilst this cross-reactivity reduces the specificity of the antibody in humans as an exact molecular probe, it should increase the sensitivity of the antibody as an agent for imaging activated endothelium in clinical inflammatory disorders.

Rheumatoid arthritis

Our initial clinical imaging focused on inflamed joints in patients with rheumatoid arthritis. After informed consent, the joints in fourteen patients were scanned following injection of 35 μg [111]Indium-labelled 1.2B6 F(ab')$_2$ fragments. Images were compared with those achieved after injection of [111]Indium-labelled polyclonal human immunoglobulin (HIG), an imaging agent that has previously been evaluated in rheumatoid arthritis [1], and which is thought to localise by non-specific diffusion across activated endothelium. Images were analysed 4 and 24 h after injection using a large field-of-view gamma camera [28].

Accumulation of anti-E-selectin was easily detected in inflamed joints of all patients, with the most obvious images being obtained after 24 h. Identification of individual joints was possible, including the small peripheral joints of the hands and feet (Fig. 6). Although the majority (around 80%) of joints imaged by mAb 1.2B6 were also imaged by HIG, E-selectin imaging of inflamed synovium was significantly more intense and more focal. Furthermore, mAb 1.2B6 imaging was also significantly more sensitive, with 22% of joints imaged by mAb 1.2B6 being negative with HIG. It was notable that mAb 1.2B6 frequently imaged additional joints that were not clinically swollen, whilst joints imaged by HIG tended to be those with clinically obvious synovial swelling.

Inflammatory bowel disease

Although radiolabelled leukocyte scanning is routinely used to identify the presence and localisation of active inflammation in inflammatory bowel disease [29, 30], this technique is not ideal, as the preparation of radiolabelled leukocytes is time-consuming and involves risks of infection for laboratory personnel. Thus white cell scanning tends to be restricted to specialist centres. It would be of great benefit if the extent and activity of inflammatory bowel disease could be defined in a minimally invasive way at any point in time in the follow-up of these patients. E-selectin expression has been demonstrated by immunocytochemistry to be upregulated in actively involved regions of the bowel in inflammatory bowel disease [31, 32], justifying studies to image inflamed bowel with mAb 1.2B6.

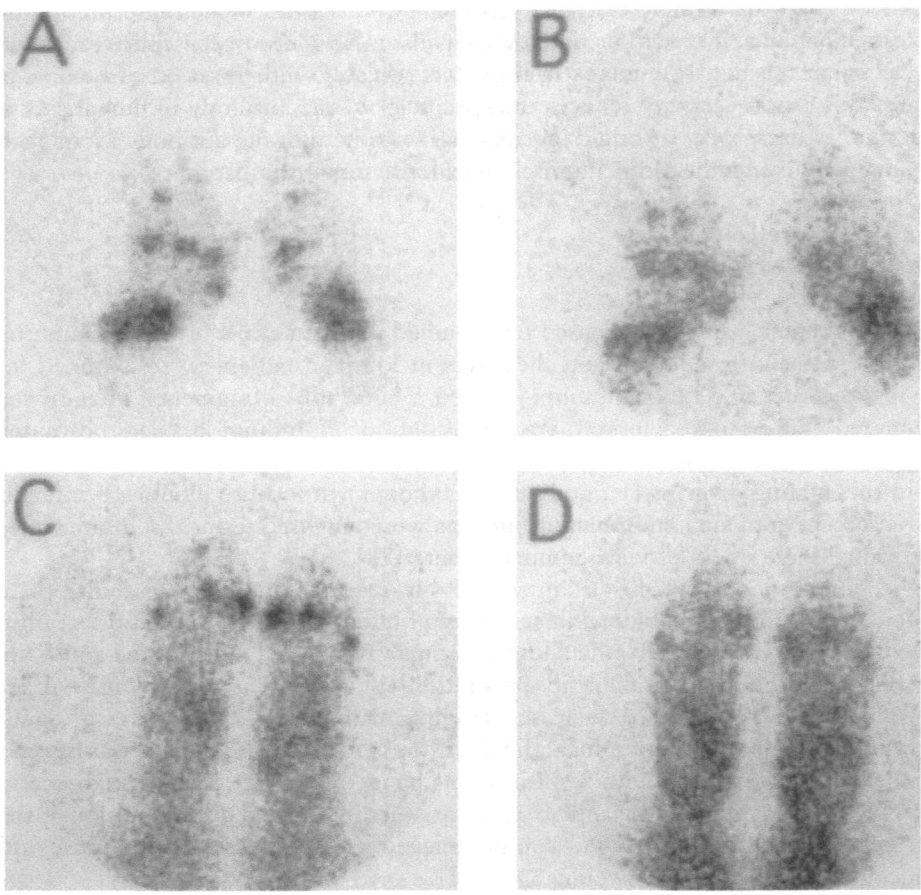

Figure 6

Gamma camera images of the hands and feet of a patient with long-standing rheumatoid arthritis, taken 24 h after intravenous injection of separately administered [111]Indium-labelled anti-E-selectin monoclonal antibody 1.2B6 (A and C) and [111]Indium-labelled poly-clonal human immunoglobulin (B and D).

Although images with both tracers demonstrate a similar distribution, uptake of 1.2B6 is clearly more intense, with a more focal pattern and a higher target to background ratio. Reproduced with permission from [28].

A pilot study in 13 patients with active inflammatory bowel disease has been undertaken [33]. After informed consent, enrolled patients received both ^{99m}Technicium-labelled leukocytes and ^{111}Indium-labelled E-selectin in sequence. In ten patients, both isotopes indicated disease in similar areas. One other patient had a positive E-selectin scan, but negative leukocyte scanning, whilst two further patients had areas of positivity with the leukocyte scanning but not with the E-selectin scan. Both scans were negative in the four patients with clinically inactive disease. Patients with positive E-selectin scans tended to have raised levels of circulating soluble E-selectin, and demonstrated E-selectin expression on immunocytochemistry of inflamed mucosa biopsied at colonoscopy.

Conclusions

A number of directions can be highlighted for further development of these techniques and for more precise interpretation of the data obtained so far. Firstly, the absolute quantification of endothelial cell antigen expression in an inflamed tissue in experimental work using tracer quantities of radiolabelled antibody is potentially complicated by variation between animals in the degree of antigen expression elsewhere, particularly in the form of circulating soluble antigen. Although this problem can be overcome by injecting saturating quantities of antibody, the size of pigs makes this solution impractical, and there are distinct advantages here in using murine models [34–36]. Secondly, experiments relating the detailed kinetics of expression of endothelial cell adhesion molecules to the kinetics of recruitment of radiolabelled leukocytes are limited by not knowing whether radiolabelled leukocytes that have localised to skin have actually transmigrated through endothelium into the tissues or are just rolling or adherent on endothelium, without necessarily being destined to transmigrate into the tissues. This issue will need to be addressed by complementary techniques such as intra-vital microscopy. Lastly, localisation of antibodies to endothelium using radiolabelling does not address the question of which vessels express the antigen, either in terms of the size of vessel or in terms of which vascular system is involved (e.g. in lung, whether pulmonary or bronchial), and complementary immunocytochemistry is required.

In spite of these technical limitations, the studies outlined in this chapter have established the principle that it is possible to quantify and image endothelial expression of inducible antigens, thereby providing a means for directly measuring the behaviour of activated endothelium in experimental models, and in patients with inflammatory disorders. Furthermore, in addition to using antibodies for this purpose, it may prove possible to target with peptides or carbohydrates derived from natural ligands, and to convey not just radioisotopes but also therapeutic agents to the site of endothelial activation [37, 38].

Acknowledgements
TYH is supported by a Garfield Weston Fellowship. The Department has support from the British Heart Foundation.

References

1   De Bois MHW, Pauwels EKJ, Breedveld FC (1995) New agents for scintigraphy in rheumatoid arthritis. *Eur J Nucl Med* 22: 1339–1346

2   Becker W (1995) The contribution of nuclear medicine to the patient with infection. *Eur J Nucl Med* 22: 1195–1211

3   Pober JS, Cotran RS (1990) Cytokines and endothelial cell biology. *Physiol Rev* 70: 427–451

4   Peters AM (1996) The choice of an appropriate agent for imaging inflammation. *Nucl Med Commun* 17: 455–458

5   Pober JS, Bevilacqua MP, Mendrick DL, Lapierre LA, Fiers W, Gimbrone MA (1986) Two distinct monokines, interleukin 1 and tumor necrosis factor, each independently induce the biosynthesis and transient expression of the same antigen on the surface of cultured human vascular endothelial cells. *J Immunol* 136: 1680–1687

6   Wellicome SM, Thornhill MH, Pitzalis C, Thomas DS, Lanchbury JSS, Panayi GS, Haskard DO (1990) A monoclonal antibody that detects a novel antigen on endothelial cells that is induced by tumor necrosis factor, IL-1 or lipopolysaccharide. *J Immunol* 144: 2558–2565

7   Tsang Y, Stevens PE, Licence ST, Haskard DO, Binns RM, Robinson MK (1995) Porcine E-selectin: cloning and functional characterization. *Immunology* 85: 140–145

8   Mason JC, Haskard DO (1994) The clinical importance of leukocyte and endothelial cell adhesion molecules in inflammation. *Vasc Med Rev* 5: 249–275

9   von Asmuth EJU, Smeets EF, Ginsel LA, Onderwater JJM, Leeuwenberg JFM, Buurman WA (1992) Evidence for endocytosis of E-selectin in human endothelial cells. *Eur J Immunol* 22: 2519–2526

10 Kuijpers TW, Raleigh M, Kavanagh T, Janssen H, Calafat J, Roos D, Harlan JM (1994) Cytokine-activated endothelial cells internalize E-selectin into a lysosomal compartment of vesiculotubular shape: a tubulin-driven process. *J Immunol* 152: 5060–5069

11 Rice GE, Bevilacqua MP (1989) An inducible endothelial cell surface glycoprotein mediates melanoma adhesion. *Science* 246: 1303–1306

12 Osborn L, Hession C, Tizard R, Vassallo C, Luhowskyj S, Chi-Rosso G, Lobb R (1989) Direct expression cloning of vascular cell adhesion molecule 1 (VCAM1), a cytokine-induced endothelial protein that binds to lymphocytes. *Cell* 59: 1203–1211

13 Thornhill MH, Haskard DO (1990) IL-4 regulates endothelial activation by IL-1, tumor necrosis factor or IFNγ. *J Immunol* 145: 865–872

14 Swerlick RA, Lee KH, Li L-J, Sepp NT, Caughman SW, Lawley TJ (1992) Regulation of

vascular cell adhesion molecule 1 on human dermal microvascular endothelial cells. *J Immunol* 149: 698–705

15 Gille J, Swerlick RA, Lawley TJ, Caughman SW (1996) Differential regulation of vascular cell adhesion molecule-1 gene transcription by tumour necrosis factor alpha and interleukin-1 alpha in dermal microvascular endothelial cells. *Blood* 87: 211–217

16 Rice GE, Munro JM, Corless C, Bevilacqua MP (1991) Vascular and nonvascular expression of INCAM-110: A target for mononuclear leukocyte adhesion in normal and inflamed human tissues. *Am J Pathol* 138: 385–393

17 Leeuwenberg JFM, Smeets EF, Neefjes JJ, Shaffer MA, Cinek T, Jeunhomme TMAA, Ahern TJ, Buurman WA (1992) E-selectin and intercellular adhesion molecule-1 are released by activated human endothelial cells *in vitro. Immunology* 77: 543–549

18 Binns RM, Licence ST, Wooding ST (1990) Phytohemagglutinin induces major short-term protease-sensitive lymphocyte traffic involving high endothelium venule-like blood vessels in acute delayed-type hypersensitivity-like reactions in skin and other tissues. *Eur J Immunol* 20: 1067–1071

19 Binns RM, Licence ST, Wooding FBP, Duffus WPH (1992) Active lymphocyte traffic induced in the periphery by cytokines and phytohemagglutinin: three different mechanisms? Eur *J Immunol* 22: 2195–2203

20 Binns RM, Pabst R (1994) Lymphoid tissue structure and lymphocyte trafficking in the pig. *Vet Immunol Immunopathol* 43: 79–87

21 Harrison AA, Stocker CJ, Chapman PT, Tsang YT, Huehns TY, Gundel RH, Peters AM, Davies KA, George AJ, Robinson MK et al (1997) Expression of VCAM-1 by vascular endothelial cells in immune- and non-immune inflammatory reactions in the skin. *J Immunol* 159: 4546–4554

22 Keelan ETM, Licence ST, Peters AM, Binns RM, Haskard DO (1994) Characterization of E-selectin expression *in vivo* using a radiolabelled monoclonal antibody. *Am J Physiol* 266: H279–H290

23 Jamar F, Chapman PT, Harrison AA, Binns RM, Haskard DO, Peters AM (1995) Inflammatory arthritis: imaging of endothelial activation with an indium-111-labeled F(ab')$_2$ fragment of anti-E-selectin monoclonal antibody. *Radiology* 194: 843–850

24 Gearing AJH, Newman W (1993) Circulating adhesion molecules in disease. *Immunology Today* 14: 506–512

25 Binns RM, Licence ST, Harrison AA, Keelan ETD, Robinson MK, Haskard DO (1966) *In vivo* E-selectin upregulation correlates with early infiltration of PMN, later with PBL-entry; mAbs block both. *Am J Physiol* 270: H183–H193

26 Keelan ETM, Harrison AA, Chapman PT, Binns RM, Peters AM, Haskard DO (1994) Imaging vascular endothelial activation: an approach using radiolabelled monoclonal antibody against the endothelial cell adhesion molecule E-selectin. *J Nucl Med* 35: 276–281

27 Chapman PT, Jamar F, Harrison AA, Binns RM, Peters AM, Haskard DO.(1994) Non-invasive imaging of E-selectin expression by activated endothelium in urate crystal-induced arthritis. *Arthritis Rheum* 37: 1752–1756

28 Chapman PT, Jamar F, Keelan ETM, Peters AM, Haskard DO (1966) Use of a radiola-
    beled monoclonal antibody against E-selectin for imaging endothelial activation in
    rheumatoid arthritis. *Arthritis Rheum* 39: 1371–1375

29 Scholmerich J, Schmidt E, Schumichen C, Billmann P, Schmidt H, Gerok W (1988)
    Scintigraphic assessment of bowel involvement and disease activity in Crohn's disease
    using technetium 99m-hexamethyl propylene amine oxime as leukocyte label. *Gas-
    troenterology* 95: 1287–1293

30 Peters AM, Danpure HJ, Osman S, Hawker RJ, Henderson BL, Hodgson HJ, Kelly JD,
    Neirinckx RD, Lavender JP (1986) Clinical experience with ^{99m}Tc hexamethylpropylene
    amine oxime for labelling leucocytes and imaging inflammation. *Lancet* 2: 946–949

31 Ohtani H, Nakamura S, Watanabe Y, Fukushima K, Mizoi T, Kimura M, Hiwatashi N,
    Nagura H (1992) Light and electron microscopic immunolocalization of endothelial leu-
    cocyte adhesion molecule-1 in inflammatory bowel disease. Morphological evidence of
    active synthesis and secretion into vascular lumen. *Virchows Arch A Pathol Anat
    Histopathol* 420: 403–409

32 Koizumi M, King N, Lobb R, Benjamin C, Podolsky DK (1992) Expression of vascular
    adhesion molecules in inflammatory bowel disease. *Gastroenterology* 103: 840–847

33 Bhatti M, Chapman P, Peters AM, Haskard DO, Hodgson H (1998) Visualizing E-
    selectin in the detection and evaluation of inflammatory bowel disease. *Gut* 43: 40–47

34 Panes J, Perry MA, Anderson DC, Manning A, Leone B, Cepinskas G, Rosenbloom CL,
    Miyasaka M, Kvietys PR, Granger DN (1995) Regional differences in constitutive and
    induced ICAM-1 expression *in vivo*. *Am J Physiol* 38: H1955–H1964

35 Eppihimer MJ, Wolitzky BA, Anderson DC, Labow MA, Granger DN (1996) Hetero-
    geneity of expression of E- and P-selectins *in vivo*. *Circ Res* 79: 560–569

36 Henninger DD, Panes J, Eppihimer M, Russell J, Gerritsen M, Anderson DC, Granger
    DN (1997) Cytokine-induced VCAM-1 and ICAM-1 expression in different organs in
    the mouse. *J Immunol* 158: 1825–1832

37 Wickham TJ, Haskard D, Segal D, Kovesdi I (1997) Targeting endothelium for gene
    therapy via receptors upregulated during angiogenesis and inflammation. *Cancer
    Immunol Immunother* 45: 149–151

38 Harari OA, Wickham TJ, Stocker CJ, Kovesdi I, Segal DM, Huehns TY, Sarraf C,
    Haskard DO (1999) Targeting an adenoviral gene vector to cytokine-activated vascular
    endothelium via E-selectin. *Gene Therapy* 5: 801–807

Leukocyte adhesion and activation in xenografts

[1]Simon C. Robson and [2]David Goodman

[1]Department of Medicine, Beth Israel Deaconess Medical Center, Research North, Rm 370H, 99 Brookline Avenue, Boston, MA 02215, USA; and [2]Department of Clinical Immunology and Nephrology, St Vincent's Hospital Melbourne, Fitzroy 3065, Australia

Introduction

Over the decade, substantial increases in transplant organ and recipient survival have been accompanied by a significant increase in the quality of life for patients with end stage organ failure. However, the increasing access to organ transplant lists, coupled with static or even falling organ donation rates, have resulted in a doubling of the waiting time for patients receiving a cadaveric kidney to around three years at many major centers. In addition, many patients waiting for a suitable heart or liver die while waiting because of the lack of effective life support systems. While living related kidney transplantation has the potential to alleviate kidney organ shortages, grafting of liver or lung from living donors has been performed in only a few specialised centres to date.

The proposed use of an unlimited supply of animal organs in clinical practice, i.e. xenotransplantation, could provide a bridge to a successful allograft, or more optimistically may even substitute for allografts and provide for long term graft survival [1–3]. Unfortunately, the clinical application of xenotransplantation, to date, has resulted in universal suboptimal results with failure when measured against the routine and effective use of allografts. This form of clinical intervention will only be feasible once the mechanisms of xenograft loss have been better determined and effective therapies tested in appropriate animal models [2, 4–6]. Indeed, recent developments in the field of xenotransplantation biology have greatly expanded our understanding of the mechanisms by which xenografts are rejected [7–10]. Novel molecular biological techniques have allowed the production of donor animals (pigs) with human transgenes directed toward amelioration of the complement (C) activation [11] and antibody interactions [12, 13] shown to be of great immediate importance in xenograft rejection. However, with these advances, it has become apparent that the rejection response directed at a discordant xenograft is composed of many separate elements that appear to have different kinetics and result in various manifestations of xenograft rejection [3, 5, 7].

Discordant porcine organs can function for several days in primates following the inhibition of C and/or removal of xenoreactive natural antibodies (XNA) that are associated with hyperacute rejection (HAR) [3, 14, 15]. However, a xenograft rejection process, characterized by humoral and cell-mediated vascular and parenchymal injury, then ensues. This acute vascular-type or delayed xenograft rejection process (AVR/DXR) and the associated antibody/cellular mediated responses in primates to porcine antigens are considered the major barrier to xenograft acceptance at this time [4, 5, 7]. This response may be initiated by natural killer (NK) cell-mediated endothelial cell (EC) activation, associated with secondary xenoreactive antibody and T cell responses [16]. Currently, the mechanisms whereby NK cells, T cells and monocytes interact with porcine endothelium and the role of co-stimulatory pathways remain undetermined but available data will be addressed in this chapter.

The scientific uncertainty regarding the mechanisms of these immune reactions has been recently coupled with public health questions regarding the importance of potential zoonoses such as porcine endogenous retroviruses (PERV) and how interspecies molecular barriers may compromise control of certain infections [17, 18] or even any associated lymphoproliferative disorders. These unresolved scientific issues, in addition to many social and potential ethical issues surrounding xenotransplantation, will require extensive debate between the appropriate regulatory bodies prior to the commencement of clinical trials in xenotransplantation. These issues are beyond the scope of this chapter but have recently been reviewed [19].

Mechanisms of discordant xenograft rejection

Hyperacute rejection (HAR)

Following transplantation of a vascularized discordant xenograft (pig to primate), pre-formed XNA are bound to the endothelial cells (EC) resulting in C activation, vascular damage, intravascular thrombosis and finally ischaemic necrosis. Depending on the species combination, HAR is either initiated by the rapid deposition of XNA from recipients within the graft and the subsequent activation of the classical pathway of C activation (e.g. pig to primate) [20] , or is mediated by direct activation of host C through the graft endothelium (e.g. guinea pig to rat combination) [21]. In addition to the activation of C, neutrophil adherence and vasoconstriction may contribute to the pathogenesis of HAR in various models of xenograft rejection [8, 22, 23]. One of the major complications that accompanies HAR relates to thrombosis of the graft microvasculature with platelet sequestration [8]. This development may be associated with ongoing inflammatory responses linked to C-activation [24, 25] or to other inflammatory mediators in certain vascular beds, such as that of the lung [26].

The activation of C on xenogeneic surfaces is largely uncontrolled by vascular complement regulatory proteins because of the functional incompatibilities between the pig and certain primate species, including man [27, 28]. Effective regulation of C activation in xenografts may be obtained using human regulatory proteins, e.g. CD55 (decay accelerating factor or DAF), CD59 and CD46 or pharmaceutical approaches with anti-complement strategies [29–31]. These approaches can successfully abrogate HAR [32, 33].

In addition, techniques to downregulate the expression of the major porcine xenoantigen for binding XNA, α-(1,3) gal, have been developed in transgenic pigs that express H-transferase or other glycosyltransferases [12, 13, 34, 35]. The EC from these animals may effectively downregulate C activation though inhibition of XNA binding, but the ability to directly inhibit NK cell interactions remains unclear [36].

Acute vascular rejection or delayed xenograft rejection (AVR/DXR)

When primate recipients are pre-treated to avert HAR either by effective blockade of C activation and/or by removing or inhibiting XNA, porcine xenografts survive for several days. Such organs are still rejected by a process designated as AVR/DXR that has been observed in several models of discordant xenotransplantation [22], such as clinically relevant pig to baboon heart and kidney xenotransplantation [3, 7, 37]. Morphologically, AVR/DXR is characterized by a progressive infiltration with mononuclear cells (MNC) occurring over 2–4 days post-transplant and a process of intravascular thrombosis. These events are paralleled by a progressive activation of EC, including the upregulation of inflammatory cytokines and evolution of a procoagulant environment [8].

The activation of EC is associated with induction of adhesion molecules, as well as stimulation of a procoagulant state through upregulation of tissue factors on monocyte-macrophages (Mo) and graft EC, and downregulation of anticoagulant molecules, including thrombomodulin, tissue factor pathway inhibitor and antithrombin [38–41]. Downregulation of thrombomodulin expression, resulting in a markedly reduced capacity of EC to bind thrombin and activate protein C, may further enhance Mo cytokine production. Activated protein C appears to have a key role in inhibition of Mo activation [42]. Fibrin generation, local hypoxia, the deleterious effects of TNF, IL-1 and other cytokines generated in response to activated C components and activated coagulation factors may cause substantial graft injury. The effects of MNC binding to EC, mediated through XNA binding, may synergize to result in the profound vascular injury observed with AVR/DXR [8, 41].

Mo and NK cells that are found at the site of rejection in recipients pretreated with the C activator and depleting agent, cobra venom factor, may recognise and bind to xenogeneic EC directly and cause cellular activation. Potential receptors have been described for both of these major cell types: Mo express carbohydrate binding factors or lectins and NK cells have receptors with specific lectin-binding domains [16, 43]. NK cells have been shown to have the potential to cause damage to endothelium [16, 44–48]. T cells do not appear to alter the principal features leading to AVR/DXR in small animal models; in addition, kinetics of host Mo and NK cell infiltration are not significantly influenced by the absence or presence of T cells [49].

Currently, it is uncertain as to what further features would emerge if AVR/DXR could be abrogated. It has been suggested that the equivalent of the T cell mediated rejection of an allograft would occur in a discordant graft. Evidence from concordant xenografting of organs in man implies that processes of xenoreactive cellular responses would be more aggressive than that of the comparable alloreactive combinations [20, 50–53]. Thus, development of an optimal therapeutic regimen that will permit long-term function of a xenograft may require not only inhibition of XNA and C but also specific interference of processes related to EC perturbation and Mo, NK and lymphocyte infiltration and activation.

Endothelial cell activation

EC activation may be a critical factor in orchestrating the immune response while balancing hemostasis [8, 54]. This process may be responsible for key elements underlying the rejection of discordant xenografts. In this fashion, the relationship of EC activation to platelet aggregation may further exacerbate the development of vascular thrombosis. Quiescent vascular EC inhibit platelet aggregation, at least in part because they express an ecto-enzyme that hydrolyzes ADP, a powerful extracellular agonist for platelet aggregation, and ATP, a potential EC agonist [55]. The presumed function of vascular ATP-diphosphohydrolase (ATPDase/CD39) is to prevent the accumulation of certain purinergic mediators and therefore modulate platelet aggregation and other inflammatory phenomena [56]. Activated EC lose ATPDase activity as a consequence of oxidative stress and thus become permissive for platelet aggregation [57].

EC activation could be triggered by the binding of low levels of XNA or of elicited xenoreactive antibodies . Alternatively, minimal C-activation to assembly of the terminal complexes and expression of IL-1α may lead to EC perturbation and upregulation of procoagulants such as tissue factor [24, 25]. Human NK cells and Mo, both of which are present in an apparently activated state in rejecting xenografts, each have the potential through TNFα to activate porcine EC in co-cultures *in vitro* [16, 43, 48, 58].

The transcription factor NF-κB appears to play a pivotal role in EC activation and many of the genes associated with EC activation have one or more NF-κB binding sites within their promoters [59]. Thrombin, which is present in many situations, activates EC in a NF-κB-dependent manner; thrombin and TNF act synergistically in this regard [60]. Reactive oxygen species are generated in many situations and would activate NF-κB thereby leading to type II EC activation ([61]; see also the chapter by Chen and Medford, this volume).

NF-κB is maintained in the cytoplasm by the inhibitory molecule Ik-Ba and only following Ik-Ba phosphorylation can NF-κB be translocated to the nucleus and contribute to transcription [62]. Overexpression of Iκ-Ba in porcine EC renders the cells resistant to activation by bacterial lipopolysaccharide [63] or by human NK cells [64]. The NF-κB pathway also contributes to the induction of anti-apoptotic genes following exposure to TNFα. Treatment of EC overexpressing Iκ-Ba results in apoptosis severely limiting this strategy to inhibit xenograft rejection [10]. A novel approach pursued by Anrather et al is based on a mutated form of NF-κB subunits [65]. This approach is not complicated by apoptosis and may be the most suitable method available for inhibiting NF-κB but further data from transgenic animals will be required.

Strategies for directly modulating EC activation and inducing protective type responses have been reviewed recently and will not be addressed in any further detail here [10].

Involvement of leukocytes in discordant xenograft rejection

Polymorphonuclear leukocytes

Polymorphonuclear leukocytes (PML) appear to represent the major leukocyte type in HAR [66-68]. PML may infiltrate xenografts more rapidly than NK cells and T cells because they adhere to P-selectin [69–72] (Fig. 1), unlike NK cells, which utilise intercellular cell adhesion molecule-1 (ICAM-1), vascular cell adhesion molecule-1 (VCAM-1) and possibly E-selectin [45, 73, 74]. The implication that neutrophils participate in xenograft rejection is further strengthened by immunohistological studies that show significant infiltrates of human leukocytes consisting predominantly of neutrophils, macrophages, and T cells, with occasional B cells and NK cells in the setting of porcine HAR [66, 75]. Despite these considerations, the role of PML in xenograft rejection is unclear and has not been a major focus of interest to date. Human neutrophils have been shown to directly recognize xenogeneic endothelium [68]. This interaction appears to be independent of XNA and C and associated with calcium-dependent immediate activation of quiescent porcine EC. Translocation of P-selectin from the Wiebel-Palade bodies to the surface of xenogeneic EC in the reported experiments was associated with enhanced expression of VCAM-1; this process also appeared to facilitate NK cytotoxicity [68].

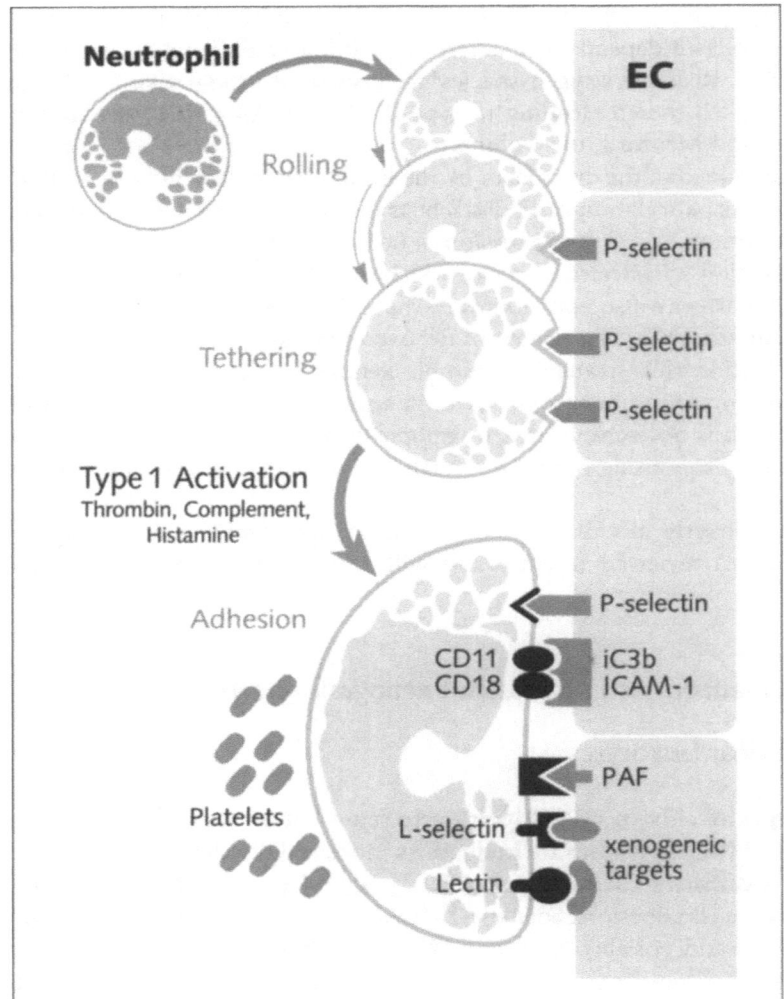

Figure 1
Interaction of neutrophils with xenogeneic endothelial cells (EC)
Human or primate neutrophil adhesion to porcine EC is modulated by type I activation responses following exposure to complement components, thrombin or even histamine. Initial and later interactions may be dictated by P-selectin interactions that are then consolidated and amplified by CD11CD18 interactions with iC3b or ICAM-1; the latter is present on both activated EC and at lower levels on quiescent EC. PAF provides a signal to neutrophils that results in activation-dependent alterations in the CD11CD18 receptors that facilitate binding to the counter-receptors as above. L-selectin and other putative lectin receptors are shown.

Monocytes

Mo are considered to be important effector cells during early xenograft rejection [41, 43, 76]. These cells may exacerbate the procoagulant potential of the graft vasculature by the heightened expression of tissue factor, thus promoting thrombotic occlusion of the vessels [77]. In addition, Mo may activate xenogeneic EC by direct cellular contact potentially by membrane bound TNFα; IL-1α may have little role in this activation response [43] (Fig. 2). Subsequent experiments have shown that the expression of a negative dominant mutant of human p55 TNF receptor by porcine EC inhibits this Mo-induced cellular activation [58].

Xenogeneic Mo-EC contacts result in upregulation of E-selectin, IL-8 and monocyte chemotactic protein-1 while increasing plasminogen activator inhibitor type-1 expression within the co-cultures [43] (Fig. 2). These cytokines and chemokines would result in further transendothelial migration of Mo and/or their activation causing inflammation, thrombosis and organ infarction [8].

Natural killer (NK) cells

Human anti-pig cellular responses may lead to xenograft rejection and NK cells appear to contribute to the human anti-porcine xenogeneic cytotoxicity [66, 74] (Fig. 2). Allogeneic as well as autologous normal cells are not susceptible to NK cell-mediated cytotoxicity because they express certain MHC class I molecules that give a negative signal to NK cells through specific inhibitory receptors [78]. It has been suggested that xenogeneic target cells may be susceptible to NK cell-mediated lysis because their MHC class I molecules are not recognised by these receptors.

Ex vivo cardiac perfusion experiments suggest that the combination of NK cells and XNA are the major cause of organ injury [45, 66]. These, and other findings in xenogeneic islet transplantation, implicate NK cells in cell-mediated xenograft rejection [49]. However, as yet no definitive proof exists that NK cells are obligatory for the evolution of this process in vascularized discordant xenografts.

Purified human NK cells have low level cytotoxic activity when tested on porcine aortic EC lines in the absence of XNA [16, 47, 74]. The addition of XNA to human NK porcine EC co-cultures promotes antibody dependent cell-mediated cytotoxicity (ADCC) [16, 48] that is mediated by the release of perforin and granzyme secreted by NK cells [74, 79] (Fig. 3). Additional work has confirmed that NK cells can activate EC by direct cell contact and that the addition of IgG xenoreactive antibodies enhances EC activation and NK cell transcription with secretion of TNFα and IFNγ [16, 64]. Depletion or adoptive transfer experiments of Mo and/or NK cells in small animal models of xenograft rejection suggest that depletion of both cell types will be required to achieve a prolongation in xenograft survival [80–82].

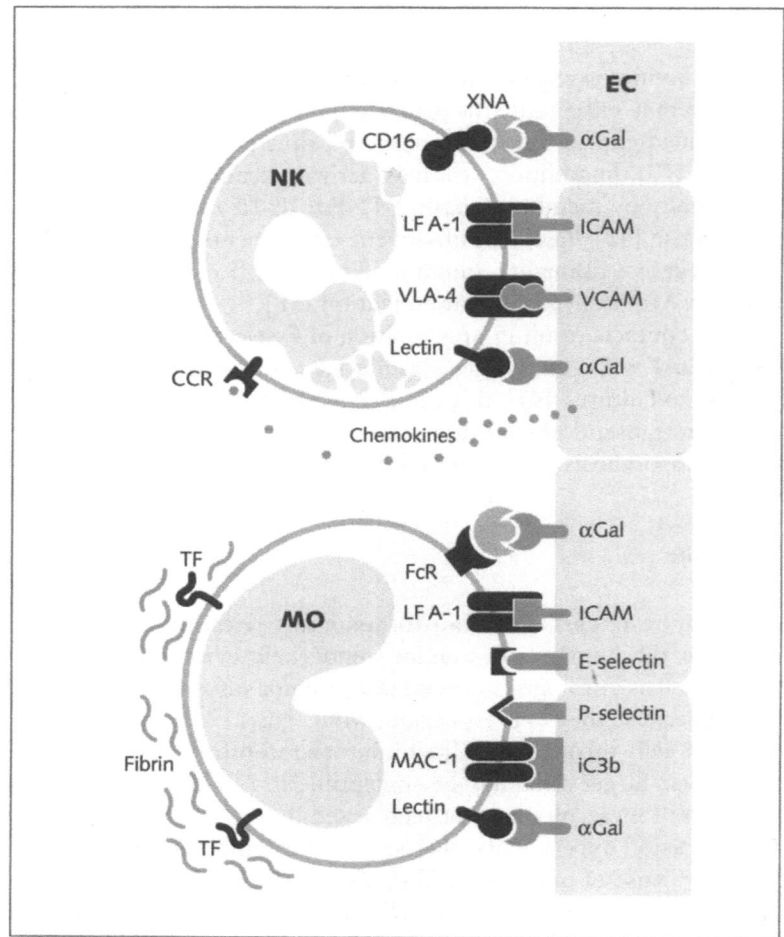

Figure 2
Interaction of NK cells and monocytes (Mo) with xenogeneic endothelial cells (EC)
The following adhesive interactions are postulated for the interaction of human NK cells with porcine EC. CD16 (Fc receptor) mediated recognition of XNA bound to EC is augmented by putative direct binding of Gal sugars by NK lectins. Direct receptor-ligand interactions such as between LFA-1/ICAM and VLA-4/VCAM are proposed. The stimulation of NK cell receptor (CCR) by chemokines may promote this process.
Putative xenogeneic Mo-EC contacts mediated via lectins and Fc receptors (in a manner analogous to NK cells) result in upregulation of E-selectin and EC activation. Release of cytokines and chemokines would result in adhesion, migration of monocytes and/or further activation augmenting inflammation and thrombosis. Central interactions include those mediated via LFA-1/ICAM and CD11bCD18 or MAC-1/iC3b.

It remains to be determined if human NK cells have specific receptors for α-Gal sugars [46, 64]. In mice and pigs the adhesion molecules required for xenoreactivity are glycosylated with α-Gal sugars [83–86]. Antibodies toward these sugars or CD11a/CD18 inhibit adhesion and subsequent cytotoxicity [36, 46]. Inhibition of human NK cell adhesion across species is specifically blocked by melibiose, the same sugar that inhibits the binding of XNA to α-Gal antigen [35], highlighting the role of α-Gal expression in the absence of XNA [46].

T and B lymphocytes

Most of the available data suggest that the direct cytotoxic response of human lymphocytes to porcine cells appears to be largely heterogeneous [20, 50–53, 87–89]. Lysis of xenogeneic targets can be significantly inhibited by anti-CD3 or anti-CD8 antibody and partially inhibited by anti-CD2 antibody; anti-CD2 or anti-CD4 antibodies had little effect in allogeneic control experiments. Human anti-pig cell-mediated cytotoxic responses appear comparable to allogeneic reactions, and have been shown to be restricted by swine leukocyte antigens (SLA) class I and class II [52, 53, 87, 88].

B cells have been detected in rejecting porcine xenografts [75]. However, little is known of the nature of elicited B cell responses to xenoantigen (α-Gal). T cell independent B cells may be central in this event but this is controversial and T cell involvement in the development of elicited xenoreactive antibodies remains a possibility [90–94].

Molecular targets recognized by xenogeneic mononuclear cells

The triggering of NK cell ADCC responses is ameliorated by depletion of XNA and promoted by functional incompatibilities between swine MHC or SLA and human NK killer inhibitory receptors (KIR) [47, 78]. Direct recognition of xenospecific oligosaccharide ligands on pig target cells by huNK cells followed by activation may be antibody-independent [46], but these avenues remain to be completely determined (see Fig. 3). In other published experiments, α-galactosidase-treated porcine EC have been used as targets in cytotoxicity experiments. Although now resistant to XNA and C, the cells did not acquire resistance to human IgG-dependent cellular cytotoxicity, despite the decrease in IgG binding [36]. However, these experiments did not titrate the amount of XNA as the number of molecules binding to trigger ADCC is much less than that required for a C-mediated lysis assay. The data also suggest that α-Gal is not the only xenoantigen. From isotype and subtype analysis, IgG1 XNA (including those which are not

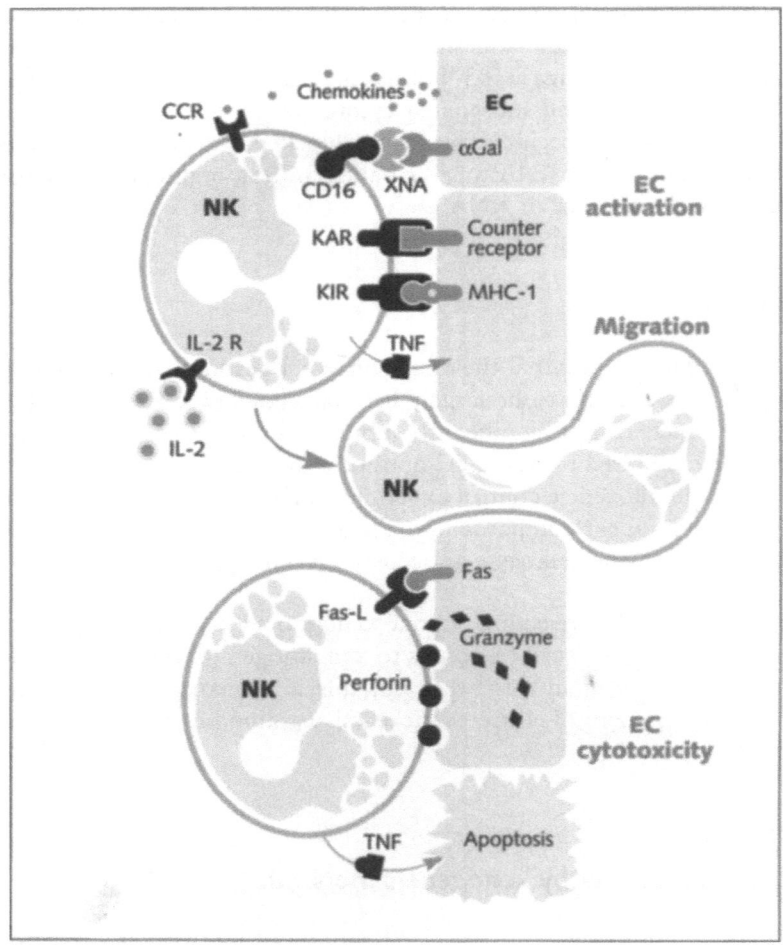

Figure 3
EC activation and cytotoxicity induced by NK cells
The effector function of NK cells in association with EC will be modulated by CD16/XNA and killer activatory receptors in counterbalance to killer inhibitory receptors that fail to fully interact with human MHC-1 and thereby downregulate NK responses. Pro-inflammatory cytokines may then be released from NK cells following these activation interactions with xenogeneic EC. This has the potential to induce EC activation causing reciprocal release of chemokines and further recruitment of leukocytes including NK cells. Retraction of EC and the associated formation of gaps between cells are associated with migration and tissue infiltration of NK cells. Cytotoxicity of EC may be mediated by three different pathways; FasL/Fas interactions, perforin/granzyme and the release of high levels of cytotoxic cytokines such as TNF.

directed at the α-galactosyl residue) appeared to be responsible for the ADCC [36].

A clearer understanding of how the specific inhibition of NK-mediated cytotoxicity fails in xenogeneic responses will be important in modulating graft injury during xenograft rejection. This phenomenon appears to occur by direct cell-cell interactions and failure to recognize self-MHC epitopes in allo-combinations. Two major groups of receptors have been characterized: (i) Ig-superfamily with classical killer inhibitory receptors (KIR) and also the related (killer) activator receptors (KAR) (Fig. 3), and (ii) C-lectin superfamily or CD94/NKG2 [74].

To evaluate KIR, human MHC class I expression on porcine immortalized EC lines has been obtained by transfection of the specific MHC cDNA; lysis by human NK cells was then examined. Three different human MHC class I allelic genes (HLA-A2, -B27, or -Cw3) were studied by Seebach and colleagues [78]. Specifically, the cytotoxic activity of several CL183(+) NK clones, that lysed untransfected porcine cells effectively, was substantially blocked by the presence of HLA-Cw3. However, even if successful *in vivo*, this approach raises concerns about inducing alloreactivity with respect to T cell responses. This latter possibility could be obviated by the use of mutant HLA molecules.

The function of costimulatory pathways across species has not been evaluated in the pig to primate model in any depth but cloning of porcine homologues of B7.1, 2 and CD40 or CD40L is underway at several centers. CTLA4.Ig has been studied to some extent and appears to be effective at blocking mixed xenogeneic lymphocyte responses [95, 96].

Sequestration and activation of mononuclear cells within xenograft vasculature

Discordant xenografts surviving the initial HAR phase may be subject to cellular rejection processes mediated by infiltrating leukocytes including T cells, NK cells and Mo [97]. The β_2 integrin molecules CD11a and CD18 play a key role in adhesion across species [45, 98, 99]. Addition of anti-CD11a or anti-CD18 reduces adhesion and cytotoxicity in the NK cell-EC coculture systems [16].

In addition, the stable adhesion of MNC to EC may relate to molecular interactions of the integrins VLA-4 and LFA-1 with their respective ligands (VCAM and ICAM-1) present on EC (Fig. 2). Human VLA-4 binds to porcine VCAM and blocking mAbs specific for porcine VCAM have been developed [97, 98]. The epitope of the antiporcine VCAM has been localized and humanized antibodies made that can inhibit adhesion of purified resting and activated human T cells to porcine EC. From the currently available data, it appears as if the blockade of human VLA-4 interaction with porcine VCAM may by itself be sufficient to impair adhesion of human leukocytes to porcine EC [97].

Putative molecular incompatibility of cytokines and modulation of actions

There are several cytokines that are documented not to function across wide species barriers. Whereas TNF and IL-1α have been shown to be fully functional across species, others may not have this lack of specificity. In this instance, certain molecular incompatibilities might be advantageous for xenograft survival. Two other human cytokines that are of potential importance in xenografting of porcine organs and are produced by the infiltrating mononuclear cells in AVR/DXR are IFNγ and IL-1β. These two human cytokines do not stimulate porcine EC [16, 76]. However, while such incompatibilities may have benefits in xenotransplantation, they could still contribute to activation of the host immune system.

The role of TNFα in apoptosis has led to an interest in mutation of the TNF receptor as a means to inhibit cellular xenograft responses [58]. The role of anti-apoptotic genes such as A20 has been demonstrated to involve inhibition of NF-κB activation and further studies will be required to evaluate the ability of transgenic expression of these genes to prevent xenograft rejection [10, 100].

Platelet adhesion and disordered thromboregulation

The enhanced potential of porcine von Willebrand factor (vWF) to associate with human platelet glycoprotein (GP)Ib through the vWF A1 domain suggests that this will represent an important barrier to xenograft acceptance [101]. Any expression of vWF in the subendothelium by the xenogeneic vasculature following EC retraction or injury could result in massive activation of circulating platelets with formation of aggregates [7]. The importance of locally synthesized C-components in promoting platelet activation and the associated thrombotic process remains undetermined [102].

Recently, several potentially important molecular incompatibilities have been recognized between activated human coagulation factors and the natural anticoagulants expressed on xenogeneic EC [7]. Such incompatibilities are analogous to cross-species alterations in function of complement regulatory proteins previously documented as being important in HAR [27, 28]. These thromboregulatory incompatibilities are potentially relevant to the progression of inflammatory events in AVR/DXR and for the development of disseminated intravascular coagulation (DIC) in this setting (unpublished observations). Pertinent examples include the inability of porcine tissue factor pathway inhibitor to adequately neutralize human factor Xa [41] and the failure of porcine thrombomodulin to bind human thrombin and hence activate human protein C [103]. These incompatibilities contribute to substantial generation of human thrombin from prothrombin by porcine EC [103]. Thrombin may initiate not only clotting but is an important mediator of EC activation (Fig. 1) and platelet aggregation [60] ; beneficial effects of thrombin inhibition have been noted in several models of discordant xenograft rejection [104, 105].

All of the above have the potential to cause substantive vascular damage, activation of platelets and coagulation with thrombosis independently of complement and antibody deposition within the xenograft vasculature and would exacerbate the problems caused by the associated loss of vascular ATPDase/CD39 [56, 57]. Inhibition of platelet aggregation by treatment of the recipient with an antagonist to the platelet fibrinogen receptor, GPIIb/IIIa [106], by the use of antagonists of P-selectin or platelet activating factor (PAF) [71, 107, 108], or by administration of a soluble ATPDase [109] has been shown to prolong graft survival in several discordant xenotransplantation models.

Additional insights from transgenic animals and knock-out mice

Major goals in breeding genetically modified animals with organs suitable for transplantation has been the reduction (or complete removal) of the α-Gal antigen and the expression of membrane bound inhibitors of human C-activation [110]. There is now increasing evidence that this combined approach of α-Gal reduction or elimination coupled with the expression of one or more C-regulatory molecules will be a minimal requirement for significant xenograft survival.

Transgenic expression of human H-transferase has been achieved in the mouse, and is being developed in the pig [12, 13, 111]. The reduction in α-Gal expression has been sufficient to demonstrate protection of murine splenocytes from lysis by human XNA and C [111]. An alternative to transgene expression of enzymes that compete with the substrates for α-Gal synthesis is the targeted deletion of α-1–3 galactosyltransferase enzyme by homologous recombination [112]. At present, embryonic stem cells are only available for selected mouse strains preventing the generation of α-Gal-deficient pigs by knock-out technology. Galactosyltransferase knock-out mice are healthy, fertile and do not express the α-Gal antigen [112]. There are concerns that any reduction in α-Gal expression may be associated with unexpected changes to other carbohydrate structures on the cell surface giving rise to neoantigens. Such perturbations in cell surface lectin binding are clearly observed in galactosyltransferase knock-out mice transgenic for human H-transferase [113]; the novel epitopes here express sialylated Tn and Forssman antigens and could possibly initiate HAR.

Transgenic mice have been generated expressing one or more membrane bound complement regulatory molecules (CD46, CD55 and CD59).The level of expression plays a critical role in the biological function of the transgenes. The use of high level endothelium-specific promoters has resulted in levels of expression several fold higher than those observed in human cells. CD55 and CD59 transgenic mice have a significant resistance to C-mediated lysis and demonstrate a prolongation in function on an *ex vivo* cardiac perfusion apparatus [114, 115]. Several groups associated with Imutran, Alexion and Nextran have published data regarding human CD55, CD59/CD55 or CD46/CD55 transgenic porcine organs and compatibility with primates [116–119]. Significant prolongation in cardiac survival has been observed albeit not to durations suitable for clinical application. The administration of immunosuppressives to primates receiving porcine transgenic organs has extended the duration of survival from days to weeks [120]. However, despite major immunosuppression, these animals still display vascular injury and inflammatory changes, highlighting the need for a greater understanding of the mechanisms contributing to AVR/DXR.

A major problem at present is the lack of a widely accepted small animal model of DXR. It is not really feasible to test multiple strategies in pig to primate models and compelling evidence of potential benefit in an appropriate small animal model could provide a useful screening . We have used α-Gal deficient mice to establish a model of cell-mediated transplant rejection. These α-Gal-deficient mice, like humans acquire antibodies to the α-Gal antigen following exposure to α-Gal antigens [93]. Transplantation of α-Gal-bearing hearts to immunized α-Gal-deficient mice results in rejection after 8–10 days. The cellular infiltrate consists of Mo and NK cells in association with marked vascular rejection (unpublished observations). This murine allograft system provides a model for testing complex genetic strategies to inhibit inflammatory mechanisms relevant to discordant xenograft rejection.

Therapeutic options and endeavours

As discussed above, xenografts are rejected even where the evidence suggests that C is blocked; we would expect the same if both C and XNA actions are abrogated. The precise definition of mechanisms that contribute to processes of xenograft rejection, including platelet activation, thrombosis, and inflammation, and development of therapeutic strategies to overcome such problems are important. We believe that one of the next steps in overcoming rejection will be to be able to effectively prevent these complications. The activation of the endothelium and also of the host MNCs that infiltrate the graft appears to contribute to rejection.

Immunosuppressive agents are associated with significant morbidity and mortality by increasing the risk of infection and the development of cancers. Despite life-threatening doses of cyclophosphamide in combination with cyclosporin, rejection of transgenic porcine organs in primates has not been halted. The possibility exists that other therapeutic agents such as FK506 or deoxyspergiulin may be more suitable to xenograft rejection. Application of such further therapeutic strategies, potentially including an approach to abrogating EC activation and involving both genetic manipulation and conventional therapeutic agents directed at specific targets in the overall rejection apparatus, will contribute to achieving long-term survival of a xenograft. It must remain of theoretical concern that accelerated chronic rejection may manifest in xenografted organs.

Conclusions

There are several proposed therapies for dealing with the problem of C-activation, XNA and elicited xenoreactive antibodies in addition to the genetic engineering approach. Adequate immunosuppression, other interventions such as plasmapheresis, anti-C therapies and the control of any resulting EC activation process following binding of xenoreactive antibodies will be of crucial importance

The concept of AVR/DXR, involving a greater understanding of the mechanisms of inflammation and thrombosis, and appreciation of molecular incompatibilities, has led to novel ideas that may translate into approaches for therapy. As the problems of HAR and AVR/DXR are overcome, it is assumed that effective therapy for subsequent graft-specific cellular responses will be necessary. However, whether all of this will lead to clinical application of discordant xenografting of immediately-vascularized organs must await the appropriate experimentation and the acceptance of clinical application by the transplant community.

References

1   Taniguchi S, Cooper D (1997) Clinical xenotransplantation – past, present and future. *Ann Royal Coll Surg* 79: 13–19

2   Platt JL, Bach FH (1991) Discordant xenografting: challenges and controversies. *Curr Opin Immunol* 3: 735–739

3   Platt JL (1996) Xenotransplantation – recent progress and current perspectives. *Curr Opin Immunol* 8: 721–728

4   Platt JL (1996) The immunological barriers to xenotransplantation. *Crit Rev Immunol* 16: 331–358

5   Parker W, Saadi S, Lin SS, Holzknecht ZE, Bustos M, Platt JL (1996) Transplantation of discordant xenografts – a challenge revisited. *Immunol Today* 17: 373–378

6   Platt JL, Bach FH (1991) The barrier to xenotransplantation. *Transplantation* 52: 937–947

7   Bach FH, Winkler H, Ferran C, Hancock WW, Robson SC (1996) Delayed xenograft rejection. *Immunol Today* 17: 379–384

8   Bach FH, Robson SC, Ferran C, Winkler H, Millan MT, Stuhlmeier KM, Vanhove B, Blakely ML, Vanderwerf WJ, Hofer E, Demartin R, Hancock WW (1994) Endothelial cell activation and thromboregulation during xenograft rejection. *Immunol Rev* 141: 5–30

9   Dalmasso AP (1992) The complement system in xenotransplantation. *Immunopharma-cology* 24: 149–60

10   Bach FH, Ferran C, Soares M, Wrighton CJ, Anrather J, Winkler H, Robson SC, Hancock WW (1997) Modification of vascular responses in xenotransplantation – inflammation and apoptosis. *Nature Med* 3: 944–948

11   Rosengard AM, Cary NR, Langford GA, Tucker AW, Wallwork J, White DJ (1995) Tissue expression of human complement inhibitor, decay-accelerating factor, in transgenic pigs A potential approach for preventing xenograft rejection. *Transplantation* 59: 1325–33

12   Sandrin MS, Fodor WL, Mouhtouris E, Osman N, Cohney S, Rollins SA, Guilmette ER, Setter E, Squinto SP, Mckenzie I (1995) Enzymatic remodelling of the carbohydrate surface of a xenogenic cell substantially reduces human antibody binding and complement-mediated cytolysis. *Nature Med* 1: 1261–1267

13   Sandrin MS, Fodor WL, Cohney S, Mouhtouris E, Osman N, Rollins SA, Squinto SP, Mckenzie I (1996) Reduction of the major porcine xenoantigen gal1-alpha(1,3)gal by expression of alpha(1,2)fucosyltransferase. *Xenotransplantation* 3: 134–140

14   Dalmasso AP, Vercellotti GM, Fischel RJ, Bolman RM, Bach FH, Platt JL (1992) Mechanism of complement activation in the hyperacute rejection of porcine organs transplanted into primate recipients. *Am J Path* 140: 1157–66

15   Platt JL, Bach FH (1991) The barrier to xenotransplantation. *Transplantation* 52: 937–947

16   Goodman DJ, Vonalbertini M, Willson A, Millan MT, Bach FH (1996) Direct activation of porcine endothelial cells by human natural killer cells. *Transplantation* 61: 763–771

17   Patience C, Takeuchi Y, Weiss RA (1997) Infection of human cells by an endogenous retrovirus of pigs. *Nature Med* 3: 282–286

18   Chapman LE (1995) Xenotransplantation and xenogeneic infections. *N Eng J Med* 333: 1498–1501

19   Bach FH, Fishman JA, Daniels N, Proimos J, Anderson B, Carpenter CB, Forrow L, Robson SC, Fineberg HV (1998) Uncertainty in xenotransplantation: individual benefit versus collective risk. *Nature Med* 4: 141–144

20   Auchincloss H (1990) Xenografting: a review. *Transplantation* 4: 14–20

21   Baldwin WMI, Pruitt SK, Brauer RB, Daha MR, Sanfilippo F (1995) Complement in organ transplantation. *Transplantation* 59: 797–808

22   Hancock WW, Blakely ML, Van der Werf W, Bach FH (1993) Rejection of guinea pig cardiac xenografts post-cobra venom factor therapy is associated with infiltration by mononuclear cells secreting interferon-gamma and diffuse endothelial activation. *Transpl Proc* 25: 2932

23   Bach FH, Robson SC, Winkler H, Ferran C, Stuhlmeier KM, Wrighton CJ, Hancock WW (1995) Barriers to xenotransplantation. *Nature Med* 1: 869–873

24   Saadi S, Holzknecht RA, Patte CP, Stern DM, Platt JL (1995) Complement-mediated regulation of tissue factor activity in endothelium. *J Exp Med* 182: 1807–1814

25 Saadi S, Platt JL (1995) Transient perturbation of endothelial integrity induced by natural antibodies and complement. *J Exp Med* 181: 21–31

26 Norin AJ, Brewer RJ, Lawson N, Grijalva GA, Vaynblatt M, Burton W, Squinto SP, Kamholz SL, Fodor WL (1996) Enhanced survival of porcine endothelial cells and lung xenografts expressing human CD59. *Transpl Proc* 28: 797–798

27 Dalmasso AP, Vercellotti GM, Platt JL, Bach FH (1991) Inhibition of complement-mediated endothelial cell cytotoxicity by decay- accelerating factor Potential for prevention of xenograft hyperacute rejection. *Transplantation* 52: 530–533

28 Dalmasso AP, Platt JL, Bach FH (1991) Reaction of complement with endothelial cells in a model of xenotransplantation. *Clin Exp Immunol* 1: 31–35

29 White D (1992) Transplantation of organs between species. *Int Arch Allergy Immunol* 98: 1–5

30 Tucker AW, Carrington CA, Richards AC, Robson SC, White D (1997) Endothelial cells from human decay acceleration factor transgenic pigs are protected against complement mediated tissue factor expression *in vitro*. *Transpl Proc* 29: 888

31 White D, Wallwork J (1993) Xenografting – probability, possibility, or pipe dream? *Lancet* 342: 879–880

32 Baldwin WM, Pruitt SK, Brauer RB, Daha MR, Sanfilippo F (1995) Complement in organ transplantation – contributions to inflammation, injury, and rejection. *Transplantation* 59: 797–808

33 Pruitt SK, Kirk AD, Bollinger RR, Marsh HC, Collins BH, Levin JL, Mault JR, Heinle JS, Ibrahim S, Rudolph AR, Baldwin WM, Sanfilippo F (1994) The effect of soluble complement receptor type 1 on hyperacute rejection of porcine xenografts. *Transplantation* 57: 363–370

34 Sandrin MS, Vaughan HA, Dabkowski PL, Mckenzie I (1993) Studies on human naturally occurring antibodies to pig xenografts. *Transpl Proc* 25: 2917–2918

35 Vaughan HA, Mckenzie I, Sandrin MS (1995) Biochemical studies of pig xenoantigens detected by naturally occurring human antibodies and the galactose-alpha(1-3)galactose reactive lectin. *Transplantation* 59: 102–109

36 Watier H, Guillaumin JM, Piller F, Lacord M, Thibault G, Lebranchu Y, Monsigny M, Bardos P (1996) Removal of terminal alpha-galactosyl residues from xenogeneic porcine endothelial cells – decrease in complement-mediated cytotoxicity but persistence of IgG1-mediated antibody-dependent cell-mediated cytotoxicity. *Transplantation* 62: 105–113

37 McCurry KR, Diamond LE, Kooyman DL, Byrne GW, Martin MJ, Logan JS, Platt JL (1996) Human complement regulatory proteins expressed in transgenic swine protect swine xenografts from humoral injury. *Transpl Proc* 28: 758

38 Conway EM, Rosenberg RD (1988) Tumour necrosis factor suppresses transcription of the thrombomodulin gene in endothelial cells. *Mol Cell Biol* 8: 5588–5592

39 Esmon CT (1993) Cell mediated events that control blood coagulation and vascular injury. *Ann Rev Cell Biol* 9: 1–26

40 Conway EM, Bach R, Rosenberg RD, Konigsberg WH (1989) Tumor necrosis factor

enhances expression of tissue factor mRNA in endothelial cells. *Thromb Res* 53: 231–241

41   Kopp CW, Siegel JB, Hancock WW, Anrather J, Winkler H, Geczy CL, Kaczmarek E, Bach FH, Robson SC (1997) Effect of porcine endothelial tissue factor pathway inhibitor on human coagulation factors. *Transplantation* 63: 749–758

42   Grey S, Tsuchida A, Orthner CL, Salem HH, Hancock WW (1994) Selective inhibitory effects of the anticoagulant activated protein C on the responses of human mononuclear phagocytes to LPS, IFN-γ or phorbol ester. *J Immunol* 153: 3664–3672

43   Millan MT, Geczy C, Stuhlmeier KM, Goodman DJ, Ferran C, Bach FH (1997) Human monocytes activate porcine endothelial cells, resulting in increased e-selectin, inter-leukin-8, monocyte chemotactic protein-1, and plasminogen activator inhibitor-type-1 expression. *Transplantation* 63: 421–429

44   Inverardi L, Samaja M, Marelli F, Bender JR, Pardi R (1992) Cellular early immune recognition of xenogeneic vascular endothelium. *Transpl Proc* 24: 459–461

45   Inverardi L, Samaja M, Motterlini R, Mangili F, Bender JR, Pardi R (1992) Early recognition of a discordant xenogeneic organ by human circulating lymphocytes. *J Immunol* 149: 1416–1423

46   Inverardi L, Clissi B, Stolzer AL, Bender JR, Sandrin MS, Pardi R (1997) Human natural killer lymphocytes directly recognize evolutionarily conserved oligosaccharide ligands expressed by xenogeneic tissues. *Transplantation* 63: 1318–1330

47   Seebach JD, Yamada K, Mcmorrow IM, Sachs DH, Dersimonian H (1996) Xenogeneic human anti-pig cytotoxicity mediated by activated natural killer cells. *Xenotransplantation* 3: 188–197

48   Malyguine AM, Saadi S, Platt JL, Dawson JR (1996) Human natural killer cells induce morphologic changes in porcine endothelial cell monolayers. *Transplantation* 61: 161–164

49   Lin Y, Vandeputte M, Waer M (1997) Natural killer cell- and macrophage-mediated rejection of concordant xenografts in the absence of T and B cell responses. *J Immunol* 158: 5658–5667

50   Auchincloss H (1988) Xenogeneic transplantation. *Transplantation* 46: 1–20

51   Moses RD, Winn HJ, Auchincloss HJ (1992) Evidence that multiple defects in cell-sur-face molecule interactions across species differences are responsible for diminished xenogeneic T cell responses. *Transplantation* 53: 203–209

52   Brevig T, Kristensen T (1997) Direct cytotoxic response of human lymphocytes to porcine PHA-lymphoblasts and lymphocytes. *Apmis* 105: 290–298

53   Yamada K, Seebach JD, Dersimonian H, Sachs DH (1996) Human anti-pig T-cell medi-ated cytotoxicity. *Xenotransplantation* 3: 179–187

54   Robson SC, Candinas D, Hancock WW, Wrighton C, Winkler H, Bach FH (1995) Role of endothelial cells in transplantation. *Int Arch Allergy Immunol* 106: 305–322

55   Von Albertini MA, Palmetshofer A, Kaczmark E, Koziak K, Stoka D, Grey ST, Stuhlmeier KM, Robson SC (1997) Extracellular ATP and ADP activate transcription

factor NF-κB and induce endothelial cell apoptosis. *Biochem Biophys Res Comm* 248: 822–829

56 Kaczmarek E, Koziak K, Sevigny J, Siegel JB, Anrather J, Beaudoin AR, Bach FH, Robson SC (1996) Identification and characterization of CD39 vascular ATP diphosphohydrolase. *J Biol Chem* 271: 33116–33122

57 Robson SC, Kaczmarek E, Siegel JB, Candinas D, Koziak K, Millan M, Hancock WW, Bach FH (1997) Loss of ATP diphosphohydrolase activity with endothelial cell activation. *J Exp Med* 185: 153–163

58 Stroka DM, Cooper JT, Brostjan C, Millan MT, Goodman DJ, Wrighton CJ, Bach FH, Ferran C (1997) Expression of a negative dominant mutant of human p55 tumor necrosis factor-receptor inhibits tnf and monocyte-induced activation in porcine aortic endothelial cells. *Transpl Proc* 29: 882

59 Baeuerle PA, Baltimore D (1988) Activation of DNA-binding activity in an apparently cytoplasmic precursor of the NF-kappaB transcription factor. *Cell* 53: 211–217

60 Anrather D, Millan MT, Palmetshofer A, Robson SC, Geczy C, Ritchie AJ, Bach FH, Ewenstein BM (1997) Thrombin activates nuclear factor-kappa-b and potentiates endothelial cell activation by TNF. *J Immunol* 159: 5620–5628

61 Ferran C, Millan MT, Csizmadia V, Cooper JT, Brostjan C, Bach FH, Winkler H (1995) Inhibition of NF-κB by pyrrolidine dithiocarbamate blocks endothelial cell activation. *Biochem Biophys Res Comm* 214: 212–223

62 Baeuerle PA, Baltimore D (1988) IkappaB: a specific inhibitor of the NF-kappaB transcription factor. *Science* 242: 541–546

63 Wrighton CJ, Hofer WR, Moll T, Eytner R, Bach FH, de Martin R (1996) Inhibition of endothelial cell activation by adenovirus-mediated expression of IkappaB alpha, an inhibitor of the transcription factor NF-kappa B. *J Exp Med* 183: 1013–1022

64 Goodman DJ, Von Albertini MA, McShea A, CJ Wrighton, and FH Bach (1996) Adenoviral-mediated overexpression of I-kappa-B-alpha in endothelial cells inhibits natural killer cell-mediated endothelial cell activation. *Transplantation* 62: 967–972

65 Anrather J, Csizmadia V, Brostjan C, Soares MP, Bach FH, Winkler H (1997) Inhibition of bovine endothelial cell activation *in vitro* by regulated expression of a transdominant inhibitor of NF-kappa-B. *J Clin Invest* 99: 763–772

66 Kirk AD, Heinle JS, Mault JR, Sanfilippo F (1993) *Ex vivo* characterization of human anti-porcine hyperacute cardiac rejection. *Transplantation* 56: 785–793

67 Robson SC, Young VK, Cook NS, Kottirsch G, Siegel JB, Lesnikoski BA, Candinas D, White D, Bach FH (1996) Inhibition of platelet GPIIbIIIa in an *ex vivo* model of hyperacute xenograft rejection does not prolong cardiac survival time. *Xenotransplantation* 3: 43–52

68 Almohanna F, Collison K, Parhar R, Kwaasi A, Meyer B, Saleh S, Allen S, Alsedairy S, Stern D, Yacoub M (1997) Activation of naive xenogeneic but not allogeneic endothelial cells by human naive neutrophils – a potential occult barrier to xenotransplantation. *Am J Path* 151: 111–120

69 Mulligan MS, Polley MJ, Bayer RJ, Nunn MF, Paulson JC, Ward PA (1992) Neutrophil-

dependent acute lung injury – requirement for P- Selectin (GMP-140). *J Clin Invest* 90: 1600–1607

70 Sugama Y, Tiruppathi C, Janakidevi K, Andersen TT, Fenton JW, Malik AB (1992) Thrombin-induced expression of endothelial P-Selectin and intercellular adhesion molecule-1 – a mechanism for stabilizing neutrophil adhesion. *J Cell Biol* 119: 935–944

71 Coughlan AF, Berndt MC, Dunlop LC, Hancock WW (1993) *In vivo* studies of P-selectin and platelet activating factor during endotoxemia, accelerated allograft rejection, and discordant xenograft rejection. *Transpl Proc* 25: 2930–1

72 Patel KD, Zimmerman GA, Prescott SM, McEver RP, McIntyre TM (1991) Oxygen radicals induce human endothelial cells to express GMP-140 and bind neutrophils. *J Cell Biol* 112: 749–759

73 Xing Z, Jordana M, Kirpalani H, Driscoll KE, Schall TJ, Gauldie J (1994) Human NK cells expressing alpha 4 beta 1/beta 7 adhere to VCAM-1 without preactivation Scand. *J Immunol* 39: 131–136

74 Seebach JD, Waneck GL (1997) Natural killer cells in xenotransplantation. *Xenotransplantation* 4: 201–211

75 Ibrahim S, Kirk AD, Sanfilippo F (1996) Phenotype of infiltrating cells in an *ex vivo* model of human antiporcine hyperacute cardiac xenograft rejection. *Transpl Proc* 28: 777

76 Bach FH, Robson SC, Ferran C, Millan M, Anrather J, Kopp C, Lesnikoski B, Goodman DJ, Hancock WW, Wrighton C et al (1995). Xenotransplantation: endothelial cell activation and beyond. *Transpl Proc* 27: 77–9

77 Nemerson Y (1992) The tissue factor pathway of blood coagulation. *Semin Hematol* 29: 170–188

78 Seebach JD, Comrack C, Germana S, Leguern C, Sachs DH, Dersimonian H (1997) HLA-CW3 expression on porcine endothelial cells protects against xenogeneic cytotoxicity mediated by a subset of human NK cells. *J Immunol* 159: 3655–3661

79 Smyth MJ, Thia K, Kershaw MH (1997) Xenogeneic mouse anti-human NK cytotoxicity is mediated via perforin. *Xenotransplantation* 4: 78–84

80 Chavin KD, Lau HT, Bromberg JS (1992) Prolongation of allograft and xenograft survival in mice by Anti-CD2 monoclonal antibodies. *Transplantation* 54: 286–291

81 Arakawa K, Akami T, Okamoto M, Akioka K, Lee PC, Sugano Y, Kamei J, Suzuki T, Nagase H, Tsuchihashi Y (1994) Prolongation of heart xenograft survival in the NK-deficient rat. *Transpl Proc* 26: 1266–1267

82 Fryer JP, Leventhal JR, Dalmasso AP, Chen S, Simone PA, Goswitz JJ, Reinsmoen NL, Matas AJ (1995) Beyond hyperacute rejection – accelerated rejection in a discordant xenograft model by adoptive transfer of specific cell subsets. *Transplantation* 59: 171–176

83 Bizouarne N, Mitterrand M, Monsigny M, Kieda C (1993) Characterization of membrane sugar-specific receptors in cultured high endothelial cells from mouse peripheral lymph nodes. *Biol Cell* 79: 27–35

84 Platt JL, Lindman BJ, Chen H, Spitalnik SL, Bach FH (1990) Endothelial cell antigens recognized by xenoreactive human natural antibodies. *Transplantation* 50: 817–22

85 Parker W, Lateef J, Everett ML, Platt JL (1996) Specificity of xenoreactive anti-gal-alpha-1-3gal IgM for alpha-galactosyl ligands. *Glycobiology* 6: 499–506

86 Holzknecht ZE, Platt JL (1995) Identification of porcine endothelial cell membrane antigens recognized by human xenoreactive natural antibodies. *J Immunol* 154: 4565–4575

87 Gonias SL (1994) Demonstration of direct xenorecognition of porcine cells by human cytotoxic T lymphocytes. *Immunology* 81: 268–272

88 Springer TA (1994) Indirect presentation of MHC antigens in transplantation. *Immunol Today* 15: 32–38

89 Sultan P, Murray AG, Mcniff JM, Lorber MI, Askenase PW, Bothwell A, Pober JS (1997) Pig but not human interferon-gamma initiates human cell-mediated rejection of pig tissue *in vivo*. *Proc Natl Acad Sci USA* 94: 8767–8772

90 Oriol R, Ye Y, Koren E, Cooper D (1993) *In vivo* depletion of xenoreactive natural antibodies with an anti-mu monoclonal antibody. *Transplantation* 56: 1427–1433

91 Stone KR, Walgenbach AW, Abrams JT, Nelson J, Gillett N, Galili U (1997) Porcine and bovine cartilage transplants in cynomolgus monkey: 1. A model for chronic xenograft rejection. *Transplantation* 63: 640–645

92 Galili U, Latemple DC, Walgenbach AW, Stone KR (1997) Porcine and bovine cartilage transplants in cynomolgus monkey: 2. Changes in anti-gal response during chronic rejection. *Transplantation* 63: 646–651

93 Galili U (1993) Interaction of the natural anti-gal antibody with alpha-galactosyl epitopes – a major obstacle for xenotransplantation in humans. *Immunol Today* 14: 480–482

94 Galili U, Tibell A, Samuelsson B, Rydberg L, Groth CG (1996) Increased anti-gal activity in diabetic patients transplanted with porcine islet cells. *Transpl Proc* 28: 564–566

95 Ibrahim S, Xu R, Burdick JF, Baldwin W, Sanfilippo F, Kittur DS (1996) CTLA4Ig inhibits humoral and cellular immune responses to concordant xenografts. *Transpl Proc* 28: 715–716

96 Lenschow DJ, Zeng Y, Thistlethwaite JR, Montag A, Brady W, Gibson MG, Linsley PS, Bluestone JA (1992) Long-term survival of xenogeneic pancreatic islet grafts induced by CTLA4lg. *Science* 257: 789–792

97 Mueller JP, Giannoni MA, Hartman SL, Elliott EA, Squinto SP, Matis LA, Evans MJ (1997) Humanized porcine vcam-specific monoclonal antibodies with chimeric IgG2/G4 constant regions block human leukocyte binding to porcine endothelial cells. *Mol Immunol* 34: 441–452

98 Carter AS, Welsh KI, Morris PJ, Fuggle SV (1996) Antibodies to human adhesion molecules and their ligands – cross-species reactivity and potential application in xenotransplantation. *Xenotransplantation* 3: 35–42

99 Vercellotti GM, Platt JL, Bach FH, Dalmasso AP (1991) Neutrophil adhesion to xenogeneic endothelium via iC3b. *J Immunol* 146: 730–734

100 Cooper JT, Stroka DM, Brostjan C, Palmetshofer A, Bach FH, Ferran C (1996) A20

blocks endothelial cell activation through a NF-kappa-B-dependent mechanism. *J Biol Chem* 271: 18068–18073

101 Schulte am Esch J, Siegel JB, Cruz M, Anrather J, Robson SC (1997) The A1 domain of von Willebrand factor expressed on cell membranes directly activates platelets. *Blood* 90: 4425–4437

102 Robson SC, Siegel JB, Lesnikoski BA, Kopp C, Candinas D, Ryan U, Bach FH (1996) Aggregation of human platelets induced by porcine endothelial cells is dependent upon both activation of complement and thrombin generation. *Xenotransplantation* 3: 24–34

103 Siegel JB, Grey ST, Lesnikoski BA, Kopp CW, Soares M, Esch J, Bach FH, Robson SC (1997) Xenogeneic endothelial cells activate human prothrombin. *Transplantation* 64: 888–896

104 Lesnikoski BA, Candinas D, Otsu I, Metternich R, Bach FH, Robson SC (1997) Thrombin inhibition in discordant xenograft rejection. *Xenotransplantation* 4: 140–146

105 Robson SC, Young VK, Cook NS, Metternich R, Kasper-Konig W, Lesnikoski BA, Candinas D, Pierson RN, Hancock WW, White DJ, Bach FH (1996) Thrombin inhibition in an *ex vivo* model of hyperacute xenograft rejection. *Transplantation* 61: 862–868

106 Candinas D, Lesnikoski BA, Hancock WW, Otsu I, Koyamada N, Dalmasso AP, Robson SC, Bach FH (1996) Inhibition of platelet integrin GPIIbIIIa prolongs survival of discordant cardiac xenografts. *Transplantation* 62: 1–5

107 Makowka L, Chapman FA, Cramer DV, Qian SG, Sun H, TE Starzl (1990) Platelet-activating factor and hyperacute rejection The effect of a platelet-activating factor antagonist, SRI 63-441, on rejection of xenografts and allografts in sensitized hosts. *Transplantation* 50: 359–65

108 Ohair DP, Roza AM, Komorowski R, Moore G, Mcmanus RP, Johnson CP, Adams MB, Pieper GM (1993) Tulopafant, a paf receptor antagonist, increases capillary patency and prolongs survival in discordant cardiac xenotransplants. *J Lipid Med* 7: 79–84

109 Koyamada N, Miyatake T, Candinas D, Hechenleitner P, Siegel J, Hancock WW, Bach FH, Robson SC (1996) Apyrase administration prolongs discordant xenograft survival. *Transplantation* 62: 1739–1743

110 Cooper DKC, Koren E, Oriol R (1994) α-Galactosyl oligosaccharides and discordant xenografting. *Xenotransplantation* 2

111 Chen CG, Fisicaro N, Shinkel TA, Aitken V, Katerelos M, Vandenderen B, Tange MJ, Crawford RJ, Robins AJ, Pearse MJ, Dapice A (1996) Reduction in gal-alpha-1,3-gal epitope expression in transgenic mice expressing human h-transferase. *Xenotransplantation* 3: 69–75

112 Tearle RG, Tange MJ, Zannettino ZL, Katerelos M, Shinkel TA, Vandenderen B, Lonie AJ, Lyons I, Nottle MB, Cox T, Becker C, Peura AM, Wigley PL, Crawford RJ, Robins AJ, Pearse MJ, Dapice A (1996) The alpha-1,3-galactosyltransferase knockout mouse – implications for xenotransplantation. *Transplantation* 61: 13–19

113 Shinkel TA, Chen CG, Salvaris E, Henion TR, Barlow H, Galili U, Pearse MJ, Dapice A (1997) Changes in cell surface glycosylation in alpha-1,3-galactosyltransferase knockout and alpha-1,2-fucosyltransferase transgenic mice. *Transplantation* 64: 197–204

114 McCurry KR, Kooyman DL, Diamond LE, Byrne GW, Logan JS, Platt JL (1995) Transgenic expression of human complement regulatory proteins in mice results in diminished complement deposition during organ xenoperfusion. *Transplantation* 59: 1177–1182

115 Byrne GW, McCurry KR, Kagan D, Quinn C, Martin MJ, Platt JL, Logan JS (1995) Protection of xenogeneic cardiac endothelium from human complement by expression of CD59 or DAF in transgenic mice. *Transplantation* 60: 1149–1156

116 Fodor WL, Williams BL, Matis LA, Madri JA, Rollins SA, Knight JW, Velander W, Squinto SP (1994) Expression of a functional human complement inhibitor in a transgenic pig as a model for the prevention of xenogeneic hyperacute organ rejection. *Proc Natl Acad Sci USA* 91: 11153–11157

117 Kennedy SP, Rollins SA, Burton WV, Sims PJ, Bothwell A, Squinto SP, Zavoico GB (1994) Protection of porcine aortic endothelial cells from complement-mediated cell lysis and activation by recombinant human CD59. *Transplantation* 57: 1494–1501

118 McCurry KR, Kooyman DL, Alvarado CG, Cotterell AH, Martin MJ, Logan JS, Platt JL (1995) Human complement regulatory proteins protect swine-to-primate cardiac xenografts from humoral injury. *Nature Med* 1: 423–427

119 Diamond LE, McCurry KR, Martin MJ, McClellan SB, Oldham ER, Platt JL, Logan JS (1996) Characterization of transgenic pigs expressing functionally active human CD59 on cardiac endothelium. *Transplantation* 61: 1241–1249

120 White, DJG (1996) hDAF transgenic pig organs: are they concordant for human transplantation. *Xenotransplantation* 4: 50–54

Control of leukocyte adhesion and activation in ischemia-reperfusion injury

Tak Yee Aw and D. Neil Granger

Department of Molecular and Cellular Physiology, Louisiana State University Medical Center, PO Box 33932, 1501 Kings Highway, Shreveport, LA 71130-3932, USA

Introduction

Ischemia, which is a marked reduction in blood flow to a vacular bed, can lead to tissue injury and organ dysfunction if it is prolonged. While early restoration of blood flow (reperfusion) to an ischemic organ is essential for prevention of hypoxic injury, there appears to be a distinct process of vascular dysfunction and parenchymal cell necrosis that can result from this abrupt reperfusion of ischemic tissues. This phenomenon, called "reperfusion injury", appears to be linked to the reintroduction of molecular oxygen and eventual recruitment of inflammatory cells into postischemic tissues. The importance of activated leukocytes in reperfusion injury is supported by several lines of evidence: (a) leukocytes accumulate in the postischemic tissues, (b) depletion of circulating leukocytes reduces reperfusion-induced tissue injury and "capillary no-reflow", (c) reagents that interfere with reperfusion-induced leukocyte-endothelial cell adhesion are also effective in blunting the microvascular dysfunction and tissue injury elicited by ischemia/reperfusion (I/R), (d) reperfusion-induced tissue injury is attenuated in animals that are genetically deficient in adhesion glycoproteins, (e) conditions that exacerbate the inflammatory responses to I/R, such as diabetes and hypercholesterolemia also lead to an enhancement of I/R-induced tissue injury, and (f) I/R-induced inflammatory responses (leukocyte adhesion, increased vascular permeability) can be mimicked *in vitro* by exposing endothelial cell monolayers to hypoxia and reoxygenation [1–5].

The recognition that leukocyte-endothelial cell adhesion is an early and rate-limiting event in the pathogenesis of reperfusion injury has led to an intensive effort to identify the factors that promote the recruitment and activation of inflammatory cells in postcapillary venules of tissues exposed to ischemia and reperfusion (I/R). This chapter explores some of the factors and mechanisms that may explain I/R-induced leukocyte-endothelial cell adhesion in postcapillary venules as well as I/R-

Vascular Adhesion Molecules and Inflammation, edited by J. D. Pearson
© 1999 Birkhäuser Verlag Basel/Switzerland

induced leukocyte-capillary plugging. Data derived from both *in vivo* (postcapillary venules) and *in vitro* (cultured endothelial cells) models of ischemia/reperfusion (anoxia/reoxygenation) are compared and contrasted.

Leukocyte-capillary plugging

Hemorrhagic shock and ischemia are conditions that are associated with capillary obstruction by circulating blood cells. In both instances, circulating blood cells (leukocytes, platelets) and/or aggregates of these cells with fibrin (microthrombi) can lodge within the capillary lumen, thereby preventing the flow of blood through these vessels [1, 6–9]. Furthermore, some of the leukocytes that become lodged in ischemic capillaries remain stuck upon restoration of perfusion pressure, causing "capillary no-reflow". A potential consequence of this capillary no-reflow is an increased resistance to blood flow in postischemic tissues and a diminished capacity to recover from the ischemic insult.

The propensity for capillary plugging with leukocytes in ischemic tissues has been attributed to a number of events, including increased stiffness of activated leukocytes, endothelial cell swelling, leukocyte-endothelial cell adhesion, and low driving pressures for leukocyte movement along the capillaries [1]. It is likely that the relative contribution of each of these factors to capillary no-reflow varies between organs. Those organs (e.g. heart) that are perfused by capillaries with small internal diameters will be more sensitive to leukocyte plugging during and following periods of hypotension. Other tissues (e.g. skin) that have large arterial-venous anastamoses, which shunt leukocytes past the capillary bed, will be less prone to leukocyte-capillary plugging. The physical restriction or trapping of leukocytes within capillaries has been implicated as a major contributor to the leukocyte accumulation observed in postischemic myocardium, liver, brain, kidney and skeletal muscle. The strong correlation between the percentage of capillaries exhibiting no-reflow and the percentage of capillaries that contain granulocytes in postischemic tissues suggests that leukocyte trapping likely accounts for capillary no-reflow [10]. Additional supportive evidence is provided by reports that demonstrate virtual elimination of capillary no-reflow in animals that are either rendered neutropenic or that receive antibodies that interfere with leukocyte-endothelial cell adhesion in postcapillary venules [7–9]. Since the level of adhesion molecule expression on capillary endothelium is quite low (compared to venular endothelium), the ability of adhesion molecule-directed antibodies to attenuate capillary no-reflow has been attributed to an action on the downstream postcapillary venules [7]. Adherent leukocytes in postcapillary venules appear to promote leukostasis in upstream capillaries by enhancing fluid and protein filtration across venular endothelium. The resulting interstitial edema raises interstitial fluid pressure to a level sufficient to occlude the capillary lumen and thereby facilitate the entrapment of leukocytes.

Leukocyte-endothelial cell adhesion in postcapillary venules exposed to I/R

The technique of intravital microscopy has been applied to several tissues to quantify the recruitment of rolling, firmly adherent, and emigrated leukocytes in postcapillary venules exposed to I/R [1, 2, 11–15]. Some investigators have employed I/R models that involve complete arterial occlusion, while others have used partial ischemia models. The latter approach allows for measurement of leukocyte-endothelial cell adhesion during both the ischemic and reperfusion periods, while the former allows for data collection only during the reperfusion period. Complete arterial occlusion elicits more profound increases (30–35-fold) in the number of firmly adherent leukocytes in postcapillary venules than partial ischemia models (2–10-fold). The magnitude of the reperfusion-induced recruitment of adherent leukocytes is dependent on the duration of the ischemic insult. The number of rolling and emigrating leukocytes also increases after reperfusion. Whole body (hemorrhage-reinfusion) I/R has been shown to yield a nearly identical increase in leukocyte-endothelial cell adhesion to that observed following local I/R, suggesting that the sympathoadrenal discharge elicited by hemorrhage has little influence on the leukocyte recruitment response [15]. A detailed morphological evaluation of mesenteric venules has revealed that most of the adherent and emigrated leukocytes are neutrophils [13].

Factors involved in the modulation of I/R-induced leukocyte-endothelial cell adhesion

A variety of factors have been implicated in the recruitment of rolling, adherent, and emigrating leukocytes in postcapillary venules exposed to I/R. While different strategies have been employed to test for the contribution of different factors in this inflammatory process, most of the available data is based on the use of pharmacological agents and monoclonal antibodies. Table 1 summarizes some of the different agents that have been applied to address potential mediators of the leukocyte-endothelial cell adhesion elicited by I/R in postcapillary venules.

Reduced venular shear rates

Low flow (partial arterial occlusion) ischemia is associated with 4–5-fold increases in the number of rolling and adherent leukocytes during the ischemic period [16–19]. A significant fraction (> 50%) of the leukocyte adherence observed during low flow ischemia can be attributed to the low venular shear rates. It has been shown that reductions in venular shear rate over a range of 800–50 s^{-1} lead to an increased number of rolling and adherent leukocytes [16]. Furthermore, the number of

223

Table 1 - Pharmacological agents and monoclonal antibodies used to identify potential mediators of I/R-induced leukocyte-endothelial cell adhesion in postcapillary venules.

Oxygen radical-directed interventions

Superoxide dismutase (scavenges superoxide anion)
Catalase (detoxifies hydrogen peroxide)
Desferrioxamine (chelates iron)
Allopurinol or oxypurinol (inhibits xanthine oxidase)

Lipid mediator-directed interventions

SC41930 (LTB$_4$ antagonist)
L663,536 (leukotriene synthesis inhibitor)
WEB 2086 (PAF receptor antagonist)

Nitric oxide-directed interventions

L-NAME, L-NMMA (NO synthase inhibitors)
NONOATEs, nitroprusside (NO donating compounds)

Mast cell-directed interventions

Lodoxamide, doxantrazole (mast cell stabilizers)
Compound 48/80 (mast cell degranulator)

Endothelial cell adhesion molecule antibodies

PB1.3 (anti-P-selectin)
RR1/1, 1A29 (anti-ICAM-1)
CL3 (anti-E-selectin)

Leukocyte adhesion molecule antibodies

IB4, WT.3 (anti-CD11/CD18)
HRL3 (anti-L-selectin)

adherent leukocytes that are recruited by an inflammatory mediator such as platelet activating factor (PAF) is far greater at low than at normal shear rates [19], suggesting that it is easier for leukocytes to create strong adhesive bonds with venular endothelial cells at low shear rates. A dependence of leukocyte adherence on shear forces has also been demonstrated using *in vitro* models that employ isolated neutrophils and monolayers of cultured endothelial cells; however, much lower shear stresses (3 vs 15 dynes/cm^2) are needed to dislodge an adherent leukocyte *in vitro* [2].

The recruitment of adherent leukocytes that is observed in postcapillary venules exposed to low shear rates has been attributed to a reduced washout of inflammatory mediators that are normally produced by endothelial and/or parenchymal cells [18]. At low shear rates these mediators accumulate within microvessels to elicit the activation and/or increased expression of leukocyte adhesion molecules. Support for this view is provided by studies that demonstrate an attenuated recruitment of adherent leukocytes in mesenteric venules at low shear rates following administration of either a leukotriene B$_4$ (LTB$_4$) (but not a PAF-) receptor antagonist or a 5-lipoxygenase inhibitor, suggesting that LTB$_4$ accumulation contributes to the recruitment of adherent leukocytes at low shear rates. The shear rate-dependent recruitment of firmly adherent leukocytes appears to involve an interaction between CD11/CD18 on leukocytes and constitutively expressed intercellular cell adhesion molecule-1 (ICAM-1) on endothelial cells [17].

Adhesion glycoproteins

There are three general lines of evidence that support a role for both leukocyte and endothelial cell adhesion molecules in the recruitment of adherent leukocytes in venules exposed to I/R: (1) the expression of these adhesion molecules is increased after I/R [20], (2) blocking antibodies directed against these adhesion molecules attenuate the recruitment of adherent leukocytes [21, 22], and (3) I/R-induced leukocyte-endothelial cell adhesion is blunted in venules of animals that are genetically deficient in leukocyte or endothelial cell adhesion molecules [4]. For example, the available data suggest that P-selectin is the dominant mediator of the rapid and sustained recruitment of rolling leukocytes. This contention is supported by data showing that I/R elicits a rapid (10–30 min) increase in P-selectin expression in the intestinal vasculature that is followed by a larger increase at 5 h after reperfusion [20]. P-selectin mRNA measurements in the same tissues suggest that the early rise in P-selectin expression likely represents mobilization of its preformed pool, while the later increase is a transcription-dependent process. Evidence of a more direct nature is provided by studies that demonstrate significant attenuation of I/R-induced leukocyte-endothelial cell adhesion in animals receiving blocking antibodies against P-selectin and in mice that are genetically deficient in P-selectin [4, 23].

Similar evidence has been presented to support a role for CD11/CD18 on leukocytes and ICAM-1 on endothelial cells in mediating recruitment of firmly adherent leukocytes in postischemic venules [3, 21]. Leukocytes obtained from venous blood draining some postischemic tissues exhibit an increased expression of CD11b/CD18, as measured by flow-cytometry. ICAM-1 expression is also increased on endothelial cells after I/R. However, a few hours are required for this transcription-dependent up-regulation of ICAM-1, while ICAM-1 blocking antibodies inhibit the firm adherence of leukocytes observed within a few minutes after the initiation of reperfusion. The latter observation has been attributed to the binding of CD11/CD18-expressing leukocytes with constitutively expressed ICAM-1 on endothelial cells . Additional support for this view is provided by the observation that ICAM-1 deficient mice exhibit a diminished accumulation of adherent leukocytes in postcapillary venules exposed to about 30 min of reperfusion [4].

Reactive oxygen metabolites

The reactive oxygen metabolites (ROM) that are produced by activated leukocytes and endothelial cells have also been implicated in I/R-induced leukocyte accumulation [12]. It is known that exposure of postcapillary venules to exogenous hydrogen peroxide or superoxide promotes leukocyte-endothelial cell adhesion [24]. The proadhesive effect of H_2O_2 can be significantly attenuated by PAF receptor antagonists as well as CD18-specific MAbs, suggesting that the oxidant elicits the formation of PAF, which in turn induces the up-regulation of CD11/CD18 on neutrophils. Direct evidence that supports a role for ROM in I/R-induced leukocyte adhesion comes from reports that demonstrate a reduction in adhesion that is associated with administration of superoxide dismutase (SOD) or catalase [25,26]. Transgenic mice that overexpress CuZn-SOD also exhibit a reduced recruitment of adherent leukocytes in terminal hepatic venules after intestinal I/R.

A likely source of the ROM that mediate I/R-induced leukocyte-endothelial cell adhesion is the enzyme xanthine oxidase [27]. This enzyme, which can generate both superoxide and hydrogen peroxide, is localized primarily in vascular endothelial cells of humans and many animal species. A role for xanthine oxidase in I/R-induced leukocyte-endothelial cell adhesion is supported by studies that show a blunted recruitment response in animal models treated with allopurinol or other agents that inhibit or inactivate the enzyme [12, 25]. Although the enzyme exists as a dehydrogenase (which cannot generate oxygen radicals) in normal tissues, conditions (such as ischemia) associated with hypoxia, acidosis and/or limited proteolysis can initiate its conversion to the radical-generating oxidase form. Since ischemia also results in the accumulation of purines from ATP, both substrates for xanthine oxidase are provided upon reperfusion, i.e., molecular oxygen and hypoxanthine, which leads to the generation of superoxide and hydrogen peroxide. The preferential localization of xanthine oxidase to vascular endothelial cells is often invoked to explain the vulnerability of the microvasculature to I/R injury [27].

Nitric oxide (NO)

It has been proposed that the relative rates of production of superoxide and nitric oxide (NO) are an important determinant of whether leukocytes adhere in post-capillary venules after I/R [28]. Nitric oxide, which reacts avidly with superoxide, is normally produced by vascular endothelium. Inhibition of NO production with analogues of L-arginine (e.g. L-NAME, L-NMMA) results in an intense leukocyte adherence response in mesenteric venules, suggesting that NO is an endogenous inhibitor of leukocyte-endothelial cell adhesion [28]. Consequently, one would predict that conditions associated with an enhanced formation of superoxide (e.g. I/R) should lead to increased leukocyte adherence by virtue of superoxide's ability to render nitric oxide biologically inactive. The contention that nitric oxide attenuates leukocyte-endothelial cell adhesion is supported by reports that demonstrate a reduced adhesion response to different inflammatory mediators following the administration of nitric oxide donors [14]. Endothelial cell production of nitric oxide appears to fall following I/R and agents that spontaneously release NO have been shown to attenuate leukocyte adhesion in mesenteric venules exposed to I/R [14].

The mechanisms that underlie the protective role of NO in I/R-induced leukocyte adhesion remain unclear. Since NO reacts with superoxide at least three times faster than SOD, it appears likely that NO simply acts to prevent the pro-adhesive effects of superoxide by scavenging the free radical [29]. Inasmuch as NO synthase inhibitors elicit the upregulation of P-selectin [29], while NO donors can attenuate I/R-induced P-selectin expression [20], it also appears likely that the protective actions of NO relate to its ability to modulate endothelial cell adhesion molecule expression. Mast cell-derived substances have also been implicated in the recruitment of adherent leukocyte after I/R (see below). Since NO donors stabilize mast cells, while NO synthase inhibitors promote mast cell degranulation, this cell population may also represent a major target for the beneficial actions of NO after I/R [23].

Lipid mediators

There are several lines of evidence that implicate the lipid inflammatory mediators, platelet activating factor (PAF) and LTB_4, in the recruitment of adherent leukocytes in postischemic venules [1, 2]. Phospholipase A_2 (PLA_2), an enzyme that can catalyze the production of both PAF and LTB_4, is activated in some tissues after I/R [1]. Since pretreatment with allopurinol or SOD can attenuate the PLA_2 activation, it has been proposed that xanthine oxidase-derived ROM may be responsible for activation of the enzyme. Furthermore, both inflammatory mediators have been shown to accumulate in postischemic tissues. Direct exposure of postcapillary venules to

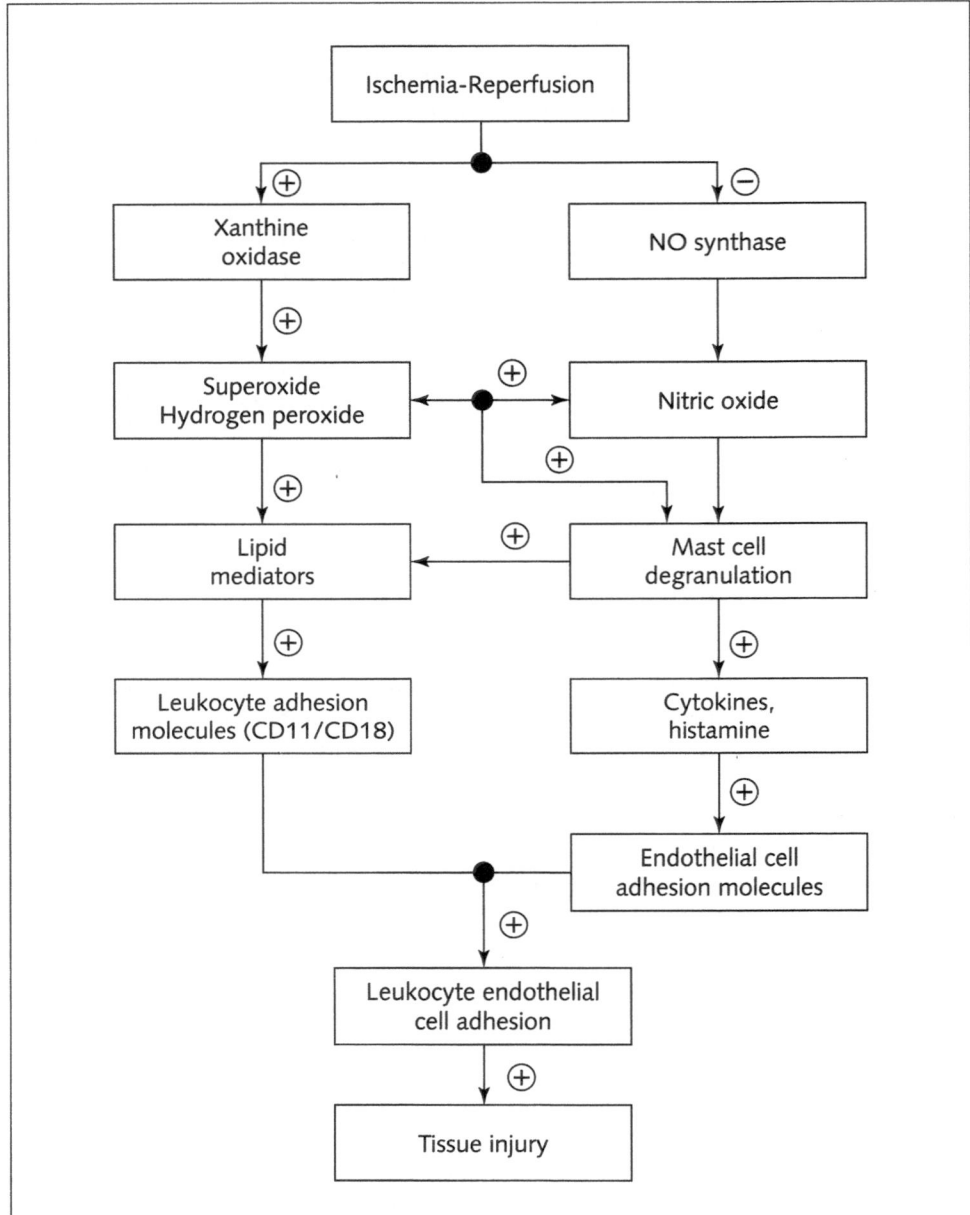

Figure 1
Mechanism proposed to explain the leukocyte-endothelial cell adhesion elicited in postcapillary venules by ischemia-reperfusion.

either PAF or LTB$_4$ elicits a rapid, CD11/CD18-ICAM-1 dependent leukocyte adhesion response similar to that observed in postischemic venules. However, the most compelling evidence in support of a role for these lipid mediators in I/R-induced leukocyte recruitment is derived from studies that demonstrate an attenuation of the inflammatory response with PAF- or LTB$_4$-receptor antagonists, or with a 5-lipoxygenase inhibitor [30–32]. While it is generally assumed that the lipid mediators primarily exert their action on the leukocytes to increase the expression of CD11b/CD18, there is some evidence to support the possibility that 5-lipoxygenase products elicit the rapid expression of P-selectin on endothelial cells exposed to I/R [20]. This observation suggests that the leukotrienes generated after reperfusion may also contribute to P-selectin dependent recruitment of rolling leukocytes in postischemic venules.

Mast cells

Mast cells are usually found closely apposed to the microvasculature, particularly surrounding postcapillary venules [23]. These cells are exquisitely sensitive to activation by a variety of stimuli, including oxygen radicals (e.g. superoxide), lipid mediators (PAF, leukotrienes), and nitric oxide synthase inhibition. Upon activation, mast cells release a number of substances that can influence the function of endothelial cells and/or leukocytes, including histamine, NO, cytokines (e.g. tumor necrosis factor (TNF), interleukin-1 (IL-1)), proteases (e.g. cathepsin G), and reactive oxygen metabolites. Ischemia and reperfusion is a potent stimulus for mast cell degranulation, with the number of degranulated cells surrounding postcapillary venules increasing as the duration of ischemia increases [14, 23]. Agents that elicit mast cell degranulation (e.g. compound 48/80) can produce many of the microvascular responses observed after I/R, including leukocyte rolling, firm adhesion, and emigration [14]. Furthermore, mast cell stabilizing agents such as lodoxamide are highly effective in blunting the leukocyte-endothelial cell adhesion elicited by I/R, suggesting that mast cell-derived inflammatory mediators contribute to the recruitment of leukocytes into postischemic tissues [31].

In summary, the available data on I/R-induced leukocyte-endothelial cell adhesion in postcapillary venules are generally consistent with the scheme outlined in Figure 1. Two key events that elicit the recruitment of leukocytes are an enhanced production of oxygen radicals and a concomitant decline in the generation and/or accumulation (due to superoxide inactivation) of nitric oxide. These events initiate the production of inflammatory mediators (PAF and LTB$_4$) that promote the expression of β_2-integrins on circulating leukocytes, and the release of mast cell products (e.g. histamine, cytokines) that enhance the expression of adhesion molecules (eg, P-selectin, ICAM-1) which mediate leukocyte rolling or firm adhesion. The firmly adherent and emigrating leukocytes subsequently mediate tissue injury by releasing proteases and oxidants.

Anoxia/reoxygenation-induced neutrophil-endothelial cell interactions: an *in vitro* model of I/R-induced microvascular dysfunction

Exposure of endothelial cell monolayers to anoxia followed by reoxygenation (A/R) has been used extensively as a model system by many investigators to simulate the microvascular dysfunction that is normally elicited by I/R. Using these *in vitro* cell models, A/R was shown to elicit several alterations in endothelial cell function similar to those produced by I/R *in vivo*, namely, (a) xanthine oxidase activation [33–35], (b) enhanced formation of superoxide and hydrogen peroxide [36, 37], (c) activation of redox-sensitive nuclear transcription factors NFκB and AP-1 [38], (d) increased expression of endothelial cell adhesion molecules [38], (e) increased adhesivity to neutrophils [39], and (f) a reduction in endothelial barrier function [40]. These *in vitro* models have provided important insights into understanding the factors, such as proteases and oxidants, that modulate anoxia-reoxygenation-induced, neutrophil-mediated endothelial cell injury [33, 41]. In addition, endothelial cell monolayers have provided a useful model for detailed characterization of the contribution of different leukocyte and endothelial cell adhesion glycoproteins to the elevated neutrophil-endothelial cell adhesion elicited by A/R [38, 39]. For instance, mechanistic studies on A/R-treated monolayers have revealed that endothelial cells produce and liberate hydrogen peroxide, which results in a PAF-dependent up-regulation of neutrophil adhesion molecules (CD11/CD18) and the subsequent engagement of these adhesion receptors to their counterparts on the endothelial cell surface [35, 36, 38, 39].

While most of the microvascular alterations elicited *in vivo* by ischemia- reperfusion can be reasonably and accurately simulated by A/R-exposed endothelial cell monolayers *in vitro*, some responses cannot. For example, the blocking effect of leukotriene biosynthesis inhibitors and LTB$_4$-receptor antagonists on the recruitment of leukocytes that is observed in mesenteric venules exposed to I/R *in vivo* [1, 41, 42] cannot be mimicked using cultured endothelial cell monolayers [39]. Similarly, while P-selectin specific monoclonal antibodies (mAbs) have been shown to be effective in attenuating leukocyte adhesion in postischemic venules [1, 41, 42], these mAbs are minimally effective in blocking neutrophil adhesion to endothelial monolayers exposed to A/R [42], indicating a difference in the contribution of selectins to the recruitment of leukocytes after reperfusion (*in vivo*) versus reoxygenation (*in vitro*).

A variety of factors is likely to contribute to the inconsistent responses of intact versus cultured endothelial cells to ischemia (anoxia)-reperfusion (reoxygenation). Importantly, the use of late passaged endothelial cells (i.e. cell passage greater than two) may explain the inability to demonstrate a role for P-selectin in some *in vitro* models of A/R-induced neutrophil-endothelial cell adhesion [39]. Since most data on neutrophil- endothelial cell adhesive interactions following A/R have been generated using static systems, the application of shear to endothelial cell monolayers could also resolve some of the discrepancies. The lack of incorporation of flow into *in vitro* adhesion assays has not allowed for simulation of the hemodynamic constraints imposed on the adhesive interactions between neutrophil and endothelial cells such as those occurring within the microcirculation. Endothelial cell monolayers exposed to shear stress appear either to reorganize their cytoskeletal elements (formation of stress fibers) to allow for greater adhesion of endothelial cells to the underlying matrix [43], to increase their constitutive expression of adhesion glycoproteins (ICAM-1), or to increase the storage pool of preformed adhesion molecules (P-selectin).

The absence of mast cells, which are known to degranulate and promote P-selectin-dependent leukocyte adhesion in postcapillary venules [23], may also contribute to a diminished role for P-selectin in *in vitro* studies. The absence of other cell types may similarly explain an inability of leukotriene-targeted reagents to attenuate neutrophil adhesion *in vitro*. While endothelial cells per se may have a limited capacity to generate leukotrienes, biosynthesis of leukotrienes occurs during coincubation of endothelial cells with platelets or neutrophils, indicating a transcellular cooperation in the production of leukotrienes when appropriate substrates are provided by other cell types. Taken together, these findings suggest that some caution is warranted in extrapolation of *in vitro* results to understanding events *in vivo*. This notwithstanding, the endothelial cell monolayer offers a simple and well defined *in vitro* cell model that allows for detailed mechanistic studies and precise delineation of the molecular events that are associated with A/R-induced leukocyte-endothelial cell interactions.

The early phase of neutrophil-endothelial cell adhesion after anoxia/reoxygenation

Studies from our laboratory and by others have demonstrated an early (10–30 min) increase in adhesive interaction between neutrophils and endothelial cells after reoxygenation *in vitro* [38, 39, 44]. The identity of the neutrophil attractant and/or activator generated by endothelial cells exposed to A/R has not been fully resolved. The possibility that endothelial cells liberate factors that result in the activation of β_2-integrins on leukocytes is supported by data derived from endothelial cell monolayers exposed to A/R [39]. Incubation of neutrophils with conditioned media obtained from endothelial cell monolayers exposed to A/R results in an increased surface expression of CD11b/CD18 and an increased adhesion of neutrophils to naive monolayers [39]. These findings indicate that A/R elicits the release of a stable, soluble inflammatory mediator(s) from endothelial cells that is capable of up-regulating the expression of CD11b/CD18 on the surface of neutrophils. The hyperadhesivity of these neutrophils is blocked by either catalase or a PAF receptor antagonist, but not by either an LTB$_4$ antagonist or a 5-lipoxygenase inhibitor [39]. These observations from our laboratory, coupled with results in the literature [1, 45], implicate a role for endothelial cell-derived reactive oxygen metabolites (ROM), including hydrogen peroxide, in enhancing the production and/or liberation of PAF. Previous evidence suggests that the enzyme xanthine oxidase is a source of the ROM [27]. The importance of PAF in mediating the neutrophil adhesion response to hypoxia-reoxygenation is supported by the finding that L659,989, a PAF-receptor antagonist, effectively blocks hypoxia-induced neutrophil hyperadhesion to cultured human umbilical vein endothelial cells (HUVECs) [46].

Using a static adhesion assay system, Yoshida et. al. [39] demonstrated that an anti-ICAM-1 specific mAb, but not mAbs against either E-selectin, L-selectin or P-selectin, attenuated the A/R-induced neutrophil adherence to an extent comparable to that observed with mAbs against either CD11a or CD11b. We have observed a basal level of expression of ICAM-1, but not E-selectin, on endothelial cell monolayers and that exposure of endothelial cell monolayers to A/R did not enhance the expression of either adhesion glycoprotein in this early phase after reoxygenation [39].

Studies by Palluy et al. [44] also demonstrated a transient increase in neutrophil adhesion, observed at 20 min after reoxygenation, in endothelial cell monolayers exposed to hypoxia (30 mmHg for 5 h), rather than anoxia. This early hyperadhesive period elicited by hypoxia/reoxygenation was associated with increased endothelial cell xanthine oxidase activity and could be ameliorated by superoxide dismutase, catalase or hydroxyl radical scavengers, indicating a role for reactive oxygen metabolites in mediating the adhesion response. There are, however, some differences in the relative contribution of various adhesion molecules to the adherence responses observed with reoxygenation after either an hypoxic or anoxic stress. The early hyperadhesivity observed following a hypoxic stress model are effectively attenuated by a mAb against P-selectin, while the same mAb has no effect following an anoxic stress. At present, there is no clear explanation for the differences in the molecular determinants of adhesion in the anoxia- versus hypoxia-reoxygenation models of ischemia/reperfusion. Possibly, the discrepancies are related to differences in magnitude and/or duration of the hypoxic insult, as well as the times at which neutrophil adhesion was monitored after reoxygenation, or both.

The late phase of anoxia-reoxygenation-induced neutrophil-endothelial cell adhesion

Palluy et al. [44] were first to report that hypoxia followed by reoxygenation results in a second phase of enhanced neutrophil adhesion that is observed at 4 h after reoxygenation. This late phase of neutrophil hyperadhesivity was accompanied by an increased endothelial cell xanthine oxidase activity and the adhesion was inhibitable by catalase, superoxide dismutase, or hydroxyl radical scavengers. This result indicates that both the early and late phase adhesion is mediated by oxidants. However, they differ in the role for adhesion molecules. Anti-E-selectin, but not anti-ICAM-1, prevented the increased neutrophil adhesion observed 4 h after reoxygenation [44]; a result that contradicts the proposed role for ICAM-1 in the early response elicited by A/R [39] and in ischemia/reperfusion-induced leukocyte adhesion in postcapillary venules [21]. This apparent discrepancy in adhesion molecule requirement suggests a fundamental difference in the molecular control of leukocyte hyperadhesivity in the early and late phases of hypoxia/reoxygenation-induced leukocyte-endothelial cell interactions.

In a recent study, we have extensively characterized the molecular mechanisms of leukocyte adhesion to cultured endothelial cells induced by anoxia followed by up to 10 h reoxygenation. We found a biphasic response for A/R-induced neutrophil adhesion to HUVECs, with peak responses at 30 min (phase 1) and 4 h (phase 2) after reoxygenation [38]. The phase 1, but not the phase 2, adhesion response was blunted by oxypurinol and catalase, indicating a role for xanthine oxidase and H_2O_2 in the early A/R-induced inflammatory response [38], which is consistent with previous observations [39]. Moreover, PAF contributed to both phases of neutrophil adhesion [38]. Further mechanistic studies revealed that this *in vitro* A/R protocol was associated with a profound upregulation of E-selectin, which peaked at 4 h after reoxygenation of the endothelial cell monolayers (Tab. 2). P-selectin mAb blocked adhesion at 30 min after reoxygenation, but both P-selectin and E-selectin mAbs were effective in attenuating the neutrophil-endothelial cell adhesion observed at 4 h after A/R (Tab. 2).

Results derived from A/R-induced E-selectin expression in HUVEC monolayers treated with the inhibitors of de novo macromolecule synthesis, cycloheximide- or actinomycin D, are consistent with a transcription-dependent process in the late phase adhesion response (Tab. 2). In this regard, we found that A/R results in the upregulation and activation of the p65/p50 heterodimer of NFκB, a transcription factor that is closely linked with upregulation of a variety of inflammatory genes associated with various exogenous stimuli such as oxidants (H_2O_2) [47, 48] or cytokines (e.g. TNF, IL-1) ([49, 50]; see also chapter by Chen and Medford, this volume). In our model system, we further demonstrated that inhibition of NFκB and AP-1 by cognate DNA sequences gave phase 2 adhesion responses that invoke a major role for both nuclear transcription factors in A/R-induced expression of E-selectin, but not P-selectin or ICAM-1 (Tab. 2) [38].

In summary, the available data indicate that A/R elicits an early and late phase neutrophil-endothelial cell adhesion response (Fig. 2). While the magnitude of leukocyte adhesion appears to be similar in both phases [38], they differ in terms of contribution of chemical mediators and endothelial cell adhesion molecules. Furthermore, this two-phase inflammatory process involves both transcription-independent (phase 1) and transcription-dependent (phase 2) components of endothelial cell adhesion molecular expression.

Table 2 - A/R-induced leukocyte adhesion, surface expression of ECAMs, and role for transcription factors

A. Leukocyte adhesion	Phase 1 (30 min reoxygenation)	Phase 2 (4 h reoxygenation)
	% adhesion	
Normoxia	6.0 ± 0.9	5.2 ± 0.7
A/R control (without inhibitors)	$15.3 \pm 0.8^{*}$	$14.0 \pm 0.2^{*}$
+ anti P-selectin (20 µg/ml)	$6.2 \pm 0.6^{**}$	$7.3 \pm 0.2^{**}$
+ anti E-selectin (20 µg/ml)	16.2 ± 0.3	$5.5 \pm 0.5^{**}$
+ cycloheximide (1 µg/ml)	14.5 ± 0.9	$9.0 \pm 0.6^{**}$
+ actinomycin D (2 µg/ml)	14.2 ± 1.1	$8.2 \pm 0.4^{**}$

B. Phase 2 ECAM surface expression	ICAM-1	P-selectin	E-selectin
		%, A/R control	
A/R control (without inhibitors)	100	100	100
+ cycloheximide (1 µg/ml)	94 ± 4	70 ± 2	$45 \pm 5^{**}$
+ actinomycin D (2 µg/ml)	82 ± 4	74 ± 8	$24 \pm 4^{**}$

C. Role for transcription factors in Phase 2 ECAM expression	ICAM-1	P-selectin	E-selectin
		% A/R control	
A/R control (without inhibitors)	100	100	100
+ κB ds-oligonucleotide (20 µmol/l)	80 ± 4	81 ± 5	$65 \pm 6^{**}$
+ AP-1 ds-oligonucleotide (20 µmol/l)	83 ± 4	$72 \pm 5^{**}$	$71 \pm 3^{**}$

$^{*}P < 0.05$ versus normoxia; $^{**}P < 0.05$ versus A/R control; ECAM, endothelial cell adhesion molecules

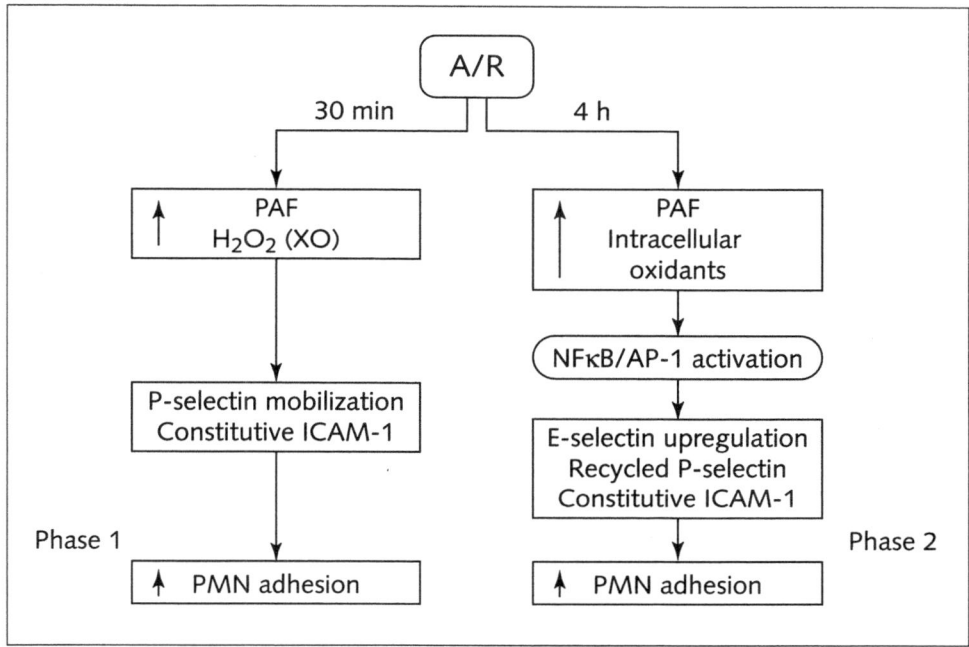

Figure 2
Two-phase leukocyte (PMN) adhesion to endothelial cells induced by anoxia/reoxygenation (A/R).

Acknowledgments
Research in the authors' laboratories was supported by grants from NIH DK43785 & HL26411 (DNG) and DK44510 (TYA) and a grant from AHA (TYA).

References

1   Granger DN, Korthuis RJ (1995) Physiologic mechanisms of postischemic tissue injury. *Ann Rev Physiol* 57: 311–332

2   Granger DN, Kvietys PR, Perry MA (1993) Leukocyte-endothelial cell adhesion induced by ischemia and reperfusion. *Can J Physiol Pharmacol* 71: 67–75

3   Jaeschke H, Farhood A, Smith CW (1990) Neutrophils contribute to ischemia/reperfusion injury in rat liver *in vivo*. *FASEB J* 4: 3355–3359

4   Horie Y, Wolf R, Anderson DC, Granger DN (1997) Hepatic leukostasis and hypoxic stress in adhesion molecule-deficient mice after gut ischemia-reperfusion. *J Clin Invest* 99: 781–788

5   Panes J, Granger DN (1998) Leukocyte-endothelial cell interactions: Molecular mechanisms and implications in gastrointestinal disease. *Gastroenterology* 114: 1–26

6   Engler RL, Schmid-Schoenbein GW, Pavelec RS. 1983 Leukocyte capillary plugging in myocardial ischemia and reperfusion in the dog. *Am J Pathol* 111: 98–111

7   Jerome SN, Akamitsu T, and Korthuis RJ (1994) Leukocyte adhesion,edema and the development of postischemic capillary no-reflow. *Am J Physiol* 267: H1329–H1336

8   Jerome SN, Smith CW, Korthuis RJ (1992). CD18-dependent adherence reactions play an important role in the development of the no-reflow phenomenon. *Am J Physiol* 263: H1637–H1642

9   Jerome SN, Dore M, Paulson JC, Smith CW, Korthuis RJ (1994) P-selectin and ICAM-1 dependent adherence reactions: role in the genesis of postischemic capillary no-reflow. *Am J Physiol* 266: H1316–H1321

10   Skalak R, Skalak TC(1995) Flow behavior of leukocytes in small tubes. In: DN Granger, GW Schmid-Schoenbein (eds): *Physiology and pathophysiology of leukocyte adhesion.* Oxford University Press, New York, 97–115

11   Erlansson M, Bergqvist D, Persson, NH, Svensjo E (1991) Modification of postischemic increase of leukocyte adhesion and vascular permeability in the hamster by iloprost. *Prostaglandins* 41: 157–168

12   Granger DN, Benoit JN, Suzuki M, Grisham MB (1989) Leukocyte adherence to venular endothelium during ischemia-reperfusion. *Am J Physiol* 257: G683–G688

13   Oliver MG, Specian RD, Perry MA, Granger DN (1991) Morphologic assessment of leukocyte-endothelial cell interactions in mesenteric venules subjected to ischemia and reperfusion. *Inflammation* 15: 331–346

14   Kurose I, Wolf R, Grisham MB, Granger DN (1994) Modulation of ischemia/reperfusion-induced microvascular dysfunction by nitric oxide. *Circ Res* 74: 376–82

15   Perry MA, Granger DN (1992) Leukocyte adhesion in local versus hemorrhage-induced ischemia. *Am J Physiol* 263: H810–H815

16   Perry MA, Granger DN (1991) Role of CD11/CD18 in shear rate-dependent leukocyte-endothelial cell interactions in cat mesenteric venules. *J Clin Invest* 87: 1798–1804

17   Bienvenu K, Granger DN (1993) Molecular determinants of shear rate-dependent leukocyte adhesion in postcapillary venules. *Am J Physiol* 264: H1504–H1508

18   Bienvenu K, Russell J, Granger DN (1992) Leukotriene B$_4$ mediates shear rate- dependent leukocyte adhesion in mesenteric venules. *Circ Res* 71: 906–911

19   Bienvenu K, Russell J, Granger DN (1993) Platelet-activating factor promotes shear rate-dependent leukocyte adhesion in postcapillary venules. *J Lipid Mediators* 8: 95–103

20   Eppihimer MJ, Russell J, Anderson DC, Epstein CJ, Laroux S, Granger DN (1997) Modulation of P-selectin expression in the post-ischemic intestinal microvasculature. *Am J Physiol* 273: G1326–G1332

21   Kurose I, Anderson DC, Miyasaka M, Tamatani T, Paulson JC, Todd RF, Rusche JR, Granger DN (1994) Molecular determinants of reperfusion-induced leukocyte adhesion and vascular protein leakage. *Circ Res* 74: 336–343

22 Kubes P, Kurose I, Granger DN (1994) NO donors prevent integrin-induced leukocyte adhesion but not P-selectin-dependent rolling in postischemic venules. *Am J Physiol* 267: H931–H937

23 Kubes P, Granger DN (1996) Leukocyte-endothelial cell interactions evoked by mast cells. *Cardiovasc Res* 32: 699–708

24 Suzuki M, Asako H, Kubes P, Jennings S, Grisham MB, Granger DN (1991) Neutrophil-derived oxidants promote leukocyte adherence in postcapillary venules. *Microvasc Res* 42: 38125–38150

25 Suzuki M, Grisham MB, Granger, DN (1991) Leukocyte-endothelial cell interactions: role of xanthine oxidase-derived oxidants. *J Leukocyte Biol* 50: 488–494

26 Suzuki M, Inauen W, Kvietys PR, Grisham MB, Meininger C, Schelling ME, Granger HS, Granger DN (1989) Superoxide mediates reperfusion-induced leukocyte-endothelial cell interactions. *Am J Physiol* 257: H1740–H1745

27 Granger DN (1988) Role of xanthine oxidase and granulocytes in ischemia-reperfusion injury. *Am J Physiol* 255: H1269–H1275

28 Kubes P, Suzuki M, Granger DN (1991) Nitric oxide: An endogenous modulator of leukocyte adhesion. *Proc Natl Acad Sci USA* 88: 4651–4655

29 Lefer AM, DJ Lefer (1996) The role of nitric oxide and cell adhesion molecules on the microcirculation in ischemia-reperfusion. *Cardiovasc Res* 32: 743–751

30 Granger DN, Kurose I, Kvietys PR (1995) Modulation of leukocyte adherence and emigration during ischemia and reperfusion. In: DN Granger, GW Schmid-Schoenbein (eds): *Physiology and pathophysiology of leukocyte adhesion.* Oxford University Press, New York, 323–338

31 Kurose I, Argenbright LW, Wolf R, Lianxi L, Granger DN (1997) Ischemia/reperfusion-induced microvascular dysfunction: role of oxidants and lipid mediators. *Am J Physiol* 272: H2976–H2982

32 Kubes P, Ibbotson G, Russell J, Wallace JL, Granger DN (1990) Role of platelet-activating factor in ischemia/reperfusion-induced leukocyte adherence. *Am J Physiol* 259: G300–G305

33 Inauen W, Granger DN, Meininger CJ, Schelling ME, Granger HJ, Kvietys PR (1990) An *in vitro* model of ischemia-reperfusion induced microvascular injury. *Am J Physiol* 259: H925–H931

34 Ratych RE, Chuknyiska RS, Bulkley GB (1987) The primary localization of free radical generation after anoxia/reoxygenation in isolated endothelial cells. *Surgery* 102: 122–131

35 Terada LS, Guidot DM, Leff JA, Willingham IR, Hanley ME, Piermattei D, Repine JE (1992) Hypoxia injures endothelial cells by increasing endogenous xanthine oxidase activity. *Proc Natl Acad Sci USA* 89: 3362–3366

36 Terada LS, Willingham IR, Rosandick ME, Leff JA, Kindt GW, Repine JE (1991) Generation of superoxide anion by brain endothelial cell xanthine oxidase. *J Cell Physiol* 148: 191–196

37 Zweier JL, Kuppusamy P, Thompson-Gorman S, Klunk D, Lutty GA (1994) Measure-

ment and characterization of free radical generation in reoxygenated human endothelial cells. *Am J Physiol* 266: C700–C708

38 Ichikawa H, Kvietys PR, Wolf R, Granger DN, Aw TY (1997) Molecular mechanisms of anoxia/reoxygenation-induced neutrophil adherence to cultured endothelial cells. *Circ Res* 81: 922–931

39 Yoshida N, Granger DN, Anderson DC, Rothlein R, Lane C, Kvietys PR (1992) Anoxia/reoxygenation induced neutrophil adherence to culture endothelial cells. *Am J Physiol* 262: H1891–H1898

40 Inauen W, Payne DK, Kvietys PR, Granger DN (1990) Hypoxia/reoxygenation increases the permeability of endothelial cell monolayers: role of oxygen radicals. *Free Rad Biol Med* 9: 219–223

41 Eppihimer MJ, Granger DN (1997) Ischemia/reperfusion-induced leukocyte-endothelial interactions in postcapillary venules. *Shock* 7: 1–10

42 Granger DN, Grisham MB, Kvietys PR (1994) Mechanisms of microvascular injury. In: LR Johnson (ed): *Physiology of the gastrointestinal tract.* Raven Press, New York, 1693–1772

43 Wechezak AR, Wright TN, Vigers RF, Sauvage LR (1989) Endothelial adherence under shear stress is dependent on microfilament reorganization. *J Cell Physiol* 139: 136–146

44 Paully O, Morliere L, Gris JC, Bonne C, Modat G (1992) Hypoxia/ reoxygenation stimulates endothelium to promote neutrophil adhesion. *Free Rad Biol Med* 13: 21–30

45 Kvietys PR, Granger DN (1997) Endothelial cell monolayers as a tool for studying microvascular pathophysiology. *Am J Physiol* 273: G1189–G1199

46 Milhoan KA, Lane TA, Bloor CM (1992) Hypoxia induces endothelial cells to increase their adherence for neutrophils: role of PAF. *Am J Physiol* 263: H956–H962

47 Lo SK, Janakidevi K, Lai L, Malik AB (1993) Hydrogen peroxide-induced increase in endothelial adhesiveness is dependent on ICAM-1 activation. *Am J Physiol* 264: L406–L412

48 Bradley JR, Johnson D, Pober JS (1993) Endothelial activation by hydrogen peroxide: selective increases of intercellular adhesion molecule-1 and major histocompatibility complex class I. *Am J Pathol* 142: 1598–1609

49 Read MA, Neish AS, Luscinskas FW, Palombella VJ, Maniatis T, Collins T(1995) The proteasome pathway is required for cytokine-induced endothelial-leukocyte adhesion molecular expression. *Immunity* 2: 493–506

50 Cobb RR, Felts KA, Parry GCN, Mackman N (1996) Proteasome inhibitors block VCAM-1 and ICAM-1 gene expression in endothelial cells without affecting nuclear translocation of nuclear factor κB. *Eur J Immunol* 26: 839–845

Control of leukocyte adhesion and activation in atherogenesis

Judith A. Berliner, Devendra K. Vora and Peggy T. Shih

Departments of Medicine and Pathology, University of California, Los Angeles, CA 90095-1732, USA

Introduction

A number of studies have suggested that atherosclerosis represents a chronic and unsuccessful inflammatory response. Studies by Gerrity et al. [1] and Ross et al. [2] showed that within one week after the feeding of a high cholesterol diet monocytes begin to enter and accumulate in the aortic wall in certain areas referred to as the areas of predilection. When these monocytes take up lipid, they form the principal cell of the fatty streak. Very few if any neutrophils enter the wall in response to the diet. Important early studies by Gerrity's group demonstrated that both monocytes and endothelial cells from hypercholesterolemic animals become more adhesive and contribute to increased monocyte endothelial interactions [3]. Studies in a number of species have shown that monocytes continue to enter at the edges of more advanced lesions. More recent studies have shown that T cells are also present in lesions and represent approximately 0.5% of the total inflammatory cells. While these lymphocytes play an important role in atherogenesis, this review will focus on the monocyte. Studies both *in vitro* and *in vivo* suggest that monocytes may play an important role in all stages of lesion development. In Apo E null, op/op mice which lack monocyte colony stimulating factor (M-CSF), fatty streak formation is significantly reduced [4, 5]. This observation suggests an important role for monocytes in initiation of the disease process. Monocytes may play an important role in modulating smooth muscle migration, replication and matrix synthesis. Evidence for this role comes from the finding that macrophages isolated from lesions or studied *in situ* produce smooth muscle regulatory cytokines [6]. Monocytes may also play an important role in plaque rupture. There is evidence that the overall macrophage content of the ruptured plaques, obtained from patients with unstable angina undergoing atherectomy, is 3–4-fold higher than that of the plaques obtained from patients with stable angina [7]. It has been proposed that MMP-1 and MMP-2 (matrix metalloproteinases) secreted by the macrophages play a direct role in causing collagen breakdown, thus leaving the plaque vulnerable to rupture [8]. Galis et

Vascular Adhesion Molecules and Inflammation, edited by J. D. Pearson
© 1999 Birkhäuser Verlag Basel/Switzerland

al. [9] demonstrated that plaque macrophages over-express several matrix metallo-proteinases and also showed actual proteolytic activity in the plaques and not in normal arteries.

Characteristics of the areas of predilection

The nature of the vessel wall determines the areas where monocytes accumulate in hyperlipidemic animals. The areas of predilection have particular flow characteristics which have been especially well studied for the coronary arteries and for the branch vessels of the abdominal aorta [10, 11]. The flow in these areas is swirling and non-laminar, while the shear stress is modest (10–30 dynes/cm^2) compared to other areas of the vessel. Gottlieb and collaborators have examined microfilament patterns as a function of shear stress in endothelial cells and have concluded that the areas of predilection are under low shear stress and shear forces differ significantly from cell to cell. Thus the lower flow rate in the areas of predilection may be a factor in monocyte entry. The areas of predilection in animals fed a high diet [1] and in young humans [10] are characterized by thickened intima with large numbers of matrix containing synthetic smooth muscle cells and undifferentiated mesenchymal cells. It has also been shown that low density lipoprotein (LDL) accumulates to a greater extent in the modified matrix of the areas of predilection [12] and this lipoprotein accumulation may contribute to the activation of the endothelium. Another determinant of monocyte accumulation in the areas of predilection may be the decreased levels of nitric oxide produced by cells exposed to low shear [13].

Monocyte adhesion molecules

The particular adhesion molecules important in causing the entry of monocytes into lesions have not been identified. However, considerable knowledge has been gained by *in vitro* studies using monocytes and monocytic cell lines.

It is now well accepted that leukocyte recruitment to the subendothelial space is a highly regulated stepwise process ([14]; see also the chapters by Ley and Smith et al., this volume). The monocytes in rapid transition in the circulation undergo a considerable but reversible slowing through the process of "rolling" which is brought about by the interaction of the selectins with their counter-ligands. L-Selectin, P-selectin glycoprotein ligand-1 (PSGL-1), sialyl Lewis^X and other molecules expressed by the monocytes have been shown to be involved in this process [15]. Of the endothelial selectins, P-selectin and to some extent E-selectin may be involved in monocyte rolling [16]. Recently, it has been reported that very late antigen-4 (VLA-4) and vascular cell adhesion molecule-1 (VCAM-1) interaction may mediate monocyte specific rolling, particularly under conditions of low shear stress [17].

The leukocytes upon slowing are exposed to activating molecules expressed by the activated endothelial cells. These activating factors stimulate the leukocytes to cause upregulation of the expression and/or the activation of the surface integrins [18]. The specificity of mononuclear cell versus neutrophil recruitment is in part mediated by the these activation signals. Certain activators like MCP-1, fractalkine, MCSF etc. act specifically on the mononuclear cells while others like Rantes/GRO, leukotriene B_4 (LTB$_4$), formyl peptides etc. have been reported to activate all leukocyte types ([19[; see also the chapter by Furie, this volume). However, a recent study has raised some interesting questions regarding the role of these activators *in vivo* [20]. This suggested that most known activator agents require incubation with leukocytes for at least several minutes. Under *in vivo* flow conditions, only the activators which are effective within seconds are likely to be important. Such rapid activators of mononuclear cells remain to be identified.

The firm adhesion of the leukocyte to endothelial cells is usually mediated by the interaction of leukocyte integrins with their endothelial ligands. Monocytes express abundant but inactive β_2 integrins LFA-1 and MAC-1 and β_1 integrin VLA-4 which are the major molecules involved in firm adhesion to the endothelium. These integrins need activation to bring about firm adhesion. The endothelial counterligands for the β_2 integrins are predominantly intercellular cell adhesion molecule-1 (ICAM-1) and possibly ICAM-2 which are constitutively expressed [21]. VLA-4 interacts with inducible endothelial VCAM-1 and with the CS-1 domain of fibronectin and this interaction may determine monocyte-specific recruitment in certain chronic inflammatory processes [22, 23]. Firm adhesion of the leukocytes to endothelial cells allows transendothelial migration which is thought to be mediated by homotypic platelet endothelial cell adhesion molecule (PECAM-1), CD18 - ICAM-1 and VLA4 - CS-1 interactions ([24]; see see also the chapter by Muller, this volume). Once in the subendothelium the monocytes have the opportunity to transform into macrophages which secrete various cytokines, chemoattractants and growth factors and thus promote further inflammation.

The role of lipoproteins and other risk factors in fatty streak formation

Monocytes enter the vessel wall within one week of high fat feeding in animal models suggesting that lipids play an important role in their entry. Lipids that accumulate in the vessel wall and also lipids that accumulate in the bone marrow may play a role in this process [3]. Lipoproteins begin to accumulate in the vessel wall before the entry of monocytes is initiated. The major lipoproteins that accumulate in cholesterol fed animals are LDL and beta VLDL [25, 26]. There is also evidence that lipoproteins accumulate in the bone marrow of cholesterol fed animals resulting in increased levels of M-CSF, monocytosis and altered monocytic phenotype [3]. These lipoproteins have been shown to become oxidized in the subendothelial space [27, 28]. There is evidence that oxidized lipids can activate endothelial cells to bind monocytes [29]. In addition, in some animal models of atherosclerosis, antioxidants inhibit lesion formation [30]. In some human clinical trials and epidemiological studies, antioxidants have also been associated with decreased clinical events [30]. The best evidence for a role of oxidized lipids is from studies showing that injection of oxidized or modified LDL into rabbits (who then make antibodies to the oxidized LDL) gives protection against lesion formation when a high fat diet is fed [31, 32]. These studies establish an important role for lipoproteins as determinants of monocyte entry both by activating the endothelium and by altering monocyte behaviour. In addition to effects of lipoproteins, other risk factors may also be important in regulating monocyte entry. Several groups have shown that glucose and advanced glycation end products (AGE) can activate endothelium to bind leukocytes [33, 34]. Fatty streak formation is also accelerated in hypertensive animals (a condition in which angiotensin levels are elevated) and lesion formation is accelerated in hypertensive humans. Angiotensin can induce monocyte binding *in vitro* [35].

In vitro regulation, by atherosclerosis risk factors, of endothelial expression of monocyte adhesion molecules

A number of studies have examined the ability of lipoproteins and lipids to activate endothelial cells to produce monocyte adhesion molecules. Native LDL at 1–2 mg/ml, in the presence of 10% serum containing the antioxidant butylated hydroxytoluene (BHT), has been shown to increase expression of VCAM-1 and monocyte binding after a two-day period of exposure [36]. However, the majority of studies have focused on the effects of short term exposure (2–4 h) to oxidation products of LDL. Treatment with minimally modified (MM)-LDL induced the binding of monocytes but not neutrophils [37]. Our group has demonstrated that MM-LDL can increase levels of molecules associated with all stages of monocyte endothelial interaction. MM-LDL mediates the accumulation of P-selectin within the Weibel Palade bodies, and release can be mediated by highly oxidized LDL [38]. MM-LDL also increases levels of MCP-1, Gro/KC and M-CSF which support monocyte activation, chemotaxis and maturation into macrophages [39–41]. Treatment of endothelial cells was also able to increase firm adhesion of monocytes without increasing expression of E-selectin, VCAM-1 or ICAM-1 [42]. We have recently shown that increased monocyte binding induced by MM-LDL is strongly inhibited by antibody to the monocyte VLA-4 integrin [43]. We have further shown that MM-LDL increased apical expression of an alternative spliced form of fibronectin containing the CS-1 peptide, previously shown to bind VLA-4.

The activities of MM-LDL on monocyte endothelial interactions have been shown to be associated with the phospholipid fraction of MM-LDL. Three different active phospholipids have been identified (active at approximately 1 μM) which each activate endothelial cells to bind monocytes but have different effects on monocyte adhesion molecules [44]. Lysophosphatidylcholine (10 μM), another oxidation product of phospholipid, also increases expression of VCAM-1 and ICAM-1 [45]. Furthermore, 13-hydroperoxyoctadecadienoic acid (13-HPODE) has been shown to increase expression of these two molecules [46]. All of these lipids accumulate in lesion areas. Treatment of endothelial cells with MM-LDL (but not native LDL) upregulates two novel molecules that mediate monocyte binding: one is blocked by antibody Ig 9 and the other by antibody LM151 [47, 48]. Recent studies from our group have shown that the major firm adhesion molecule increased by MM-LDL is an alternatively spliced form of fibronectin that binds to VLA-4 ligand [43]. Thus *in vitro* oxidized lipids have been found to be capable of inducing endothelial expression of ligands for rolling, activation and firm adhesion of monocytes. Injection of highly oxidized LDL into animals upregulates P-selectin and PAF expression [49].

Several other risk factors for atherosclerosis have also been found to activate endothelial cells to bind monocytes. Long term treatment of endothelial cells with high glucose increases monocyte binding without increasing levels of E-selectin or VCAM-1 [50]. AGE treatment of endothelial cells for 4 h increased expression of VCAM-1, ICAM-1 and monocyte chemotactic activity [33, 34]. Angiotensin II, which is elevated in hypertension, increased monocyte binding to both large and small vessel endothelial cells [35]. In capillary endothelium the effect was mediated by E-selectin, whereas in large vessel endothelium the binding molecule is not known. This increased binding is blocked by treating the monocytes with blocking antibody to β_2 integrin but not by treatment of endothelial cells with anti-ICAM-1.

Increased adhesiveness of monocytes in hypercholesterolemia and activation of monocytes *in vitro* by lipoproteins

Monocytes from hypercholesterolemic swine and human have been shown to be more adhesive to endothelial cells when tested *ex vivo* [1, 51]. Monocytes from both species are more adhesive to untreated endothelial cells in culture and to non-predilection areas of vessels. Studies by Gerrity's group showed that monocytes from hypercholesterolemic swine were also more adhesive to endothelium covering the areas of predilection [3]. The basis for this increase in monocyte adhesiveness has not been identified. However, treatment of monocytes in culture with oxidized LDL results in activation of CD11b/CD18 [52]. Furthermore, antibody to CD18 blocked the increased adhesion of oxidized LDL-treated monocytes to endothelial cells [53].

Role of nitric oxide (NO) in monocyte adhesion

NO donors, in animal models, have significant anti-atherogenic effects [54]. There are several mechanisms by which decreased levels of NO may contribute to monocyte entry into atherosclerotic lesions. Flow modeling studies have shown that the areas of predilection are areas of low NO production. In addition, hypercholesterolemia has been shown to impair endothelial vasodilator function, largely due to reduced activity of endothelium-derived NO [55]. This reduction in nitric oxide action is believed to be due to quenching of the NO by oxy-radicals generated in the vessel wall in response to oxidized lipids during atherogenesis. Several mechanisms have been proposed for NO's antiatherogenic effects. NO has been shown to inhibit cytokine induced monocyte chemotaxis and adhesion *in vitro* [56]. De Caterina et al. [57] showed that the inhibition of cytokine induced leukocyte adhesion by NO is the result of inhibition of the transcription of several adhesion molecules and cytokines (VCAM-1, E-selectin, ICAM-1, IL-6 and IL-8). They further showed that these effects are probably mediated by the inhibition of NFκB activation by NO. It has been reported that hypercholesterolemic humans and animals have increased monocyte adhesiveness [58, 59]. *In vitro* treatment of monocytes with NO donors, or dietary L-arginine supplementation, were shown to reduce monocyte adhesiveness in hypercholesterolemic patients suggesting that NO can directly act on the monocytes to reduce their adhesiveness [50]. The mechanism involved is not clear but there is some evidence that NO donors decrease integrin-dependent leukocyte binding to activated EC [60].

Role of infection in monocyte recruitment

In the late 1970s it was proposed that viral infection may play an important role in the pathogenesis of atherosclerosis. Since atherosclerosis is so common, some of the ubiquitous viruses such as the herpes simplex type 1 and 2 (HSV1 and HSV2) and cytomegalovirus (CMV) were considered as potential candidates. Study of human pathology specimens has confirmed the presence of HSV and CMV genomes and antigens in the arterial wall. In the ARIC study, individuals with asymptomatic carotid wall thickening had a higher probability of having positive titres for CMV antibodies, although the association was only modest [61]. Recently, another ubiquitous infectious agent, *Chlamydia pneumoniae*, has attracted a lot of attention. Kuo et al. [62] reported increased levels of antibodies against *C. pneumoniae* in 60% of patients with myocardial infarction (MI) or severe coronary artery disease (CAD). Grayston and colleagues [63] have observed that up to 86% of plaques were positive for *C. pneumoniae* by immunocytochemistry. When more specific tests were used the results were less convincing. The detection of *C. pneumoniae* DNA by PCR was positive in 40% of the plaques and electron microscopy identified *Chlamydia-*

like structures in 35% of the plaques. In a similar study Muhlestein et al. [64] found that 73% of the atherectomy specimens from atherosclerosis patients were positive by direct immunofluorescence for *C. pneumoniae* while coronary specimens from cardiac transplant recipients with transplant coronary artery disease were negative for *C. pneumoniae*. These studies suggest that, like peptic ulcer disease, CAD could primarily be initiated by an infectious agent which sets up a mononuclear specific inflammatory reaction in the artery wall. Once the monocytes are recruited to the arterial subendothelium the presence of hyperlipidemia and other risk factors could help propagate the development of lesions. Although this seems to be a plausible hypothesis, whether *C. pneumoniae* is a bystander or has a direct causative role in atherogenesis remains to be determined.

Expression of monocyte adhesion molecules in lesions of animal models and humans

Expression of adhesion molecules has been examined in cholesterol-fed rabbits and mice at various times after the initiation of the high fat diet. In addition, human lesions at various stages have been examined. It is generally accepted, based on animal studies, that the majority of monocytes recruited during early atherogenesis in humans enter the vessel wall across the luminal endothelium. Mononuclear cells continue to be recruited as the lesion evolves. There is some suggestion that during the later stages of the lesion development inflammatory cells can also be recruited via the vasa vasorum. Studies in humans have examined both endothelial beds. There is strong evidence for increased expression of P-selectin on luminal endothelium of human lesions [38, 65]. E-Selectin has not been consistently observed on animal lesions and only weak staining of human lesions has been reported [66]. Animal studies have consistently found expression of VCAM-1 on the luminal endothelium of rabbits [67] and mice [68] even before the entry of monocytes into the lesion. However, in early and late human lesions, luminal surface expression is at best infrequent and inconsistent [69]. Increased expression of ICAM-1 on luminal endothelium has been shown in non-human primate and in advanced human lesions [70]. We have recently reported that staining for the CS-1 peptide, an alternative ligand for the monocyte specific integrin VLA-4, is increased in human fibro-fatty lesions [43]. In a recent study Duplaa et al. [71] reported the development of a new antibody, 3MA-B38, which recognizes mature macrophages. Using this antibody they were able to identify ten lesions out of a total of 41 which contained immature macrophages (HAM-56 +ve and 3MA-B38 −ve). Endothelial cells overlying lesions with immature macrophages showed significantly increased expression of ICAM-1, E-selectin and VCAM-1, suggesting that the expression of these adhesion molecules in such areas may have played a role in fresh mononuclear recruitment to the plaques. The study included only a small number of immature macrophage positive specimens and the results will have to be validated in a larger number of specimens. It has been reported that VCAM-1, ICAM-1 E-selectin and P-selectin are highly expressed in the vasa vasorum of complicated lesions, but the contribution of vasa vasorum in the mononuclear recruitment to lesions remains to be established [66].

A number of monocyte activators have also been detected in both animal and human lesions. Endothelial cells and monocytes in rabbit lesions express MCP-1 and M-CSF [72,73]. Gro/KC is expressed on monocytes and endothelium of mouse lesions and in endothelium on human lesions [40, 74]. Studies have also shown expression of IL-8 and Rantes in human lesion monocytes [75]. Though Gro and IL-8 are not normally thought of as monocyte activators, it has been shown that levels of receptor for these molecules are upregulated on both mouse and human lesions [74]. Thus there is a growing list of chemokines that are present in atherosclerotic lesions. Levels of PAF, another monocyte activator, have been shown to be increased in endarterectomy specimens from human patients [76].

Evidence from animal and human studies for the importance of particular adhesion molecules in mediating atherosclerosis

Nie et al. [77] investigated the role of ICAM-1 and lymphocyte function-associated antigen-1 (LFA-1) in an animal model by injecting monoclonal antibodies against ICAM-1 and LFA-1 into rats fed a high cholesterol diet. Using *en face* double immunohistochemical staining, they were able to visualize the cells and count them. They observed that anti-ICAM-1 treatment reduced macrophage recruitment to the intima by 42%, while the anti-LFA-1 reduced adhesion by 31%. Together, these two antibodies were able to produce a 58% inhibition of macrophage numbers. Further studies, by Patel et al [78], again investigated the role of ICAM-1 and in addition α_4 integrins and E-selectin in atherosclerosis prone ApoE –/– mice. In this study, the mice were pre-treated with antibodies before the injection of *ex vivo* labelled macrophages. Results in this study revealed that the ICAM-1 and α_4 antibodies reduced macrophage adhesion by 65% and 75% respectively. Antibodies against E-selectin, however, did not reduce macrophage recruitment. The role of various adhesion molecules has also been studied in genetically engineered mice. Mice harboring mutations for ICAM-1, P-selectin, CD18, ICAM-1/CD18 or ICAM-1/P-selectin on the atherosclerosis susceptible C57BL/6J background have been described [79–81]. All mutant strains maintained on an atherogenic diet demonstrated a reduction in the development of fatty streaks as compared to wild type C57BL/6J mice. Mice with the single mutations demonstrated 47, 63 and 63% reductions (CD18 and P-selectin and ICAM-1 respectively) in lesion area as compared to wild type C57BL6J, while mice with combination mutations demonstrated a 76 and 71% reduction (ICAM-1/CD18 and ICAM-1/P-selectin respectively) in lesion area size [82].

Boisvert et al. [74] generated an atherosclerosis prone mouse that was null for the production of the IL-8 receptor (IL-8R). LDLr $-/-$ mice were irradiated to destroy their pre-existing bone marrow before repopulating with cells from either an IL-8R $-/-$ or $+/+$ mouse. Mice that received IL-8R $+/+$ cells exhibited dense accumulation of macrophages in the atherosclerotic lesions while mice receiving IL-8R $-/-$ had significantly less staining for macrophages. This suggests that IL-8R plays an important role in the development of atherosclerosis. Studies to test the role of MCP-1 are also in progress in several different laboratories and it was recently reported that ApoE $-/-$ mice with the CCR_2 chemokine receptor (which binds MCP-1) also knocked out, showed decreased lesion formation [83].

The importance of particular monocyte adhesion molecules in human atherosclerosis has not been addressed experimentally. However, studies have examined the relative levels of soluble adhesion molecules in plasma. In a recent article Hackman et al. [84] reported increased blood levels of soluble adhesion molecules in a small number of patients with hyperlipidemia. Patients with hypertriglyceridemia had significantly higher levels of soluble VCAM-1 (sVCAM-1) as compared to patients with hypercholesterolemia or control subjects, while patients with hypercholesterolemia had higher levels of soluble E-selectin (sE-selectin). The authors speculate that the levels of the soluble adhesion molecules may be an indirect marker of coronary artery disease in patients with hyperlipidemia. Peter et al. [85] studied 52 patients with peripheral vascular disease. Total atherosclerosis burden was quantified by angiography of the abdominal aorta, pelvic and leg vessels. They found a statistically significant correlation with sVCAM-1 levels and extent of atherosclerosis but not with sICAM-1, sE-selectin or sP-selectin levels. Hwang et al. [86] recently reported their results on 792 ARIC patients. Levels of sVCAM-1 were not statistically different amongst patients with coronary heart disease (CHD), carotid atherosclerosis (CAA) and control subjects. However, sE-selectin and sICAM-1 levels were significantly higher in CHD and CAA patients as compared to the controls. After adjusting for the influence of the established risk factor variables only elevated sICAM-1 levels remained an independent predictor of CHD and CAA. Thus, multiple studies which evaluated the association between soluble adhesion molecule levels and severity or incidence of CHD have reached differing conclusions. Large scale studies in different populations will be necessary to understand fully if these observations will be clinically useful. In one such study, Ridker et al. [87] recently reported that when sICAM-1 levels at baseline from 474 participants of the Physician's Health Study who had a myocardial infarction (MI) during nine years of follow-up were compared to those of matched 474 control participants, the risk of MI was 80% higher in participants with the highest quartile of sICAM-1 levels independent of other variables, suggesting that sICAM-1 levels can predict future MI. Another way to examine the importance of particular molecules in human lesions is to compare biopsies from unstable versus stable angina. In a small study of such samples, increased expression of CD11b/CD18 was observed in patients with unstable angina [88].

Summary

Observations in animal and human atherosclerotic lesions suggest that monocytes play an important role in the disease process. There is also evidence that inhibition of monocyte entry may be beneficial at all stages of lesion development. Studies in knockout mice and using blocking antibodies suggest that fatty streak formation can be inhibited by preventing monocyte entry. In rabbit and in human lesions expansion is inhibited by regression diets . The major change in these non-expanding lesions is a decrease in the number of monocyte/macrophages [89,90]. Finally, as discussed above, monocyte adhesion molecules are increased in unstable versus stable angina.

There are several ways in which monocyte entry into the vessel wall could be targeted:

(1) Block the effects of mediators of monocyte entry. A number of mediators of monocyte entry may be involved in lesion formation and these may differ between individuals and at various stages of the disease. Native and especially oxidized lipoproteins, angiotensin, AGE, and infectious agents all have been shown to act as potential mediators. In addition, cytokines produced by monocyte/macrophages in the vessel wall such as IL-l may be important in sustaining monocyte entry. Inhibitors to target receptors for these mediators may be useful agents in controlling atherogenesis.

(2) Block the binding between monocytes and endothelial cells by targeting adhesive ligands on the endothelium or the monocyte. The particular monocyte adhesion molecules on endothelium responsible for the various stages of atherogenesis are not yet certain and may differ between human and animal models. Furthermore, they may differ between luminal endothelium and endothelium of the vasa vasorum. The majority of evidence in both human and animal models suggests an important role for the rolling molecule P-selectin at all stages with little evidence for a role of E-selectin. Human lesions have been shown to contain several different monocyte activators, including MCP-1, IL-8, MIP-1 and Rantes. Any or all of these or other chemokines yet to be identified may be potential targets. VCAM-1, CS-1 containing fibronectin and ICAM-1 all may have a role as firm adhesion molecules at different stages of atherosclerosis. However, VCAM-1 appears to be more important on the endothelium of the vasa vasorum. The majority of evidence suggests that sICAM-1 is increased in patients who have heart attacks. However, these studies should be interpreted with caution since it is not clear that the soluble adhesion molecules come from atherosclerotic vessels. There is evidence that inhibition of the corresponding monocyte integrins can block fatty streak formation in animal models. In order to develop effective human therapies, there is a major need for better information as to which monocyte adhesion molecules are present and important in the various stages of

human lesion development. Recently, several pharmacological inhibitors of individual adhesion molecule function have been identified. These may be useful especially if they could be targeted to atherosclerotic lesions.

(3) General anti-inflammatory molecules could be employed. One example of this approach is the use of nitric oxide. Other agents that inhibit activation of NFκB may also prove useful since it has been reported that NFκB activation is increased in atherosclerotic lesions [91]. The use of general anti-inflammatory agents may prove useful especially in prevention of monocyte entry into lesions of unstable angina and may be useful at other stages if one could specifically target the endothelium of the lesions. Thus the current information on monocyte adhesion molecules in atherosclerosis obtained from animal studies, *in vitro* studies, and human observations suggests several important potential therapeutic targets.

References

1   Gerrity RG (1981) The role of the monocyte in atherogenesis: I. Transition of blood-borne monocytes into foam cells in fatty lesions. *Am J Pathol* 103: 181–190

2   Ross R (1995) Cell biology of atherosclerosis. *Ann Rev Physiol* 57: 791–804

3   Gerrity RG, Goss JA, Soby L (1985) Control of monocyte recruitment by chemotactic factor(s) in lesion-prone areas of swine aorta. *Arteriosclerosis* 5: 55–66

4   Smith JD, Trogan E, Ginsberg M, Grigaux C, Tian J, Miyata M (1995) Decreased atherosclerosis in mice deficient in both macrophage colony-stimulating factor (op) and apolipoprotein E. *Proc Natl Acad Sci USA* 92: 8264–8268

5   Qiao JH, Tripathi J, Mishra NK, Cai Y, Tripathi S, Wang XP, Imes S, Fishbein MC, Clinton SK, Libby P, Lusis AJ, Rajavashisth TB (1997) Role of macrophage colony-stimulating factor in atherosclerosis: studies of osteopetrotic mice. *Am J Pathol* 150: 1687–1699

6   Tipping PG, Hancock WW (1993) Production of tumor necrosis factor and interleukin-1 by macrophages from human atheromatous plaques. *Am J Pathol* 142: 1721–1728

7   Moreno PR, Falk E, Palacios IF, Newell JB, Fuster V, Fallon JT (1994) Macrophage infiltration in acute coronary syndromes. Implications for plaque rupture. *Circulation* 90: 775–778

8   Shah PK, Falk E, Badimon JJ, Fernandez-Ortiz A, Mailhac A, Villareal-Levy G, Fallon JT, Regnstrom J, Fuster V (1995) Human monocyte-derived macrophages induce collagen breakdown in fibrous caps of atherosclerotic plaques. Potential role of matrix-degrading metalloproteinases and implications for plaque rupture. *Circulation* 92: 1565–1569

9   Galis ZS, Sukhova GK, Kranzhofer R, Clark S, Libby P (1995) Macrophage foam cells from experimental atheroma constitutively produce matrix-degrading proteinases. *Proc Natl Acad Sci USA* 92: 402–406

10   Cornhill JF, Herderick EE, Stary HC (1990) Topography of human aortic sudanophilic lesions. *Monogr Atheroscler* 15: 13–19

11   Asakura T, Karino T (1990) Flow patterns and spatial distribution of atherosclerotic lesions in human coronary arteries. *Circ Res* 66: 1045–1066

12   Schwenke DC, St Clair RW (1993) Influx, efflux, and accumulation of LDL in normal arterial areas and atherosclerotic lesions of white Carneau pigeons with naturally occurring and cholesterol-aggravated aortic atherosclerosis. *Arterioscler Thromb* 13: 1368–1381

13   Tsao PS, Buitrago R, Chan JR, Cooke JP (1996) Fluid flow inhibits endothelial adhesiveness. Nitric oxide and transcriptional regulation of VCAM-1. *Circulation* 94: 1682–1689

14   Butcher EC (1991) Leukocyte-endothelial cell recognition: three (or more) steps to specificity and diversity. *Cell* 67: 1033–1036

15   Jutila MA, Berg EL, Kishimoto TK, Picker LJ, Bargatze RF, Bishop DK, Orosz CG, Wu NW, Butcher EC (1989) Inflammation-induced endothelial cell adhesion to lymphocytes, neutrophils, and monocytes. Role of homing receptors and other adhesion molecules. *Transplantation* 48: 727–731

16   Walter UM, Issekutz AC (1997) Role of E- and P-selectin in migration of monocytes and polymorphonuclear leucocytes to cytokine and chemoattractant-induced cutaneous inflammation in the rat. *Immunol* 92: 290–299

17   Berlin CR, Bargatze F, Campbell JJ, von Andrian UH, Szabo MC, Hasslen SR, Nelson RD, Berg EL, Erlandsen SL, Butcher EC (1995) Alpha 4 integrins mediate lymphocyte attachment and rolling under physiologic flow. *Cell* 80: 413–422

18   Kishimoto TK, Larson RS, Corbi AL, Dustin ML, Staunton DE, Springer TA (1989) The leukocyte integrins. *Adv Immunol* 46: 149–182

19   Luster AD (1998) Chemokines – chemotactic cytokines that mediate inflammation. *N Engl J Med* 338: 436–445

20   Campbell JJ, Hedrick J, Zlotnik A, Siani MA, Thompson DA, Butcher EC (1998) Chemokines and the arrest of lymphocytes rolling under flow conditions. *Science* 279: 381–384

21   Carlos TM, Harlan JM (1994) Leukocyte-endothelial adhesion molecules. *Blood* 84: 2068–2101

22   Luscinskas FW, Gimbrone MA Jr (1996) Endothelial-dependent mechanisms in chronic inflammatory leukocyte recruitment. *Ann Rev Med* 47: 413–421

23   Elices MJ, Tsai V, Strahl D, Goel AS, Tollefson V, Arrhenius T, Wayner EA, Gaeta FC, Fikes JD, Firestein GS (1994) Expression and functional significance of alternatively spliced CS1 fibronectin in rheumatoid arthritis microvasculature. *J Clin Invest* 93: 405–416

24   Meerschaert J, Furie MB (1995) The adhesion molecules used by monocytes for migration across endothelium include CD11a/CD18, CD11b/CD18, and VLA-4 on monocytes and ICAM-1, VCAM-1, and other ligands on endothelium. *J Immunol* 154: 4099–4112

25 Mora R, Lupu F, Simionescu N (1989) Cytochemical localization of beta-lipoproteins and their components in successive stages of hyperlipidemic atherogenesis of rabbit aorta. *Atherosclerosis* 79 : 183–195

26 Napoli C, D'Armiento FP, Mancini FP, Postiglione A, Witztum JL, Palumbo G, Palinski W (1997) Fatty streak formation occurs in human fetal aortas and is greatly enhanced by maternal hypercholesterolemia. Intimal accumulation of low density lipoprotein and its oxidation precede monocyte recruitment into early atherosclerotic lesions. *J Clin Invest* 100: 2680–2690

27 Witztum JL, Steinberg D (1991) Role of oxidized low density lipoprotein in atherogenesis. *J Clin Invest* 88: 1785–1792

28 Lynch SM, Frei B (eds) (1994) *Antioxidants as antiatherogens: Animal studies.* Academic Press, Orlando, FL

29 Berliner JA, Navab M, Fogelman AM, Frank JS, Demer LL, Edwards PA, Watson AD, Lusis AJ (1995) Atherosclerosis: basic mechanisms. Oxidation, inflammation, and genetics. *Circulation* 91: 2488–2496

30 Berliner JA, Heinecke JW (1996) The role of oxidized lipoproteins in atherogenesis. *Free Radic Biol Med* 20: 707–727

31 Palinski W, Miller E, Witztum JL (1995) Immunization of low density lipoprotein (LDL) receptor-deficient rabbits with homologous malondialdehyde-modified LDL reduces atherogenesis. *Proc Natl Acad Sci USA* 92: 821–825

32 Ameli S, Hultgardh-Nilsson A, Regnstrom J, Calara F, Yano J, Cercek B, Shah PK, Nilsson J (1996) Effect of immunization with homologous LDL and oxidized LDL on early atherosclerosis in hypercholesterolemic rabbits. *Arterioscler Thromb Vasc Biol* 16: 1074–1079

33 Schmidt AM, Yan SD, Brett J, Mora R, Nowygrod R, Stern D (1993) Regulation of human mononuclear phagocyte migration by cell surface-binding proteins for advanced glycation end products. *J Clin Invest* 91: 2155–2168

34 Vlassara H, Fuh H, Donnelly T, Cybulsky M (1995) Advanced glycation endproducts promote adhesion molecule (VCAM-1, ICAM-1) expression and atheroma formation in normal rabbits. *Mol Med* 1: 447–456

35 Kim JA, Berliner JA, Nadler JL (1996) Angiotensin II increases monocyte binding to endothelial cells. *Biochem Biophys Res Commun* 226: 862–868

36 Lin JH, Zhu Y, Liao HL, Kobari Y, Groszek L, Stemerman MB (1996) Induction of vascular cell adhesion molecule-1 by low-density lipoprotein. *Atherosclerosis* 127: 185–194

37 Berliner JA, Territo MC, Sevanian A, Ramin S, Kim JA, Bamshad B, Esterson M, Fogelman AM (1990) Minimally modified low density lipoprotein stimulates monocyte endothelial interactions. *J Clin Invest* 85: 1260–1266

38 Vora DK, Fang ZT, Liva SM, Tyner TR, Parhami F, Watson AD, Drake TA, Territo MC, Berliner JA (1997) Induction of P-selectin by oxidized lipoproteins. Separate effects on synthesis and surface expression. *Circ Res* 80: 810–818

39 Cushing SD, Berliner JA, Valente AJ, Territo MC, Navab M, Parhami F, Gerrity R, Schwartz CJ, Fogelman AM (1990) Minimally modified low density lipoprotein induces

monocyte chemotactic protein 1 in human endothelial cells and smooth muscle cells. *Proc Natl Acad Sci USA* 87 : 5134–5138

40   Schwartz D, Andalibi A, Chaverri-Almada L, Berliner JA, Kirchgessner T, Fang ZT, Tekamp-Olson P, Lusis AJ, Gallegos C, Fogelman AM et al (1994) Role of the GRO family of chemokines in monocyte adhesion to MM-LDL-stimulated endothelium. *J Clin Invest* 94: 1968–1973

41   Rajavashisth TB, Andalibi A, Territo MC, Berliner JA, Navab M, Fogelman AM, Lusis AJ (1990) Induction of endothelial cell expression of granulocyte and macrophage colony-stimulating factors by modified low-density lipoproteins. *Nature* 344: 254–257

42   Kim JA, Territo MC, Wayner E, Carlos TM, Parhami F, Smith CW, Haberland ME, Fogelman AM, Berliner JA (1994) Partial characterization of leukocyte binding molecules on endothelial cells induced by minimally oxidized LDL. *Arterioscler Thromb* 14: 427–433

43   Shih PT, Elices MJ, Fang ZT, Ugarova TP, Strahl D, Territo MC, Frank JS, Kovach NL, Cabanas C, Berliner JA et al (1999) Minimally modified low-density lipoprotein induces monocyte adhesion to endothelial connecting segment-1 by activating β1 integrin. *J Clin Invest* 103: 613–625

44   Watson AD, Leitinger N, Navab M, Faull KF, Horkko S, Witztum JL, Palinski W, Schwenke D, Salomon RG, Sha W, Subbanagounder G, Fogelman AM, Berliner JA (1997) Structural identification by mass spectrometry of oxidized phospholipids in minimally oxidized low density lipoprotein that induce monocyte/endothelial interactions and evidence for their presence *in vivo*. *J Biol Chem* 272: 13597–13607

45   Kume N, Cybulsky MI, Gimbrone MA Jr (1992) Lysophosphatidylcholine, a component of atherogenic lipoproteins, induces mononuclear leukocyte adhesion molecules in cultured human and rabbit arterial endothelial cells. *J Clin Invest* 90: 1138–1144

46   Ku G, Thomas CE, Akeson AL, Jackson RL (1992) Induction of interleukin 1 beta expression from human peripheral blood monocyte-derived macrophages by 9-hydroxyoctadecadienoic acid. *J Biol Chem* 267: 14183–14188

47   Calderon TM, Factor SM, Hatcher VB, Berliner JA, Berman JW (1994) An endothelial cell adhesion protein for monocytes recognized by monoclonal antibody IG9. Expression *in vivo* in inflamed human vessels and atherosclerotic human and Watanabe rabbit vessels. *Lab Invest* 70: 836–849

48   McEvoy LM, Sun H, Tsao PS, Cooke JP, Berliner JA, Butcher EC (1997) Novel vascular molecule involved in monocyte adhesion to aortic endothelium in models of atherogenesis. *J Exp Med* 185: 2069–2077

49   Lehr HA, Seemuller J, Hubner C, Menger MD, Messmer K (1993) Oxidized LDL-induced leukocyte/endothelium interaction *in vivo* involves the receptor for platelet-activating factor. *Arterioscler Thromb* 13: 1013–1018

50   Kim JA, Berliner JA, Natarajan RD, Nadler JL (1994) Evidence that glucose increases monocyte binding to human aortic endothelial cells. *Diabetes* 43: 1103–1107

51   Stragliotto E, Camera M, Postiglione A, Sirtori M, Di Minno G, Tremoli E (1993) Func-

tionally abnormal monocytes in hypercholesterolemia. *Arterioscler Thromb* 13: 944–950

52 Lehr HA, Krombach F, Munzing S, Bodlaj R, Glaubitt SI, Seiffge D, Hubner C, von Andrian UH, Messmer K (1995) *In vitro* effects of oxidized low density lipoprotein on CD11b/CD18 and L-selectin presentation on neutrophils and monocytes with relevance for the *in vivo* situation. *Am J Pathol* 146: 218–227

53 Weber C, Erl W, Weber PC (1995) Enhancement of monocyte adhesion to endothelial cells by oxidatively modified low-density lipoprotein is mediated by activation of CD11b. *Biochem Biophys Res Commun* 206: 621–628

54 Cooke JP, Singer AH, Tsao P, Zera P, Rowan RA, Billingham ME (1992) Antiatherogenic effects of L-arginine in the hypercholesterolemic rabbit. *J Clin Invest* 90: 1168–1172

55 Keaney JF Jr, Vita JA (1995) Atherosclerosis, oxidative stress, and antioxidant protection in endothelium-derived relaxing factor action. *Prog Cardiovasc Dis* 38: 129–54

56 Bath PM, Hassall DG, Gladwin AM, Palmer RM, Martin JF (1991) Nitric oxide and prostacyclin. Divergence of inhibitory effects on monocyte chemotaxis and adhesion to endothelium *in vitro*. *Arterioscler Thromb* 11: 254–260

57 De Caterina R, Libby P, Peng HB, Thannickal VJ, Rajavashisth TB, Gimbrone MA Jr, Shin WS, Liao JK (1995) Nitric oxide decreases cytokine-induced endothelial activation. Nitric oxide selectively reduces endothelial expression of adhesion molecules and proinflammatory cytokines. *J Clin Invest* 96: 60–68

58 Gerrity RG, Naito HK, Richardson M, Schwartz CJ (1979) Dietary induced atherogenesis in swine. Morphology of the intima in prelesion stages. *Am J Pathol* 95: 775–792

59 Theilmeier G, Chan JR, Zalpour C, Anderson B, Wang BY, Wolf A, Tsao PS, Cooke JP (1997) Adhesiveness of mononuclear cells in hypercholesterolemic humans is normalized by dietary L-arginine. *Arterioscler Thromb Vasc Biol* 17: 3557–3564

60 Kubes P, Kurose I, Granger DN (1994) NO donors prevent integrin-induced leukocyte adhesion but not P-selectin-dependent rolling in postischemic venules. *Am J Physiol* 267: H931–H937

61 Sorlie PD, Adam E, Melnick SL, Folsom A, Skelton T, Chambless LE, Barnes R, Melnick JL (1994) Cytomegalovirus/herpesvirus and carotid atherosclerosis: the ARIC Study. *J Med Virol* 42: 33–37

62 Kuo CC, Coulson AS, Campbell LA, Cappuccio AL, Lawrence RD, Wang SP, Grayston JT (1997) Detection of *Chlamydia pneumoniae* in atherosclerotic plaques in the walls of arteries of lower extremities from patients undergoing bypass operation for arterial obstruction. *J Vasc Surg* 26: 29–31

63 Grayston JT, Kuo CC, Coulson AS, Campbell LA, Lawrence RD, Lee MJ, Strandness ED, Wang SP (1995) *Chlamydia pneumoniae* (TWAR) in atherosclerosis of the carotid artery. *Circulation* 92: 3397–3400

64 Muhlestein JB, Hammond EH, Carlquist JF, Radicke E, Thomson MJ, Karagounis LA, Woods ML, Anderson JL (1996) Increased incidence of *Chlamydia* species within the

coronary arteries of patients with symptomatic atherosclerotic versus other forms of cardiovascular disease. *J Am Coll Cardiol* 27: 1555–1561

65 Poston RN, Johnson-Tidey RR (1996) Localized adhesion of monocytes to human atherosclerotic plaques demonstrated *in vitro*: implications for atherogenesis. *Am J Pathol* 149: 73–80

66 O'Brien KD, McDonald TO, Chait A, Allen MD, Alpers CE (1996) Neovascular expression of E-selectin, intercellular adhesion molecule-1, and vascular cell adhesion molecule-1 in human atherosclerosis and their relation to intimal leukocyte content. *Circulation* 93: 672–682

67 Cybulsky MI, Gimbrone MA Jr (1991) Endothelial expression of a mononuclear leukocyte adhesion molecule during atherogenesis. *Science* 251: 788–791

68 Qiao JH, Welch CL, Xie PZ, Fishbein MC, Lusis AJ (1993) Involvement of the tyrosinase gene in the deposition of cardiac lipofuscin in mice. Association with aortic fatty streak development. *J Clin Invest* 92: 2386–2393

69 O'Brien KD, Allen MD, McDonald TO, Chait A, Harlan JM, Fishbein D, McCarty J, Ferguson M, Hudkins K, Benjamin CD et al (1993) Vascular cell adhesion molecule-1 is expressed in human coronary atherosclerotic plaques. Implications for the mode of progression of advanced coronary atherosclerosis. *J Clin Invest* 92: 945–951

70 Poston RN, Haskard DO, Coucher JR, Gall NP, Johnson-Tidey RR (1992) Expression of intercellular adhesion molecule-1 in atherosclerotic plaques. *Am J Pathol* 140: 665–673

71 Duplaa C, Couffinhal T, Labat L, Moreau C, Petit-Jean ME, Doutre MS, Lamaziere JM, Bonnet J (1996) Monocyte/macrophage recruitment and expression of endothelial adhesion proteins in human atherosclerotic lesions. *Atherosclerosis* 121: 253–266

72 Yla-Herttuala S, Lipton BA, Rosenfeld ME, Sarkioja T, Yoshimura T, Leonard EJ, Witztum JL, Steinberg D (1991) Expression of monocyte chemoattractant protein 1 in macrophage-rich areas of human and rabbit atherosclerotic lesions. *Proc Natl Acad Sci USA* 88: 5252–5256

73 Rosenfeld ME., Yla-Herttuala S, Lipton BA, Ord VA, Witztum JL, Steinberg D (1992) Macrophage colony-stimulating factor mRNA protein in atherosclerotic lesions of rabbits and humans. *Am J Pathol* 140: 291–300

74 Boisvert WA, Santiago R, Curtiss LK, Terkeltaub RA (1998) A leukocyte homologue of the IL-8 receptor CXCR-2 mediates the accumulation of macrophages in atherosclerotic lesions of LDL receptor-deficient mice. *J Clin Invest* 101: 353–363

75 Liu Y, Hulten LM, Wiklund O (1997) Macrophages isolated from human atherosclerotic plaques produce IL-8, and oxysterols may have a regulatory function for IL-8 production. *Arterioscler Thromb Vasc Biol* 17: 317–323

76 Mueller HW, Haught CA, McNatt JM, Cui K, JM Gaskell JM, Johnston DA, Willerson JT (1995) Measurement of platelet-activating factor in a canine model of coronary thrombosis and in endarterectomy samples from patients with advanced coronary artery disease. *Circ Res* 77: 54–63

77 Nie Q, Fan J, Haraoka S, Shimokama T, Watanabe T (1997) Inhibition of mononuclear

cell recruitment in aortic intima by treatment with anti-ICAM-1 and anti-LFA-1 mono-clonal antibodies in hypercholesterolemic rats: implications of the ICAM-1 and LFA-1 pathway in atherogenesis. *Lab Invest* 77: 469–482

78 Patel SS, Thiagarajan R, Willerson JT, Yeh ET (1998) Inhibition of alpha4 integrin and ICAM-1 markedly attenuate macrophage homing to atherosclerotic plaques in ApoE-deficient mice. *Circulation* 97: 75–81

79 Sligh JE Jr, Ballantyne CM, Rich SS, Hawkins HK, Smith CW, Bradley A, Beaudet AL (1993) Inflammatory and immune responses are impaired in mice deficient in intercel-lular adhesion molecule 1. *Proc Natl Acad Sci USA* 90: 8529–8533

80 Mayadas TN, Johnson RC, Rayburn H, Hynes RO, Wagner DD (1993) Leukocyte rolling and extravasation are severely compromised in P selectin-deficient mice. *Cell* 74: 541–554

81 Wilson RW, Ballantyne CM, Smith CW, Montgomery C, Bradley A, O'Brien WE, Beaudet AL (1993) Gene targeting yields a CD18-mutant mouse for study of inflamma-tion. *J Immunol* 151: 1571–1578

82 Nageh MF, Sandberg ET, Marotti KR, Lin AH, Melchior EP, Bullard DC, Beaudet AL (1997) Deficiency of inflammatory cell adhesion molecules protects against atheroscle-rosis in mice. *Arterioscler Thromb Vasc Biol* 17: 1517–1520

83 Boring L, Gosling J, Cleary M, Charo IF (1998) Decreased lesion formation in CCR2-/-mice reveals a role for chemokines in the initiation of atherosclerosis. *Nature* 394: 894–897.

84 Hackman A, Abe Y, Insull W Jr, Pownall H, Smith L, Dunn K, Gotto AM Jr, Ballantyne CM (1996) Levels of soluble cell adhesion molecules in patients with dyslipidemia. *Cir-culation* 93: 1334–1338

85 Peter K, Nawroth P, Conradt C, Nordt T, Weiss T, Boehme M, Wunsch A, Allenberg J, KublerW, Bode C. (1997) Circulating vascular cell adhesion molecule-1 correlates with the extent of human atherosclerosis in contrast to circulating intercellular adhesion mol-ecule-1, E-selectin, P-selectin, and thrombomodulin. *Arterioscler Thromb Vasc Biol* 17: 505–512

86 Hwang SJ, Ballantyne CM, Sharrett AR, Smith LC, Davis CE, Gotto AM Jr, Boerwin-kle E (1997) Circulating adhesion molecules VCAM-1, ICAM-1, and E-selectin in carotid atherosclerosis and incident coronary heart disease cases: the Atherosclerosis Risk In Communities (ARIC) study. *Circulation* 96: 4219–4225

87 Ridker PM, Hennekens CH, Roitman-Johnson B, Stampfer MJ, Allen J (1998) Plasma concentration of soluble intercellular adhesion molecule 1 and risks of future myocar-dial infarction in apparently healthy men. *Lancet* 351: 88–92

88 Mazzone A, De Servi S, Ricevuti G, Mazzucchelli I, Fossati G, Pasotti D, Bramucci E, Angoli L, Marsico F, Specchia G et al (1993) Increased expression of neutrophil and monocyte adhesion molecules in unstable coronary artery disease. *Circulation* 88: 358–363

89 Kita T, Nagano Y, Yokode M, Ishii K, Kume N, Ooshima A, Yoshida H, Kawai C (1987) Probucol prevents the progression of atherosclerosis in Watanabe heritable hyperlipi-

demic rabbit, an animal model for familial hypercholesterolemia. *Proc Natl Acad Sci USA* 84: 5928–5931

90 Blankenhorn DH, Hodis MJ (1993) Atherosclerosis – reversal with therapy. *West J Med* 159: 172–179

91 Brand K, Page S, Rogler G, Bartsch A, Brandl R, Knuechel R, Page M, Kaltschmidt C, Baeuerle PA, Neumeier D (1996) Activated transcription factor nuclear factor-kappa B is present in the atherosclerotic lesion. *J Clin Invest* 97: 1715–22

Index

α-actinin 14
acute vascular rejection (AVR) 198
adherens junction 109
advanced glycosylation endproduct of proteins (AGE) 168, 169
allopurinol 226
angiotensin II (Ang II) 167, 168
anoxia/reoxygenation 230
antibody 197
7H6 antigen 111
AP-1 230
armadillo repeat 112
arteriole 18
arthritis, experimental 189
arthritis, rheumatoid 191
ATP-diphosphohydrolase (ATPDase/CD39) 200

B lymphocyte 205
bacterial toxin 84
basal lamina 129, 130
blood-brain barrier 109
bond force 16
bond formation 12
bond strength 12
bradykinin 84

cadherin 111
Calcium ion (Ca^{2+}) 4
capillary no-reflow 222
capture 11, 12, 15, 18

catalase 232
catenin 112
CD11/CD18 225
CD11/CD18 integrin 81
CD24 21
CD31 125
CD34 22
cell-cell adhesion 109
chemoattractant 12, 66
chemokine 12, 14, 65–69, 71–74
chemokine receptor 70–72
chemotaxis 1
cingulin 111
complement 197
complement regulatory protein 208
core 2 oligosaccharide 20
critical velocity 11, 12
cyclic AMP 113

delayed-type hypersensitivity (DTH) 187
delayed xenograft rejection (DXR) 198
diapedesis 125, 129, 32
disseminated intravascular coagulation 208
Duffy antigen receptor for chemokines (DARC) 71, 72

ear chamber 3
eosinophil 13
E-selectin 13–16, 17, 19–23, 179
E-selectin ligand 23
E-selectin ligand-1 (ESL-1) 21, 23

fatty acid hydroperoxide 167
fibronectin, CS-1 domain of 241
flow velocity profile 16
fractalkine 66, 68, 73
fucosyl transferase VII (FTVII) 20, 23
fucosylation 20

glycosaminoglycan (GAG) 72, 73
glycosylation-dependent cell adhesion
    molecule-1 (GlyCAM-1) 21, 22
granulocyte 15
GRO chemokine 68, 70, 71, 73

heterologous desensitization 82
histamine 18, 84
homologous desensitization 82
hydrodynamic velocity 11
hyperacute rejection (HAR) 198

imaging 179
in vitro adhesion assay 4
inflammatory bowel disease (IBD) 191
integrin 12, 15
α_4 integrin 50
β_2 integrin 18, 81, 87, 128
β_7 integrin 17
interleukin-1 (IL-1) 15, 179
interleukin-1α (IL-1α) 84
interleukin-1β (IL-1β) 163, 165, 171
interleukin-8 (IL-8) 14, 18, 19, 67–69, 70,
    72–74
intracellular adhesion molecule-1 (ICAM-1)
    20, 43, 128, 130, 131, 225, 241

juxtacrine signaling by platelet activating factor
    (PAF) 81, 91
juxtacrine signaling molecule 81

knockout mouse 17

leukocyte adhesion deficiency 7
leukocyte integrin 81

leukocyte-capillary plugging 222
leukocyte-leukocyte interaction 17
leukotriene B$_4$ (LTB$_4$) 225
LFA-1 43
lipopolysaccharide (LPS) 163, 165, 169, 179
load-bearing bond 16
low density lipoprotein (LDL) 168, 240
L-selectin 13, 15–18, 21, 23, 240
L-selectin ligand 20
lymphocyte 14–17, 141, 185
lymphotactin 66, 71
lysophosphatic acid 114

MAC-1 43, 241
margination 11, 15
mast cell 18, 227, 229
megakaryocyte 14
metalloproteinase 14
microprocess 14
minimally modified low density lipoprotein
    (MM-LDL) 242
model membrane 89
monocyte 14, 126, 130, 131, 133, 198, 203,
    239
monocyte chemoattractant protein-1 (MCP-1)
    67, 68, 70, 72–74, 161, 163, 164, 168, 170
monocyte chemoattractant protein-1α
    (MCP-1α) 68, 71–73
monocyte chemoattractant protein-1β
    (MCP-1β) 68, 71–73
monocyte chemoattractant protein-3 (MCP-3)
    68, 70, 72
monocyte colony stimulating factor (M-CSF)
    239
mucosal adressin adhesion molecule-1
    (MAdCAM-1) 21, 23
multistep adhesion paradigm 7
myeloid leukocyte 81

NAD(P)H oxidase 162–165, 167, 168, 171
natural killer (NK) cell 14, 126, 130, 131, 133,
    198, 203

neutrophil 13, 17, 81, 126, 130–133, 136, 185

neutrophil aggregate 41

neutrophil count 19

nitric oxide (NO) 169, 170, 227, 244

nuclear factor κB (NF-κB) 161, 164, 165, 168, 170, 171, 200, 233

occludin 110

off-rate 17

on-rate 15

outside-in signaling 81

oxidant 84

oxidatively modified low density lipoprotein (LDL) (oxLDL) 166, 167, 169, 170

p120^{cas} 112

parallel-plate flow chambers 12

peripheral lymph node 17

peripheral node addressin (PNAd) 22

Peyer's patch 17, 23

pig 180

platelet 14, 18, 93, 208

platelet activating factor (PAF) 81, 227

platelet activating factor (PAF) acetylhydrolase 82

platelet activating factor (PAF) receptor 81

platelet activating factor (PAF) receptor antagonist 90

platelet activating factor (PAF) receptor homologous desensitization 90

platelet factor 4 (PF4) 70, 72, 73

platelet/endothelial cell adhesion molecule-1 (PECAM) 125

polymorphonuclear leukocyte (PMN) 81, 201

polymorphonuclear leukocyte (PMN) adhesion 81

postcapillary venular endothelium 83

postcapillary venule 11

post-translational modification 20

P-selectin 13–18, 21, 93, 225

P-selectin deficient mouse 18

P-selectin glycoprotein ligand-1 (PSGL-1) 21–23, 240

rab13 111

reactive oxygen metabolite 226, 232

reactive oxygen species (ROS) 161, 162, 165, 171

recirculation 141

recruitment of leukocytes 65–67, 73, 74

regulated on activation, normal T expressed and secreted (RANTES) 67–70, 72–74, 241

reperfusion injury 221

rheumatoid arthritis (RA) 191

rho protein 114

rolling 12, 15

rolling, spontaneous leukocyte 18

rolling velocity 18, 19

selectin 12, 13, 16, 20

selectin-deficient mouse 19

SH2 domain 126, 135

shear rate 223

shear stress 170

shedding 14

sialyl Lewis^x 20, 23

sialyl transferase 23

sialylation 20

skipping 18

sulfatide 22

sulfidopeptide leukotriene 84

superoxide dismutase (SOD) 226

symplekin 111

T cell response 198

T lymphocyte 205

tethering 11, 12

thrombin 18, 84

thrombomodulin 208

tight junction 109

trafficking 141

transendothelial migration 54, 126, 131

transgenic animal 209
transit time 11, 12
transmigration assay 127, 129
tumor necrosis factor α (TNFα) 15, 17, 18,
    84, 163, 165, 19
tyrosine phosphorylation 114
tyrosine sulfation 20

vascular cell adhesion molecule-1 (VCAM-1)
    128, 130, 161, 163, 164, 166–169, 171,
    179, 240
velocity 18

venule 18
VLA-4 ($\alpha_4\beta_1$, CD49d/CD29) 50, 128, 240
von Willebrand factor (vWF) 208

Weibel-Palade body 14, 18

xanthine oxidase 226
xenoreactive natural antibody (XNA) 198
xenotransplantation 197

zonula occludens-1 (ZO-1) 110
zonula occludens-2 (ZO-2) 110